THE
BENZODIAZEPINES
CURRENT STANDARDS
FOR
MEDICAL PRACTICE

THE
BENZODIAZEPINES
CURRENT STANDARDS
FOR
MEDICAL PRACTICE

Edited by D.E.Smith and D.R.Wesson

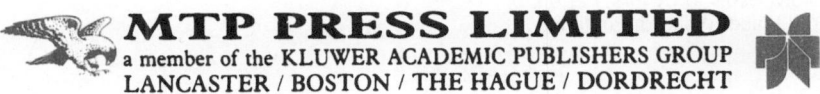

MTP PRESS LIMITED
a member of the KLUWER ACADEMIC PUBLISHERS GROUP
LANCASTER / BOSTON / THE HAGUE / DORDRECHT

Published in the UK and Europe by
MTP Press Limited
Falcon House
Lancaster, England

British Library Cataloguing in Publication Data

The Benzodiazepines: current standards for
  medical practice.
  1. Benzodiazepines
  I. Smith, David E. (David Elvin) II. Wesson, D.R.
  615′ .7882   RM666.B42

Published in the USA by
MTP Press
A division of Kluwer Boston Inc
190 Old Derby Street
Hingham, MA 02043, USA

Library of Congress Cataloging in Publication Data

Main entry under title:

The Benzodiazepines: current standards for medical
  practice.

  Includes bibliographies and index.
  1. Benzodiazepines. 2. Psychopharmacology.
  3. Medication abuse. I. Smith, David E. (David Elvin),
  1939–   . II. Wesson, Donald R., 1941–   . [DNLM:
  1. Benzodiazepine Tranquilizers—therapeutic use.
  2. Benzodiazepines—therapeutic use.   QV 77.9 B479017]
  RC483.5.B48B46   1984   615′.78   84-26126
ISBN-13: 978-94-010-8663-9   e-ISBN-13: 978-94-009-4886-0
DOI: 10.1007/978-94-009-4886-0

Copyright © 1985 MTP Press Limited

Softcover reprint of the hardcover 1st edition 1985

Phototypesetting by First Page Ltd.
Carey Place, Watford, England.

Contents

List of Contributors

S. CAMBER MA
Research Coordinator
Merritt Peralta Institute
Chemical Dependency Recovery Hospital
Oakland, California
USA

D. J. GREENBLATT MD
Chief, Division of Clinical Pharmacology
Professor of Psychiatry and Associate
    Professor of Medicine
Tufts University School of Medicine and
    New England Medical Center Hospital
Box 1007, 171 Harrison Avenue
Boston, MA 02111
USA

R. R. GRIFFITHS PhD
Departments of Psychiatry and
    Neuroscience
The Johns Hopkins University School of
    Medicine
720 Rutland Avenue
Baltimore, MD 21205
USA

W. E. HAEFELY MD
Pharmaceutical Research Department
F. Hoffman–La Roche & Co Ltd
CH-4002 Basel
Switzerland

L. E. HOLLISTER MD
Senior Medical Investigator
Veterans Administration Medical Center
3801 Miranda Avenue
Palo Alto, CA 94304 and
Professor of Medicine, Psychiatry and
    Pharmacology
Stanford University School of Medicine
Palo Alto, California,
USA

A. KALES MD
Professor and Chairman
Department of Psychiatry;
Director, Sleep Research and Treatment
    Center
Pennsylvania State University College of
    Medicine
Hershey Medical Center
Hershey, PA 17033
USA

W. LING MD
Associate Professor of Psychiatry
University of California, Los Angeles
Los Angeles
USA

J. MARKS MA, MD, FRCP, MPCPysch
Fellow, Tutor and Director of Medical
    Studies
Girton College
Cambridge CB3 0JG
United Kingdom

B. H. MEDD MD
Assistant Vice President and Director
Professional and Marketing Services
Roche Laboratories
Nutley, NJ 17110
USA

K. RICKELS MD
Stuart and Emily Mudd Professor of
    Human Behaviour;
Professor of Psychiatry and Pharmacology
University of Pennsylvania
Suite 203, Piersol Building
Hospital of University of Pennsylvania
3400 Spruce Street
Philadelphia, PA 19104
USA

J. D. ROACHE PhD
Department of Psychiatry
The Johns Hopkins University School of
  Medicine
720 Rutland Avenue
Baltimore, MD 21205
USA

R. I. SHADER MD
Chief, Division of Clinical Pharmacology;
Professor of Psychiatry and Associate
  Professor of Medicine
Tufts University School of Medicine and
  New England Medical Center Hospital
171 Harrison Avenue
Boston, MA 02111
USA

D. F. SMITH MD
Research Director, Merritt Peralta Institute
Chemical Dependency Recovery Hospital
Oakland, California;
Director and Founder of the Haight-
  Ashbury Free Medical Clinic
409 Clayton Street
San Francisco, CA 94117
USA

C. R. SOLDATOS MD
Chief, Sleep Research Unit, Department of
  Psychiatry
University of Athens School of Medicine
Athens, Greece;
Clinical Professor, Department of
  Psychiatry and Sleep Treatment Center
Pennsylvania State University College of
  Medicine
Hershey, Pennsylvania,
USA

A. VELA-BUENO MD
Director, Sleep Disorders Unit
Department of Clinical Neurophysiology
Hospital Clinico San Carlos
University of Madrid
Madrid, Spain;
Clinical Professor, Department of
  Psychiatry and Sleep Research and
  Treatment Center
Pennsylvania State University College of
  Medicine
Hershey, Pennsylvania
USA

J. WARD BA
Medical Information
Pharmaceutical Division
F. Hoffmann–La Roche & Co Ltd
CH-4002 Basel
Switzerland

U. WEIERSHAUSEN PharmD
Goedecke Research Institute
Mooswaldallee 1-9
D-7800 Freiburg
West Germany

D. R. WESSON MD
Department of Pschiatry
San Francisco Veterans Administration
  Medical Center
4150 Clement Street, 116F
San Francisco, CA 94121
USA

J. H. WOODS PhD
Departments of Pharmacology and
  Psychology
M6322 Medscience Building
University of Michigan Medical School
Ann Arbor, MI 48109
USA

Acknowledgements

In the Fall of 1982, the Haight-Ashbury Benzodiazepine Training and Research Project staged a conference on benzodiazepines in San Francisco. Following the conference, our English colleague, Dr. John Marks, internationally known for his writings on benzodiazepines, and David Bloomer, Managing Director of MTP Press, encouraged us to write a book on benzodiazepines from an international perspective. The proceedings of the conference, published in the Spring of 1983 issue of the *Journal of Psychoactive Drugs*, was the foundation on which we began this book. Some chapters of this book are revisions of papers presented at the conference, and the journal editors, E. Lief Zerkin and Jeffrey H. Novey, kindly allowed us use of many graphics and diagrams which appeared in the journal. We either wrote or solicited from other authors new manuscripts to cover recent clinical advances and new applications of benzodiazepines.

The production of the book would have been impossible without the perseverance of Susan Camber who coordinated the flow of manuscripts, compiled the appendices, assisted in manuscript editing, and badgered the editors into maintaining a production schedule. To her, we express our thanks and gratitude.

David E. Smith
Donald R. Wesson

Introduction

Since their introduction to medical practice in 1960, benzodiazepines have become among the most commonly prescribed medications and have, to a great extent, replaced prescriptions of short-acting barbiturates and other sedative–hypnotics. The discovery of their psychoactive properties was almost missed. During a cleaning of their laboratory in April of 1957, Earl Reeder called to Leo Sternbach's attention several hundred milligrams of a substance and its hydrochloride salt they had synthesized in 1955 which had not been submitted for pharmacological testing. They sent the hydrochloride salt, later given the generic designation of chlordiazepoxide (Librium), for animal testing to the pharmacology department, which was under the direction of Lowell Randall. Six tests, used for preliminary screening of tranquilizers and sedatives, were conducted. Dr. Randall phoned Dr. Sternbach a few days later to report that the compound possessed interesting psychotropic properties in animals (Sternback, 1983). Subsequently over 3000 1,4 benzo- and heterodiazepines have been synthesized (Sternbach, 1983), and more is known about the mechanism of action of this class of medications than any other psychotropic drug class (Haefely, 1983).

Used for treatment of anxiety, insomnia, muscle spasticity, convulsive disorders, anesthesia adjuncts and alcohol detoxification, the benzodiazepines have significant advantages over their predecessor medications: the short-acting barbiturates, meprobamate and methaqualone. Of significance is their high lethal/therapeutic ratio, of importance in cases of overdose; their failure to activate liver microsomal enzymes, responsible for many of the metabolic drug interactions observed with short-acting barbiturates, meprobamate and other minor tranquilizers; and their lower abuse potential.

The benzodiazepines have also become important neurochemical probes for the study of basic brain neurophysiology. The discovery of benzodiazepine receptor sites in the brain and the subsequent search for an endogenous benzodiazepine-like substance that may serve as the brain's own mechanism for modulating anxiety and sleep patterns is an exciting frontier of brain research.

1

When benzodiazepines became clinically available, they were viewed by the medical profession as safer alternatives to short-acting barbiturates and other available sedatives. The perceived safety resulted in a liberal attitude among physicians regarding their prescription and resulted in the benzodiazepines becoming embroiled in controversy concerning the "overmedicated society" and in feminist concerns about the way female patients are treated by a male-dominated medical system. Although benzodiazepines are currently at the center of the controversy, benzodiazepines did not create the controversy as the notion of the overmedicated society developed before the introduction of benzodiazepines (Morgan, 1983).

Introduction of benzodiazepines to medical practice coincided with developing space travel and widespread enthusiasm for new technological achievements. The uncritial acceptance of medicinals declined when unpredicted side effects to medications became apparent. The frequent failure of high technology products resulted in heightened legal interest in product liability and medicinals evolved as a focus of peoples' anger and resentment that common human problems failed to yield to technological solution.

Increasingly, concern about the abuse potential of benzodiazepines arose. In the early 1960's, Hollister experimentally induced physical dependence at doses several times that of therapeutic levels in human subjects who then experienced classic sedative–hypnotic withdrawal seizures on abrupt cessation of the drug. This dose-related, sedative–hypnotic-type dependence was well established, although it is rarely seen in its pure form in a clinical population. There is increasing data suggesting that theapeutic doses of benzodiazepines when taken chronically can produce physical dependence. Awareness of this possibility parallels increasing international concern about drug abuse. Both the public and media focus on the benzodiazepines shifted from their scientific and clinical importance to their contribution to substance abuse. In particular, diazepam (Valium^R) has become the target of media attention and Valium^R addiction in the 1970's became more "fashionable" than emotional disorders.

The media disproportionately focused on the abuse potential of benzodiazepines, and as a consequence, conflicting opinions exist about the role of benzodiazepines in medicine and research: Will they lead to a major scientific breakthrough in understanding fundamental brain chemistry? Are they safe and effective clinical tools for the physician to use in treating a wide variety of pathological conditions? Or are they chemical tools with which physicians unwittingly induce addiction, particularly in their female patients?

In an attempt to clarify confusion and establish objective information for physicians, consumers, substance abuse treatment programs, and regulatory agencies who are attempting to pass new legislation and enforce legal guidelines in the midst of a morass of conflicting opinion. the Benzodiazepine Research and Training Project. an activity of the Haight-Ashbury Clinic in San Francisco held a conference entitled. "The Benzodiazepines Today: Two Decades of Research and Clinical Experience". Held in San Francisco, October 8–11. 1982, the proceedings of the conference were published in a special issue of the *Journal of Psychoactive Drugs*(Vol. 15, Jan-June, 1983).

This book, intended for practicing clinicians, includes some clinical papers presented at the conference and distills the social and regulatory issues of practical clinical importance. Additional chapters have been written to cover clinical topics not addressed at the conference. Our goal has been to codify current standards of medical practice utilizing benzodiazepines and to provide an index to the clinically relevant literature developed through experience with the benzodiazepines during the past 20 years.

References

Haefely W: The biological basis of benzodiazepine actions. *J Psychoactive Drugs* 1983;15:19-39.

Morgan JP: Cultural and medical attitudes toward benzodiazepines: conflicting metaphors. *J Psychoactive Drugs* 1983;15:115-120.

Sternbach LH: The benzodiazepine story. *J Psychoactive Drugs* 1983;15:15-17.

I. Clinical Pharmacology

1. Clinical Pharmacology

1
The Biological Basis of Benzodiazepine Actions

Willy Haefely, MD

In spite of intensive research during the decade following the introduction of chlordiazepoxide into clinical medicine, the mechanism(s) of actions of benzodiazepines remained obscure. An important breakthrough occurred with the discovery of the role of gamma-amino-butyric acid (GABA) as the main inhibitory neurotransmitter in the mammalian central nervous system (CNS). Demonstration that there was a close association between benzodiazepine actions and GABAergic mechanisms (Polc, Möhler & Haefely, 1974; Costa, Guidotti & Mao, 1975; Haefely *et at.*, 1975) led to massive amounts of research which clarified the relationship between GABA and benzodiazepines and resulted in a number of fundamental neurochemical discoveries. This chapter reviews current understanding of the biological basis of benzodiazepine actions and builds on earlier comprehensive reviews (Haefely, 1977, 1978, 1980, 1983b; Haefely *et al.*, 1975,1978, 1981, 1983a).

THE PHARMACOLOGICAL PROFILE OF BENZODIAZEPINES

Benzodiazepines have a broad spectrum of pharmacological activities, which are summarized in Table 1. A remarkable feature of benzodiazepines is their selective action on the CNS. In usual doses, benzodiazepines produce no effects which are not accounted for by actions within the CNS.

Anticonvulsant Activity

Benzodiazepines are potent anticonvulsants. They prevent or abolish seizures induced by chemical convulsants, most potently those induced by drugs that interfere with normal GABAergic mechanisms (e.g., by inhibiting GABA synthesis). They are also effective in animal models of genetic, hyperbaric and high oxygen-induced epilepsy as well as in the so-called kindling epilepsy. Most benzodiazepines are less potent and some (e.g., thienotriazolodiazepines) are even ineffective (unpublished observations of this laboratory) in preventing electroshock-induced convulsions, in spite of very potent activity on pentylenetetrazol-induced seizures. The anti-convulsant effect of benzodiazepines is due primarily to the prevention of the propagation and generalization of epileptiform activity within the CNS and a depression of motor effector systems; abnormal paroxysmal electrical activity within a chronic epileptic focus is usually little affected. The clinical uses of benzodiazepines in treating epilepsy are reviewed in Chapter 9.

Table 1 Main pharmacologic actions and therapeutic uses of benzodiazepines

Pharmacologic action	Therapeutic use
'Anti-conflict', 'anti-punishment', 'anti-frustration' activity, behavioral disinhibition	Anxiety. Phobia. Anxious depression. Pathologic behavioral inhibition
Anticonvulsant action	Various forms of epileptiform activity (epilepsies, intoxications with convulsants)
Reduction of arousal and alertness. 'Anti-stress' effect. Facilitation of sleep	Hyperemotional states Schizophrenia (*) Insomnia
Attenuation of centrally mediated autonomic and endocrine responses to emotions and excessive afferent stimuli	Psychosomatic disorders (cardiovascular, gastrointestinal, urogenital, hormonal)
Central muscle relaxation	Somatic and psychogenic muscle spasms, tetanus
Potentiation of the activity of centrally depressant agents. Anterograde amnesia	Balanced anaesthesia for surgical and diagnostic interventions

* See Chapter 11

Behavioral Effects Related to Antianxiety Action

The effects of benzodiazepines on animal behavior, thought to reflect their antianxiety action in humans, have been investigated in great detail. Reviews of the vast and widely dispersed literature on the effects of benzodiazepines on animal behavior are found in Thiébot & Soubrié 1983; Gray, 1982; Kilts, Commissaris & Rech, 1981; Simon & Soubrié, 1979; Sepinwall & Cook, 1978; Dantzer, 1977. Put in the simplest terms, benzodiazepines reduce or abolish the inhibitory effect of punishment, fear of punishment, frustrative nonreward, novelty and innate fear or aversion of ongoing unconditioned or conditioned behavior (Gray, 1982; Haefely, 1982, 1978). The release by benzodiazepines of behavior depressed by fear or frustration superficially resembles a behavioral stimulant effect and yet, it is not observed with true stimulant drugs, such as amphetamine. *It is often called an anticonflict or antipunishment effect* or, even more broadly, a *behavioral disinhibitory or behavioral antisuppressant action.*

Animal tests most frequently used to screen for 'anxiolytics' (Dantzer, 1978; Thiébot & Soubrie, 1983) are variations of the 'classic' conflict test of Geller and Seifter (1960), in which sessions of food-reinforced lever pressing have interspersed segments, during which responding is simultaneously rewarded with food and punished by electric footshock. Prior conditioning is unnecessary in the so-called water-lick test, in which thirsty animals are allowed to drink water from a bottle whose metallic nipple is constantly or intermittently electrified. The innate drive to explore the environment of an animal put onto a platform may be depressed by punishing any transgressing of the safe platform with footshock, normally leading to a passive avoidance behavior; benzodiazepines reduce this passive avoidance behavior. Exploratory activity in a novel, unfamiliar surrounding seems to be the result of curiosity and neophobia, and benzodiazepines reduce the inhibitory effect of fear of novelty and thereby increase exploratory activity. A similar disinhibitory effect may underlie the increased consumption of unfamiliar or unpalatable food under the effect of benzodiazepines. It is, of course, impossible to know if an antianxiety action accounts for all the behavioral disinhibitory effects of benzodiazepines observed in these various test situations. However, only drugs with proven anxiolytic effect in humans, namely barbiturates, meprobamate and ethanol (in motor incapacitating doses), produce behavioral disinhibition in animals. Antipsychotics do not release behavior inhibited by punishment or fear.

Benzodiazepines reduce some forms of *aggressive behavior* and induce aggression in other situations. The former type of aggression appears to be 'defensive' or fear-induced, the latter ('paradoxical') aggression may occur after drug-induced attenuation of fear.

Sedative or Psychosedative Effects

The sedative or psychosedative effects of benzodiazepines comprise a

9

variety of ill-defined and difficult-to-test changes in the *level of arousal, vigilance and attention* (Haefely *et al.*, 1981). In treatment of anxiety, sedation may be a desired effect (i.e., the reduction toward a normal level of a pathologically increased state of arousal) or an undesired side effect (i.e., the decrease of arousal or vigilance to a suboptimal level that interferes with normal performance). An increased level of arousal or attention (hyperexcitability) may be caused by various internal and external factors. It also typically accompanies anxiety (Gray, 1982) and one may wonder whether a strictly non-sedative anxiolytic can be found and would have satisfactory therapeutic effects in human anxiety. Simple methods for quantifying a psychosedative effect in animals are non-specific. As an example reduction of spontaneous and forced locomotor performance may reflect psychosedation, but may also be caused by other effects (e.g., muscle relaxation). Benzodiazepines, in spite of muscle relaxant effects, may increase locomotor activity and induce a state of behavioral hyperactivity, particularly in cats. Measurements of startle responses and of EEG arousal reactions may be more meaningful than locomotor activity, but are rarely used.

Benzodiazepines are the most frequently used drugs to treat insomnia (i.e., to shorten sleep latency, to increase sleep duration and to reduce awakenings). It is unlikely that facilitation of sleep by benzodiazepines reflects a selective action on physiological mechanisms involved in the control of sleep. This 'hypnotic' effect is more likely due to the antianxiety and psychosedative actions and consists in the attenuation of the influence of endogenous and exogenous stimuli that inhibit physiological sleep mechanisms. Undisturbed sleep in animals is improved only exceptionally by benzodiazepines (e.g., in the rabbit or, at extremely low doses, in the cat). The usual effect of benzodiazepines, particularly in cats, is to reduce or disturb physiological sleep. The situation is drastically different in animal models of insomnia, where benzodiazepines have a remarkable normalizing effect (Scherschlicht *et al.*, 1981). A considerable part of the confusion created by sleep laboratory studies in the literature on benzodiazepines is due to the failure to distinguish clearly between the results on normal and disturbed sleep in humans as well as in animals.

Benzodiazepines in high doses produce *anterograde amnesia* (Bonetti *et al.*, 1982). This effect occurs with all psychosedatives and probably reflects impaired information acquisition by a reduction of the level of arousal and attention.

Effects on the Autonomic Nervous and Endocrine Systems

Benzodiazepines affect many autonomic nervous and endocrine functions by a central action (Haefely *et al.*, 1981). Under non-stressed circumstances autonomic effects of benzodiazepines are either absent or not significant, however under stressed conditions, the autonomic and endocrine *responses* to emotional stimuli are markedly attenuated (e.g., the hyperactivity of the sympathoadrenal system). Benzodiazepines reduce the occurrence of stress-induced gastric ulcer and arterial hypertension. Autonomic dysfunctions are well known to often be the only objective symptoms of emotional disorders, and psychosomatic complaints are an important indication for pharmacotherapy with benzodiazepines.

Muscle Relaxant Effects

Benzodiazepines reduce normal and, in particular, pathologically elevated skeletal muscle tone. However, a significant muscle relaxant effect usually occurs only in sedative doses. At high doses, motor coordination is impaired and ataxia occurs.

Toxicity of Benzodiazepines

The toxicity of benzodiazepines is very low (Haefely *et al.*, 1981; Hines, 1981). There are, indeed, only very few other classes of drugs with similar high safety. Several hundred and even thousand times higher doses are required to kill animals than are necessary to produce pharmacological effects. Extensive use of benzodiazepines for more than 20 years has not revealed specific organ toxicity after long lasting intake. In spite of many questionable anecdotal reports, benzodiazepines are apparently free of mutagenic and carcinogenic activity.

Tolerance, Physical Dependence and Drug-Seeking Behavior

Tolerance to some effects of benzodiazepines may occur on repeated administration (i.e., doses that produce a given effect initially become ineffective, and higher doses have to be given to obtain an effect of the initial magnitude). To date, the problem of tolerance has been investigated only sporadically. Most reports deal with the development of tolerance to the sedative and muscle relaxant effects of benzodiazepines. Various factors contribute to this phenomenon.

The most important factor appears to be pharmacodynamic in nature, based on an increasing biological adaptation of the CNS to constant concentrations of drugs. There are also psychological factors, such as the influence of the environment (File, 1982). The terms 'drug-experience' or 'drug-sophistication' have been coined to describe the surprising fact that a single exposure to a benzodiazepine (or other tranquilizer) may alter the response of an animal to subsequent dosing in intervals that exclude any biological adaptation mechanism (Sepinwall, Gradsky & Cook, 1978).

Pharmacokinetic tolerance may occur when extremely high doses are administered repeatedly. Such highly artificial schedules may result in accelerated metabolic inactivation of certain benzodiazepines. Whether tolerance also develops to effects other than sedation is less clear. Differential tolerance to the anticonvulsant action has been reported, meaning that the protective effect against some convulsants remained stable, but disappeared with respect to other convulsants. These findings have not remained uncontested. The development of tolerance to the anticonflict effect of benzodiazepines has so far not been demonstrated convincingly. On the contrary, with development of tolerance to the sedative effect, the anticonflict effect usually becomes clearer and the amplitude of behavioral disinhibition increases.

Physical or physiological dependence can be induced in animals with all known benzodiazepines, provided they are administered in sufficiently high doses, in intervals adjusted to their duration of action and over a sufficiently long period (Martin, McNichols & Cherian, 1982; Woods, 1982; Yanagita, 1981). The dependence state is a new dynamic equilibrium of physiological functions produced by the action of the drug on the organism and the compensatory countermechanisms of the organism. In the presence of the drug, the dependent organism functions as it did before exposure to the drug. Accordingly, the presence of physical dependence is not determined directly, but assessed indirectly by the occurrence of withdrawal symptoms after abrupt discontinuation of drug administration (i.e., abstinence) or by precipitation with benzodiazepine receptor antagonists such as Ro 15-1788 (Cumin *et al.*, 1982; Lukas & Griffiths, 1982; McNicholas & Martin, 1982; Rosenberg & Chiu, 1982). Benzodiazepines generally produce less severe abstinence symptoms than short-acting barbiturates. The spectrum of abstinence symptoms and the intensity of individual symptoms vary markedly in the different animal species. As an example, rats are very insensitive to withdrawal-induced seizures (Cumin *et al.*, 1982).

When withdrawal is produced by stopping a chronically administered drug, the severity of abstinence signs or symptoms does not accurately reflect the severity of physiological dependence. The reason for this is that the abstinence syndrome is markedly affected by the rate of disappearance of a drug. Because tissue levels of the long-acting benzodiazepines will decline slowly, abstinence from a very long-acting benzodiazepine results in a delayed and attenuated withdrawal reaction when compared with a short-acting benzodiazepine, although the true dependence state (i.e. the symptom-free equilibrium between drug effects and compensatory mechanisms of the organisms) may be identical. A widely held view, that short-acting drugs are more liable to induce physiological dependence, is incorrect: short-acting drugs are less likely to induce a state of dependence (Cumin *et al.*, 1982), but once dependence has developed, the abstinence syndrome is more spectacular.

Precipitated withdrawal reactions with benzodiazepine receptor antagonists will probably help to define estimations of the physical dependence liability of different benzodiazepines. However, caution must be exercised when comparing antagonist-precipitated withdrawal with that occurring by drug abstinence. The availability of specific benzodiazepine receptor blockers may lead to an overestimation of the severity of benzodiazepine dependence, as compared to the dependence on other hypno-sedatives for which no specific antagonists exist. Indeed, the almost instantaneous blockage of receptors by an antagonist produces such a highly unnatural, dramatic and rapid shift in the state of the CNS that it can reasonably be expected to produce symptoms of rebound even in individuals who are not in a severe state of physical dependence. A seemingly paradoxical finding has recently been published by Martin, McNicholas & Cherian (1982): that the precipitated withdrawal syndrome induced by the benzodiazepine receptor blocker Ro 15-1788 in rats made dependent on diazepam was less severe than the abstinence syndrome. These researchers suggest a possible reason for this unexpected finding: their use of very high doses of diazepam (above 100 mg/kg/day) likely produced additional dependency effects unrelated to benzodiazepine receptors and these nonspecific effects would not be reversed by the specific receptor blocker.

The liability of benzodiazepines to induce *drug-seeking behavior* (responsible, among other factors, for abuse, addiction and psychological dependence in humans) is modeled in animals by measuring the drug's reinforcing properties: the animal's ability to initiate and maintain responses that are rewarded by parenteral or intragastric self-administration (Woods, 1982; Griffiths & Ator, 1981; Yanagita, 1981). The methods and findings of many of these studies are reviewed by Woods in Chapter 14 and by Griffiths and Roach in Chapter 15.

THE GABA SYNAPSE AS THE BASIS OF BENZODIAZEPINE ACTION

In Search of a Transmitter for Benzodiazepines

About the time when chlordiazepoxide became available for therapeutic use in 1960, many investigators were pursuing studies of the effects of psychotropic drugs, e.g., reserpine, monoamine oxidase inhibitors, and neuroleptics, on brain monoamine neurotransmitters (dopamine, norepinephrine and serotonin). The effects of benzodiazepines on the monoamines, the central transmitters then accessible to experiments, were either absent or too weak to explain the action of benzodiazepines.

Schmidt, Vogel & Zimmermann (1967) studied the effect of diazepam on a particular type of synaptic inhibition in the spinal cord, the so-called presynaptic inhibition. Diazepam was found to enhance presynaptic

inhibition in the cat spinal cord and the investigators suggested that this effect might explain, at least in part, the muscle relaxant action of diazepam. The significance of this finding was not realized immediately. In the early 1970s, enough evidence had been accumulated to indicate the neurotransmitter role of GABA in presynaptic inhibition. This raised the possibility that benzodiazepines might interact with GABAergic synaptic transmission. Experiments to test this hypothesis (Polc & Haefely, 1976; Polc, Möhler & Haefely, 1974) led Haefely *et al.* (1975) and Costa, Guidotti & Mao (1975) to propose that the primary action of benzodiazepines is to enhance GABAergic transmission. This proposal found ample confirmation in the years that followed.

The Role of GABA

GABA is now recognized as the most important inhibitory neurotransmitter in the CNS (Cooper *et al.*, 1982). Its synthesis in GABAergic neurons from glutamic acid is catalyzed by the enzyme glutamic acid decarboxylase. GABA is stored in vesicles in the axon terminals. It is released into the synapse by the effect of calcium ions that flow into the terminal during the action potential. GABA released into the synaptic cleft is either taken up by GABAergic nerve terminals and glial cells and metabolically inactivated by the enzyme GABA-transaminase or interacts with specific receptors in the subsynaptic membrane of target neurons.

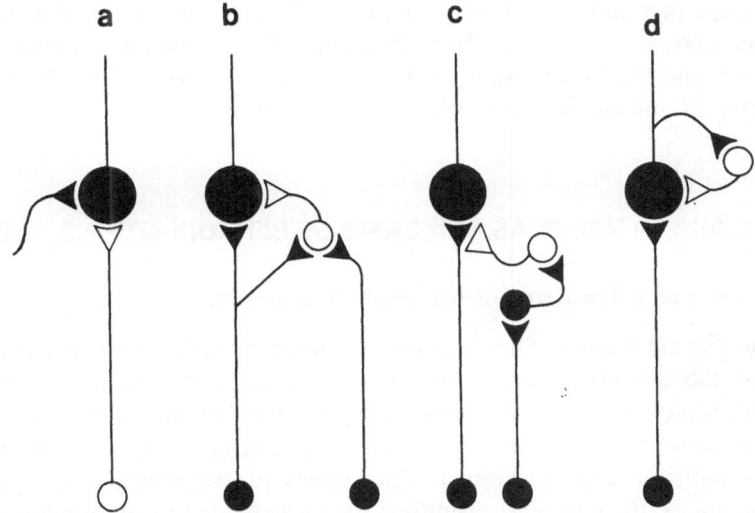

Figure 1. Wiring diagrams showing four types of arrangements of GABAergic neurons in neuronal circuits: inhibitory GABAergic neurons are shown in white, excitatory neurons in black; a, b and c are examples of feedforward inhibition. d shows the case of feedback inhibition; presynaptic inhibition is represented in c, in the other three diagrams the type of inhibition is postsynaptic.

GABA receptors are associated mainly with chloride channel proteins, and receptor activation results in the opening of chloride channels and, hence, in an increase of the membrane conductance for chloride ions (Jackson *et al.*, 1982). Chloride ions flow passively through the opened channels down their electrochemical gradient. In many neurons, the concentration of chloride is smaller in the cytoplasm than in the extracellular space and the equilibrium potential for chloride (E_{Cl}) is more negative than the resting membrane potential (E_M). The ensuing driving force results in an influx of the negatively charged chloride ions and, accordingly, to *hyperpolarization* of the membrane. In other neurons, the intracellular chloride concentration is higher, and activation of the GABA receptor leads to an efflux of chloride ions and *depolarization*. The GABA-induced chloride conductance has an overall inhibitory effect, whether producing hyperpolarization or depolarization, as will become apparent when considering a few typical GABAergic synapses.

Most GABAergic neurons are interneurons, which affect neuronal activity in their close proximity. A few pathways also exist with GABAergic neurons that have long axons impinging on neurons in structures distant from their site of origin. It is helpful for understanding the operation of GABA to consider some typical arrangements of GABAergic neurons in complex neuronal networks (Figure 1). In the circuits labeled a, b and c, the GABAergic neuron operates in a way that is called *feedforward inhibition:* signals arriving from neurons originating in a given area (on the bottom of the diagram) produce inhibition in GABAergically innervated neurons in another area irrespective of the momentary or immediately preceding activity of these GABAergic target neurons. In the case depicted 'a,' a GABAergic projection neuron carries the signals that are directly inhibitory. In the situation labeled 'b,' the signals traveling from one structure to another are excitatory, but impinge on a GABAergic interneuron that converts the signals into an inhibitory command for its target neuron. In the case marked 'c,' a similar transformation of excitatory signals into inhibitory commands takes place, however the target of the GABAergic interneuron is not the principal neuron, but the terminal of an afferent to the principal neuron. In the circuit labeled 'd', the GABAergic interneuron operates in the way of *feedback inhibition*: each action potential fired by the principal neuron (in response to its afferents from the bottom or from any other excitatory input) excites, via a recurrent axon collateral, a GABAergic interneuron that impinges on the principal neuron. In this situation and in contrast to feedforward inhibition, it is the activity of the target cell of GABAergic neurons itself which determines the amount of feedback inhibition it obtains. The GABAergic synapses in the circuits a, b and d are said to produce *postsynaptic inhibition*, meaning that they depress synaptic excitation of the principal neuron through an action on this neuron itself.

The GABAergic interneuron in the circuit c mediates *presynaptic inhibition*, meaning that it depresses synaptic excitation of the principal neuron not by a direct action on this neuron, but by reducing its excitation by depressing the release of transmitter at the excitatory input synapse. While this presynaptic type of synaptic inhibition selectively reduces distinct excitatory inputs onto a neuron without altering its responsiveness to other inputs, postsynaptic inhibition reduces the excitability of the neuron to all its afferents. GABA released in the axo-axonal synapses, mediating presynaptic inhibition of spinal motoneurons, induces a depolarization of the membrane of nerve endings of primary afferents from muscle spindles. This depolarization (and increased conductance) reduces the amplitude of action potentials invading the primary afferent nerve endings and, thereby (and perhaps additionally by decreasing the influx of calcium ions or increasing the efflux of potassium ions), reduces the amount of excitatory transmitter that can be released.

Several agents (e.g., muscimol) mimic the action of GABA at its receptors and are, therefore, called GABA mimetics or agonists. Bicuculline (and perhaps pentylenetetrazol and penicillin) block more or less specifically GABA receptors and are, therefore, *GABA receptor antagonists*. The convulsant, picrotoxin, is a representative of a group of compounds that block the chloride channel coupled to the GABA receptor and hence, indirectly, antagonize the effects of GABA mimetics.

GABA receptors are most probably not uniform. One type of GABA receptor ($GABA_A$ receptor) is activated by GABA and other mimetics, but not by the central muscle relaxant, baclofen, and is blocked by bicuculline. Another type of GABA receptor ($GABA_B$ receptor) is activated by baclofen, in addition to GABA, but is not blocked by bicuculline (Bowery et al., 1984). The $GABA_B$ receptor seems to be associated with a voltage-dependent potassium and/or calcium channel.

The Effect of Benzodiazepines on GABAergic Transmission

The effects of benzodiazepiness on GABAergic inhibitory transmission and on the action of exogenous GABA applied to neurons have been reviewed in detail (Haefely & Polc, 1983; Haefely, 1982, 1980, 1979, 1978, 1977; Haefely et al., 1983a, 1981, 1978). In the *spinal cord*, benzodiazepines potently and consistently enhance presynaptic inhibition and the late part of recurrent Renshaw inhibition (Polc & Haefely, 1982) of motoneurons (an example of recurrent postsynaptic inhibition). Spontaneously occurring inhibitory postsynaptic potentials in cultured spinal cord neurons were found to be increased by chlordiazepoxide. Flurazepam and midazolam were reported to shift to the left the dose–response curve of GABA for depolarization of frog dorsal roots. Studies of cultured spinal cord cells provided the most in-depth view into the mechanism by which the action of GABA is enhanced by benzodiazepines (see Haefely and Polc, 1985).

In the *brain stem*, diazepam was found to enhance both pre- and postsynaptic inhibition of cuneo-thalamic relay cells in the dorsal column nuclei and to enhance the depolarizing action of GABA on terminals of dorsal column afferents. The blockade by picrotoxin of GABAergic inhibition of neurons in the lateral vestibular nucleus of Deiters, mediated by cerebellar Purkinje cells, was reversed by benzodiazepines. The reduction of the spontaneous firing rate of noradrenergic neurons in the nucleus locus coeruleus, of serotoninergic cells in the dorsal raphé nucleus and of dopaminergic neurons in the substantia nigra (Laurent, Mangold & Haefely, 1983), reflected by a decrease of the turnover of the respective monoamines, is strong indirect evidence for the facilitatory action of benzodiazepines on the GABAergic input onto these monoaminergic neurons.

In the *cerebellar cortex*, whose only output neurons, the Purkinje cells, as well as probably three types of interneurons, are GABAergic, benzodiazepines enhanced synaptic inhibition and potentiated the depressant effect of GABA on spontaneous cell discharge. The firing of Purkinje cells was dose-dependently reduced by various benzodiazepines.

In the *cerebral cortex*, various benzodiazepines were found to enhance GABAergic recurrent inhibition (see Figure 1, case d), to depress the spontaneous firing rate and to enhance the depressant effect of micro-iontophoretically applied GABA.

Pyramidal cells in the *hippocampus* and granule cells in the *dentate gyrus* are under a strong recurrent collateral inhibitory influence. Recurrent inhibition was found by several investigators to be enhanced by benzodiazepines, as was the depressant action of GABA and the spontaneous firing rate.

Similar results on recurrent inhibition were obtained in the *hypothalamus*. Benzodiazepines were reported to fail to enhance the action of GABA on peripheral neurons, such as spinal ganglion cells, sympathetic ganglion cells, adrenergic nerve terminals or on lobster muscle. Recently, a GABA potentiation was observed in rat cervical ganglion cells with chlordiazepoxide and flurazepam (Little, 1984).

Mechanisms of the GABA-Facilitating Action of Benzodiazepines

Electrophysiological methods have not only been indispensable for identifying the type of synapses primarily affected by benzodiazepines, but have also revealed possible molecular mechanisms by which this facilitation is achieved. Theoretically, facilitation of GABAergic transmission could be due to a number of different mechanisms and sites of action. Benzodiazepines could act on GABAergic neurons themselves by increa-

17

sing their responsiveness to excitatory inputs, thus increasing GABAergic neuron activity. They could also affect the excitation–secretion coupling for GABA release at GABAergic nerve endings or increase the availability of GABA for release. Although some observations could support such an action of benzodiazepines on the *GABAergic neuron itself*, the evidence is not compelling.

Most of the evidence available suggests that benzodiazepines are acting on the subsynaptic membrane of GABAergic target neurons, affecting the *GABA receptor–effector mechanisms*. Electrophysiological studies on cultured spinal cord neurons carried out by two groups of investigators (Choi, Farb & Fischbach, 1981; Study & Barker, 1981) using intracellular recording, voltage clamp and fluctuation analysis have provided the following results. Benzodiazepines selectively enhance the chloride conductance increase produced by GABA without affecting the actions of other inhibitory amino acids, such as glycine, β-alanine and taurine, or that of excitatory amino acids. They produce a parallel shift to the left of the dose–response curve for the chloride conductance generation of GABA without altering the maximum of the curve. They do not alter resting membrane potential or conductance nor do they alter the conductivity or ion selectivity of single GABA-activated chloride channels and they have no relevant effect on the average single channel lifetime. Their only effect seems to be an *increase in the frequency of single channel openings* in response to a given concentration of GABA. These findings could be explained if benzodiazepines increased the affinity of GABA receptors for GABA, facilitated the conformational change induced in the GABA receptor by binding to GABA (receptor activation), or if they improved the coupling between the activated GABA receptors and chloride channels. An increase in the number of available chloride channels is unlikely because the drugs failed to increase the maximum of the GABA-induced conductance change. How these electrophysiological findings fit into the picture that emerged from biochemical studies will be considered below.

Primary and Secondary Target Neurons of Benzodiazepines

From the identification of the GABAergic synapse as the primary site of action of benzodiazepines, it follows logically that the *primary target neurons* of these drugs (i.e., those neurons immediately affected by their GABA facilitating action) are those neurons that are innervated by GABAergic neurons. Given the widespread distribution of GABAergic neurons within the CNS, there is hardly any type of neuron that could not be a primary target neuron of benzodiazepines (Haefely, 1978). In addition, many primary target neurons are interconnected with other neurons and thereby influence these, which thus act as *secondary target neurons* of benzodiazepines (see Figure 2). It is not surprising, therefore, that changes in the activity of virtually all presently identified neurotransmitter and some neuromodulatory systems (e.g., catecholamines, serotonin, acetylcholine, GABA itself, enkephalin and prostaglandins) have been erroneously interpreted as evidence against the primary GABA-directed action of benzodiazepines. The reasons why benzodiazepines produce specific somatic and behavioral effects, in spite of the fact that nearly all central neurons are potential primary or secondary target neurons, will be discussed below.

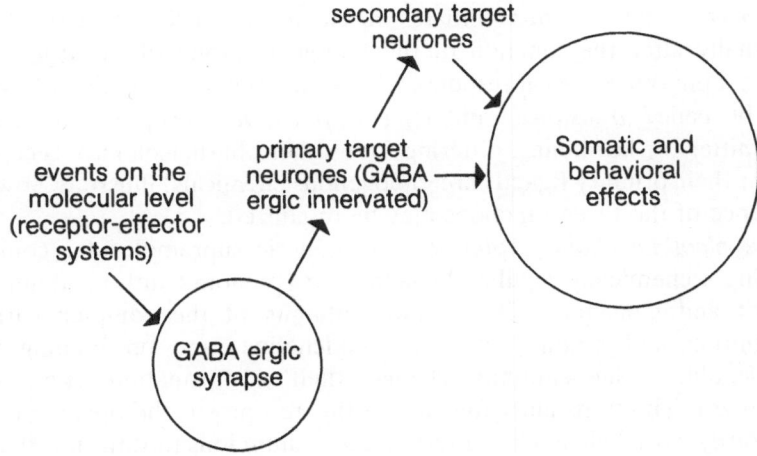

Figure 2 Overview on the different levels at which the actions of benzodiazapines are studied.

It should be briefly mentioned that *mechanisms other than GABA potentiation* have been proposed to underlie the CNS activity, in particular the sedative effects, of benzodiazepines (Phillis & Wu, 1982). Benzodiazepines have, indeed, been found to inhibit the cellular uptake and, therefore, to increase the activity of adenosine, which seems to be tonically released from CNS cells and strongly depresses neuronal activity, mainly by reducing the release of neurotransmitters. The relative potency of benzodiazepines as inhibitors of adenosine uptake is, however, not well correlated with their sedative and antianxiety activity. This mechanism is, therefore, unlikely to be essential for the CNS actions of these drugs, but may be an additional mechanism of action for some derivatives.

BENZODIAZEPINE RECEPTORS

Pharmacological receptors are large proteins or glycoproteins on the target cells with which many drugs have to interact in order to induce their effects. Membrane receptors may be enzymes, ion channels, macro-molecules coupled to enzymes or channels, or structural macromolecules. Pharmacological receptors exert several functions, one of which is to provide specificity (i.e., to recognize and bind specific ligands). This property is provided by a particular domain on the surface of the receptor molecule that has a characteristic spatial arrangement of functional groups, usually called the recognition or *binding site*.

A binding site alone does not make a drug receptor. The receptor macromolecule has to be able to undergo a change in its function when it has bound an active ligand (drug), thereby transducing the event of binding a ligand into a new chemical message. This (conformational) change or *pharmacological stimulus* initiates a chain of further processes that eventually alter the function of the biological target of the drug (i.e., induce a pharmacological response). This initiation or triggering of events may be called *transducer* and *effector function*. Receptors for neuro-transmitters or hormones, differing from other pharmacological receptors in that their primary ligands are endogenous chemicals, illustrate how the sequence of the three functions may be organized.

The *nicotinic cholinoceptor* is a pentameric supramolecular complex forming a chemically regulated channel for (predominantly) sodium ions (Popot and Changeux, 1984). Two subunits of the complex carry a recognition and binding site for acetylcholine, and on binding with acetylcholine, the subunits change their conformation (i.e., they isomerize). The transducer function of this receptor is the opening of the previously closed channel, permitting the sodium ions to flow into the cell down their electrochemical gradient. This effector function (channel opening) produces a perturbation in elements (sodium ions) that are not themselves part of the receptor–effector complex and which results in a membrane conductance increase and in the depolarization of the cell.

The β-*adrenoceptor* is even more complex (Cerione *et al.*, 1984): the macromolecule carrying the binding site may be separated most of the time from an effector part. Activation of the receptor protein by β-adrenergic agonists enables the receptor to interact with a modulatory or coupling nucleotide binding protein (N_S-protein) of the enzyme adenylate cyclase. This interaction alters the N_S-protein in such a way that it becomes able to activate the previously inactive catalytic unit of the enzyme. If adenosine triphosphate (ATP) is present at the active site of the catalytic unit, it will be transformed into cyclic adenosine $3',5'$-monophosphate (cyclic AMP), which in turn interacts with various intracellular target molecules, in particular, protein kinases. While binding of the β-adrenergic ligand occurs at the outer site of the cell membrane, the active site of the catalytic unit of the cyclase (the effector part) is located on the inner side of the membrane. It will be helpful to keep in mind the operation of these two neurotransmit-ter receptors in the following discussion of benzodiazepine receptors.

Specific Benzodiazepine Binding Sites

The pronounced structure–activity relations within the class of benzodiazepines and related compounds (Haefely *et al.*, 1985) suggested very early that these drugs produced their effects by interacting with specific pharmacological receptors. Electrophysiological experiments had clearly indicated that benzodiazepine receptors had to be closely associated – probably in a complex fashion – with the GABA receptor–effector complexes, since benzodiazepines produce their effects only in the presence of GABA in GABAergic synapses. The simplest approach for the further analysis of potential benzodiazepine receptors was to adapt the *radioligand technique* previously used in probing hormone and transmitter receptors.

Using tritiated diazepam of high specific radioactivity, three groups of investigators almost simultaneously demonstrated the presence of specific binding sites for benzodiazepines in the brain (Bosmann, Case & Di Stefano, 1977; Braestrup, Möhler, Okada & Squires, 1977; Squires & Braestrup, 1977). Briefly, the procedure for identification of receptor sites is as follows: Brain homogenates or brain membrane preparations are incubated with an increasing concentration of the radioligand in the absence or presence of high concentrations of an unlabeled benzodiazepine. After equilibrium has been reached, the membranes are rapidly washed to remove the unbound radioligand, and the amount of radioligand bound to the membranes is determined. Radioactivity retained in the presence of a cold ligand is considered to be nonspecifically bound, whereas that part of the totally bound radioactivity that is displaced by a pharmacologically active cold ligand represents the radioligand bound to specific saturable binding sites. Analysis of equilibrium binding curves allows the calculation of the *affinity of a ligand* for the binding sites and the *total number of binding sites* in a given amount of tissue. An immense number of papers dealing with benzodiazepine binding has appeared in the past five years. The most relevant findings are briefly discussed (for reviews see Braestrup, 1981; Haefely *et al.*, 1981; Tallman, Paul & Gallager, 1980; Braestrup & Nielsen, 1983; Haefely *et al.*, 1985).

Benzodiazepine binding sites are present in greatly differing *densities* in most areas of the CNS. The highest densities occur in the cerebral cortex, in structures of the limbic system, and in the cerebellar cortex; the lowest densities are found in the thalamus and lower brain stem. Benzodiazepine binding sites are glycoproteins located on the neuronal membranes. Their phylogenetic and ontogenetic development has been studied. Invertebrates apparently lack specific benzodiazepine binding sites. *Autoradiographic visualization* (see Figure 3) of the sites has enabled their detailed mapping (Young & Kuhar, 1980). Combining electron microscopic autoradiography and immunocytochemical methods, at least some benzodiazepine binding sites were shown to be located at GABAergic synapses (Möhler, Wu & Richards, 1981).

The *affinity* of pharmacologically active benzodiazepine derivatives for central benzodiazepine binding sites is very high at low temperatures (K_D values in the order of a few nanomol/l), and K_D is still in the order of 50–100 nanomol/l at 37 °C, where the dissociation rate increases markedly. There is, on the whole, a reasonably good correlation between relative binding affinities in vitro and pharmacological potencies in vivo. Striking exceptions are readily explained by pharmacokinetic or metabolic peculiarities. A high affinity for the benzodiazepine binding sites seems to be the most important determinant of pharmacological potency. As will be discussed later on, binding does not provide any information on the efficiency of ligands.

The benzodiazepine binding sites in the CNS have a high *specificity* in recognizing benzodiazepines; they do not bind barbiturates or other hypnosedatives. On the other hand, several non-benzodiazepines also bind to these sites. The latter are agonists or antagonists at benzodiazepine receptors and will be discussed below.

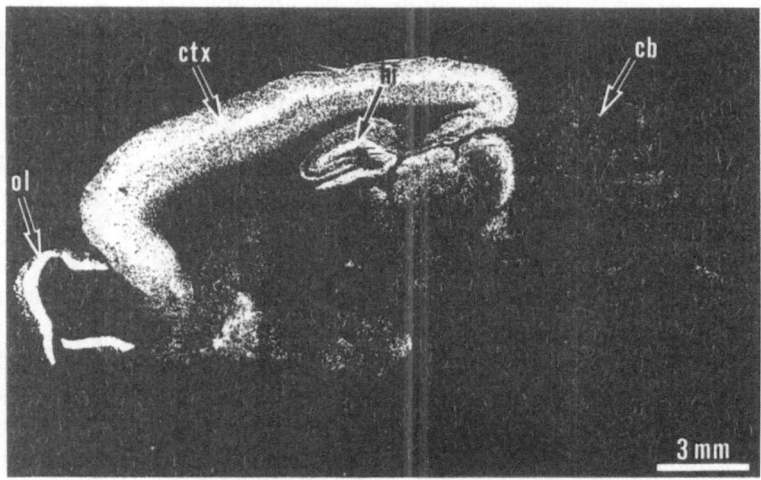

Figure 3 Distribution of specific benzodiazepine binding sites in the rat brain. Autoradiographic visualization of specific high affinity binding sites for ^{3}H-flunitrazepam in a parasagittal section of rat brain in vitro. White areas correspond to the presence of the radioligand. Note the high density of binding in the olfactory bulb (ol), cerebral cortex (ctx), hippocampus (hi) and cerebellum (cb). Courtesy of Dr. J. G. Richards.

Several specific ligands can be coupled covalently to benzodiazepine binding sites. Tritiated benzodiazepines with a nitro group in position 7, such as flunitrazepam and clonazepam, are used as photoaffinity labels. Under the influence of ultraviolet light, their reversible binding is changed into a covalent binding (Möhler, Battersby & Richards, 1980). This *photoaffinity labeling* is useful in the isolation of benzodiazepine binding sites.

Specific binding of benzodiazepines to their sites in the CNS can be demonstrated in brain tissues after their *in vivo* administration using ^{3}H-flunitrazepam for example. *In vivo binding* has been used to determine the kinetics of receptor occupation as a function of dose, time and plasma concentrations (Mennini & Garattini, 1982). The use of flunitrazepam labeled with the positron–emitting ^{11}C (very short half-life) made it possible to follow atraumatically the distribution and displacement of the label in the brain of the anesthetized baboon (Hantraye *et al.*, 1984).

The high-affinity binding of benzodiazepines to central binding sites has been used for the establishment of a *radioreceptor assay* (Lund, 1981; Hunt, Husson & Raynaud, 1979). Using brain membranes, the concentration of benzodiazepines in body liquids can be measured by their inhibition of a radioligand binding to the membranes. The test detects, of course, only drugs and their metabolites with affinity for the receptors.

Benzodiazepine binding sites are not a uniform population. Two clearly separate classes are the so-called *central (neuronal) and peripheral (or nonneuronal) types* of sites. In addition to CNS receptors, Braestrup & Squires (1977) found high-affinity binding sites for ^{3}H-diazepam in peripheral organs, and it is now well established that the adrenal cortex, the kidneys, circulating blood cells and a number of other tissues contain varying densities of binding sites. The specificity of these sites is, however, very different from that originally found in the brain. Benzodiazepine derivatives exist (e.g., Ro 5-4864: the 4'-chloro derivative of diazepam) that lack the characteristic central actions and affinity for brain binding sites but have a high affinity for the binding sites outside the CNS. Most of the potent centrally active compounds, such as clonazepam, are poor ligands in the periphery. No receptor function for this peripheral type of binding site has yet been found, hence these binding sites appear to be functionally silent or *acceptors* (Richards, Möhler & Haefely, 1982). Paradoxically, this peripheral type of binding site also occurs in the CNS. However, the location is clearly different from the usual central type, as it is present in high density, for example, in the choroid plexus, the ependyma, in the olfactory nerve and in glomerular layers of the olfactory bulb and, in low equal density, throughout the CNS (probably on glial cells). The specific benzodiazepine receptor blocker, Ro 15-1788 (see below), which blocks all pharmacological effects of benzodiazepine tranquilizers, does not displace ligands of the nonneuronal type, further suggesting the pharmacological irrelevance of this type of binding sites.

Even the neuronal binding sites for benzodiazepines may be an inhomogeneous population of binding sites. Evidence for this is the finding that, after photoaffinity binding with ^{3}H-flunitrazepam, proteins differing slightly in their apparent molecular weight could be separated after solubilization by SDS-polyacrylamide gel electrophoresis (Sieghart & Karobath, 1980). Other findings suggesting *multiplicity of benzodiazepine binding sites* were differences in heat stability (Squires *et al.*, 1979) and in the affinity of some triazolopyridazines (Klepner *et al.*, 1979). The latter authors have proposed the existence of *type I and type II benzodiazepine receptors:* type I would be present virtually uncontaminated by the other type in the cerebellar cortex, whereas in other brain areas, such as the cerebral cortex and hippocampus, both type I and type II are assumed to exist. Triazolopyridazines and beta-carbolines (see below) have a greater affinity for type I than for type II, whereas most benzodiazepines do not distinguish between the two types. Two different functions have been claimed to be mediated by the two types: type I mediating antianxiety action, type II sedative and other actions. This highly speculative view is poorly supported by functional studies. A more probable explanation for the heterogeneity of binding is that benzodiazepine receptors are a single species of molecules that can, however, exist in different conformational states.

A large number of investigations were aimed at studying the possibility that alterations in the affinity or density of specific benzodiazepine binding sites may account for functional disorders in the brain or for the development of tolerance to these drugs. While it is obvious that loss of neurons by various lesions is accompanied by a decrease of binding sites, there is so far no convincing evidence that a specific *pathology of benzodiazepine binding sites* may be causally related to functional disorders or that a 'down–regulation' of these sites occurs with the prolonged administration of benzodiazepines.

To summarize this point, specific benzodiazepine binding sites have been found both within and outside the CNS. The ligand specificity of the peripheral (or nonneuronal) type of binding sites strongly suggests that they are not part of a pharmacological receptor, but rather pharmacologically inert acceptor sites. The neuronal binding sites in the CNS have a ligand specificity that is compatible with the notion that they are the recognition sites of pharmacological benzodiazepine receptors. Whether all these binding sites or only a fraction of them are parts of true receptors and, if so, how large this fraction might be, is presently an open question. Since an unknown fraction of these sites may be only acceptors, the use of the terms 'binding sites' and 'receptors' as synonyms should be avoided until their identity is demonstrated. Attempts to isolate the specific binding sites, currently under way in various laboratories, will hopefully clarify this situation in the near future. The same is true for the proposed molecular heterogeneity of true benzodiazepine receptors.

Benzodiazepine Receptor Antagonists

Various drugs have been found or claimed to block some effect of benzodiazepines, including GABA receptor blockers, inhibitors of GABA synthesis, chloride channel blockers, methylxanthines, cholinesterase inhibitors, potassium channel · blockers (e.g., 4-aminopyridine), and naloxone (Haefely, 1983; Haefely *et al.*, 1983). They are *nonspecific antagonists* of benzodiazepines: they do not block benzodiazepine receptors, but interact in various ways with primary or secondary target neurons for benzodiazepines or depress GABAergic mechanisms which are the primary site of attack of benzodiazepines.

Recently, however, various compounds have been found that block benzodiazepine receptors with high selectivity. The best investigated representative of these compounds is the imidazobenzodiazepinone derivative *Ro 15-1788* (see Figure 4), which virtually lacks benzodiazepine-like or other actions up to high doses, yet very potently and highly selectively prevents or abolishes in a competitive manner all known pharmacological effects of benzodiazepine tranquilizers or other non-benzodiazepine agonists of benzodiazepine receptors (Bonetti *et al.*, 1982; Hunkeler *et al.*, 1981; Möhler *et al.*, 1981; Polc *et al.*, 1981). The compound also exerts the expected benzodiazepine antagonist activity in humans (Darragh *et al.*, 1982a, 1982b, 1981a, 1981b).

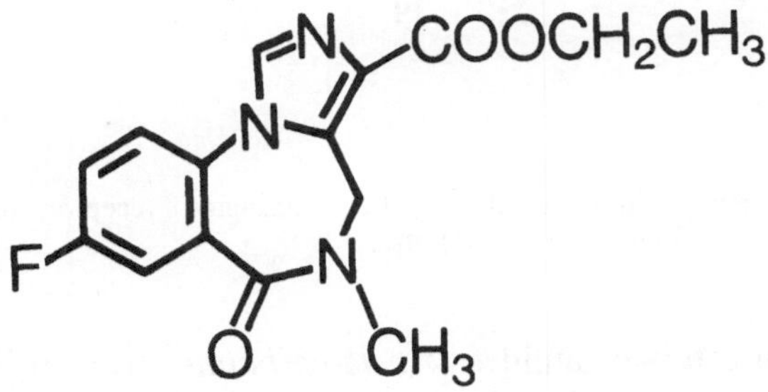

Figure 4 Structural formula of the specific benzodiazepine receptor blocker Ro 15-1788 (ethyl 8-fluoro-5,6-dihydro-5-methyl-6-oxo-4H-imidazo [1,5-a] [1,4] benzodiazepine-3-carboxylate)

Ro 15-1788 is for benzodiazepine tranquilizers what naloxone is for opiate agonists. The compound inhibits the binding of benzodiazepine derivatives to the neuronal binding sites in the CNS, but not to the nonneuronal binding sites in the CNS and in the periphery (Richards, Möhler & Haefely, 1982; Möhler & Richards, 1981). Although Ro 15-1788 interacts with the binding proteins for benzodiazepine agonists, it remains to be shown whether or not the antagonist and agonists bind to the same site on the receptor molecule. The thermodynamics of Ro 15-1788 binding and agonists differ (Möhler & Richards, 1981) and suggest that the antagonist is unable to induce the conformational change in the receptor that represents its activation by agonists. A further difference is that GABA and GABA mimetics enhance binding of benzodiazepine agonists, while they do not affect binding of Ro 15-1788 (Möhler & Richards, 1981).

The chemical structure of another benzodiazepine receptor blocker, *CGS 8216*, chemically a phenylpyrazoloquinolinone (Czernik *et al.*, 1982) is shown in Figure 5. The compound, in addition to blocking benzodiazepine receptors, also blocks adenosine receptors (as do methylxanthines (such as caffeine). This suggests that the compound might have central stimulant activity.

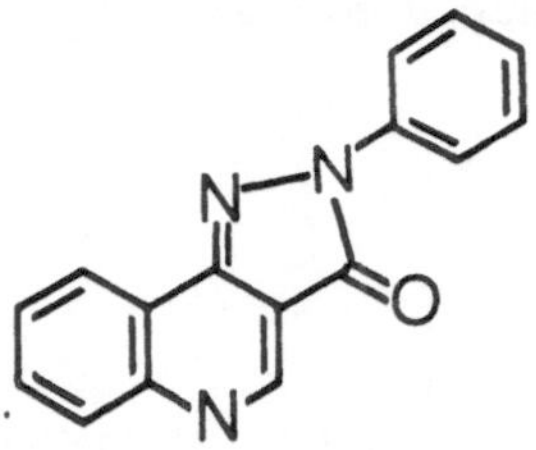

Figure 5 Structural formula of the benzodiazepine receptor blocker CGS 8216 (2-phenylpyrazolo[4,3-c]quinolin-3(5H)-one)

A series of esters or amides of *beta-carboline-3-carboxylate* (see Figure 6) have been described as benzodiazepine antagonists. The ethyl ester (β-CCE) was first detected in human urine and initially considered to be the endogenous ligand of benzodiazepine receptors (Braestrup & Nielsen, 1980). This turned out to be a methodological artifact. Nevertheless, derivatives of β-carboline-3-carboxylate are of great theoretical interest. Whereas the propyl ester (β-CCPr) behaves as a pure benzodiazepine antagonist, others such as β-CCE, the methyl ester (β-CCM) and, in particular, the dimethoxy-4-ethyl-β-carboline-3-carboxylate (DMCM) are

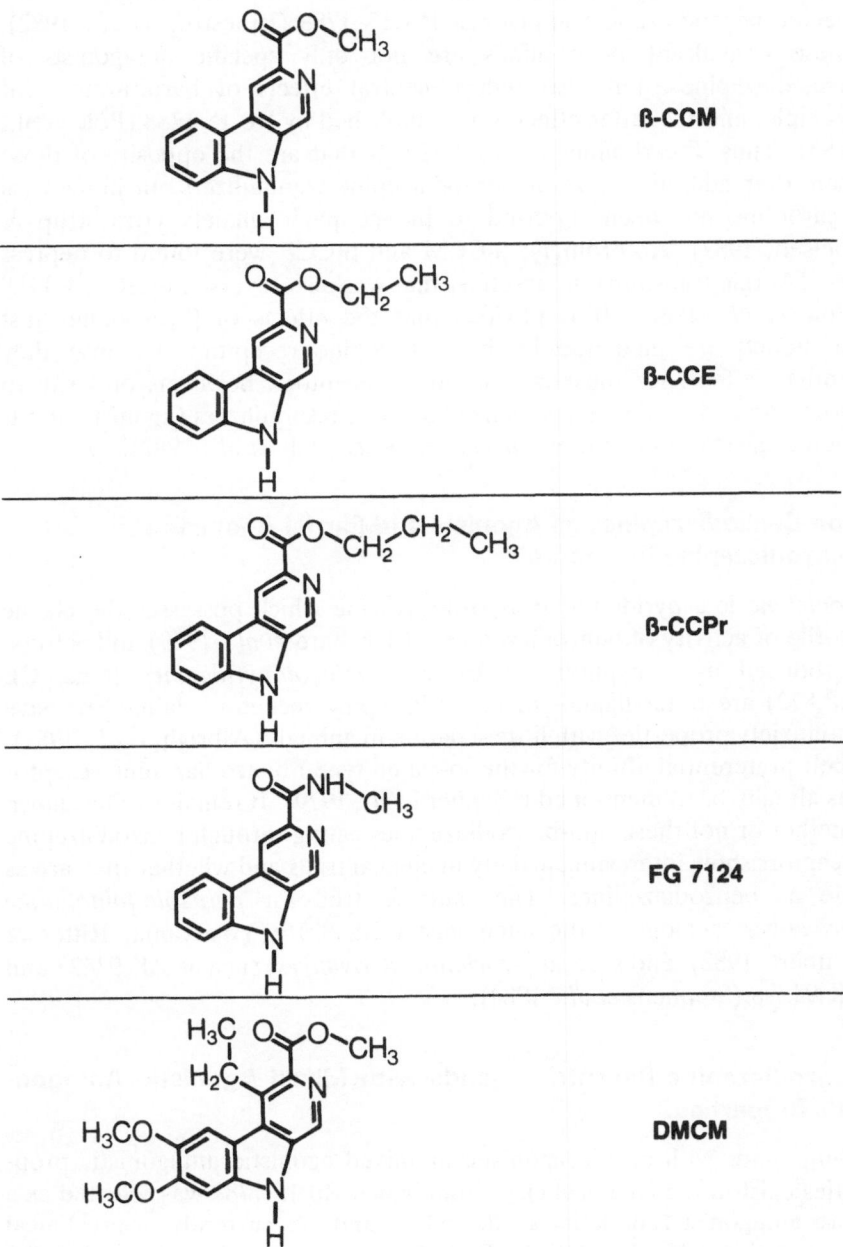

Figure 6 Structures of five ß-carboline-3-carboxylate derivatives: ß-CCM (methyl ester); ß-CCE (ethyl ester); ß-CCPr (propyl ester); FG 7142 (methylamide); DMCM (methyl 6,7-dimethoxy-4-ethyl-ß-carboline-3-carboxylate)

proconvulsants and/or convulsants. Their convulsant activity is antagonized by classic benzodiazepines, but also surprisingly by the specific benzodiazepine antagonist Ro 15–1788 (Braestrup *et el.*, 1982). These convulsant β-carbolines are not only specific antagonists of benzodiazepines, but also reduce central effects of barbiturates, for example, and the latter effect is also abolished by Ro 15-1788 (Polc et al., 1983). Thus, β-carbolines produce effects that are the opposite of those seen after administration of benzodiazepine tranquilizers. In humans, a β-carboline has been reported to induce panic anxiety (Braestrup & Nielsen, 1982). Accordingly, β-CCM and β-CCE were found to depress GABAergic transmission, an effect that was also reversed by Ro 15–1788 (Polc *et al.*, 1982). It is obvious that the effects of β-carbolines just mentioned are mediated by benzodiazepine receptors. Because they produce effects via the benzodiazepine receptors, however, opposite to those induced by the classic benzodiazepine tranquilizers (agonist), it has been suggested to call them *inverse agonists* (Polc *et al.*, 1982).

Non-Benzodiazepines as Agonists and Partial Agonists at Benzodiazepine Receptors

Zopiclone is a pyridodihydropyrrolopyrazine which possesses the classic profile of activity of benzodiazepines (Blanchard *et al.*, 1979) and is to be introduced as a hypnotic in Europe. *Triazolopyridazines* (e.g., CL 218.872) are other ligands of benzodiazepine receptors claimed to have antianxiety properties with little sedation in animals (Albright *et al.*, 1981). Their preferential affinity for the so-called type I benzodiazepine receptor has already been mentioned (Klepner *et al.*, 1979). It remains to be shown whether or not these non-benzodiazepines acting through benzodiazepine receptors show interesting activity in clinical trials and whether they are as safe as benzodiazepines. The same is true for *pyrazoloquinolinone derivatives*, analogs of the antagonist CGS 8216 (Yokoyama, Ritter & Neubert, 1982), and several β-*carboline derivatives*, such as ZK 93423 and ZK 91296 (Stephens *et al.*, 1984).

Benzodiazepine Receptor Ligands with Mixed Agonistic–Antagonistic Properties

Compounds with partial agonistic or mixed agonistic–antagonistic properties exist in the chemical class from which Ro 15-1788 was selected as a pure antagonist (Hunkeler *et al.*, 1981), and are currently in preclinical investigations (Haefely, 1984). Partial agonists were also reported in the series of phenylpyrazoloquinolinones related to the antagonist CGS 8216 (Yokoyama, Ritter & Neubert, 1982), and among β-carboline derivatives, e.g., ZK 91296 (Stephens *et al.*, 1984). Mixed agonist–antagonists of benzodiazepine receptors have a great therapeutic potential. For example, they may show profiles of activity different from full agonists. Just as pure benzodiazepine antagonists have their analog in pure opiate antagonists, partial benzodiazepine agonists remind one of the partial opiate agonists (e.g., pentazocine), some of which have advantages over full opiate agonists. An explanation for the existence of mixed agonist–antagonists has been proposed, assuming a single receptor type, submaximal efficacy and differing receptor reserve (spare receptors) on individual neurons (Haefely, 1985).

Endogenous Ligands of Benzodiazepine Receptors

In analogy to the situation with opiates, it was proposed that benzodiazepines could be exogenous synthetic ligands for receptors that are affected physiologically or in pathological conditions by endogenous compounds of the brain. The latter could be either agents that produce anxiety and other symptoms, and would be antagonized by benzodiazepines or, alternatively, normal compounds acting similarly to benzodiazepines, the lack of which could be responsible for anxiety and other disorders that are improved by benzodiazepines. A number of small molecules and peptides were identified in extracts of brain and other tissues by their (usually very low) affinity for benzodiazepine binding sites. As already mentioned, β-carbolines and yet undiscovered congeners are believed by some authors to be candidates for endogenous ligands (Haefely *et al.*, 1985). However, the evidence to date for any of them is poor (Möhler, 1981) and there is not even an a *priori* necessity for the existence of endogenous ligands.

Proposed Model of the Benzodiazepine Receptor

What has been said to this point about the synaptic actions of benzodiazepines and their receptors clearly indicates that the interaction of benzodiazepines which their receptors does not directly induce changes in the function of the CNS, but requires the presence of ongoing GABAergic synaptic activity. As mentioned before, the electrophysiological studies suggest that benzodiazepines may modulate the operation of the GABA receptor– chloride channel complex. Biochemical studies point in the same direction. Indeed, as first proposed by Costa, Guidotti & Toffano (1978) and also reported by Skerritt, Willow & Johnston (1980), benzodiazepines seem to increase the binding of GABA to its low affinity binding sites. Although these effects are seen in highly unphysiological in vitro conditions, they may offer a clue to the understanding of benzodiazepine action on the molecular level. Further insights into the function of benzodiazepine receptors have been provided by the discovery of specific benzodiazepine antagonists and convulsant ligands of benzodiazepine receptors.

The following diagram (Figure 7) is proposed to explain the facts that have been elaborated to date (Haefely *et al.*, 1985). A supramolecular complex with a molecular weight of about 200,000 (Chang & Bernard, 1982) consisting of the *GABA receptor, the benzodiazepine receptor and a chloride channel protein* (Olsen, 1982) is accepted by most workers in the field. There is no doubt about the association of the GABA receptor with the chloride channel that it regulates; similarly, the macromolecule operating as the benzodiazepine receptor is identical with the GABA receptor molecule. In this model, the benzodiazepine receptor is assumed to be a particular domain of the GABA receptor and the channel protein. Activation of the GABA receptor by GABA and GABA mimetics is transmitted to the channel domain, which results in the open state of the channel. The change induced in the benzodiazepine receptor domain by an *agonist* ligand increases the affinity of the GABA receptor for GABA and/or facilitates the channel gating function of the GABA receptor (increases the gain of the GABA receptor–channel function). Either effect alone or both effects of benzodiazepine receptor agonists in conjunction would nicely explain the increase in the probability of chloride channel opening events in response to GABA in the absence of any changes in the channel properties (single channel conductance, mean open time). *Inverse benzodiazepine receptor agonists* decrease GABAergic transmission (Polc *et al.*, 1982). It is assumed that they produce a change in the benzodiazepine receptor which has functional consequences opposite to those of agonists, namely a decrease in the gain of the GABA receptor–channel function.

Pure specific benzodiazepine receptor blockers, represented by Ro 15–1788, are proposed to act in the classic way ascribed to *competitive antagonists*, namely by binding to the specific benzodiazepine receptor domain without inducing a functional change in the receptor. By blocking the binding site, they abolish the effects of both agonists and inverse agonists.

The model also explains the complex interaction between barbiturates, β-carbolines and Ro 15-1788 (Polc *et al.*, 1982). Barbiturates (at low and medium doses) are thought to interact with a site on the channel domain (Olsen, 1982) to change the dynamics of the channel by increasing the average open channel half-life (Study & Barker, 1981). Hence, their pharmacological activity at these doses depends on ongoing GABA receptor activation. Ro 15-1788 fails to alter the effect of barbiturates, just as it fails to depress normal GABAergic transmission. However, convulsant β-carbolines antagonize barbiturate effects by depressing the gating function of the GABA receptor. This barbiturate antagonistic effect of inverse agonists is abolished by Ro 15-1788.

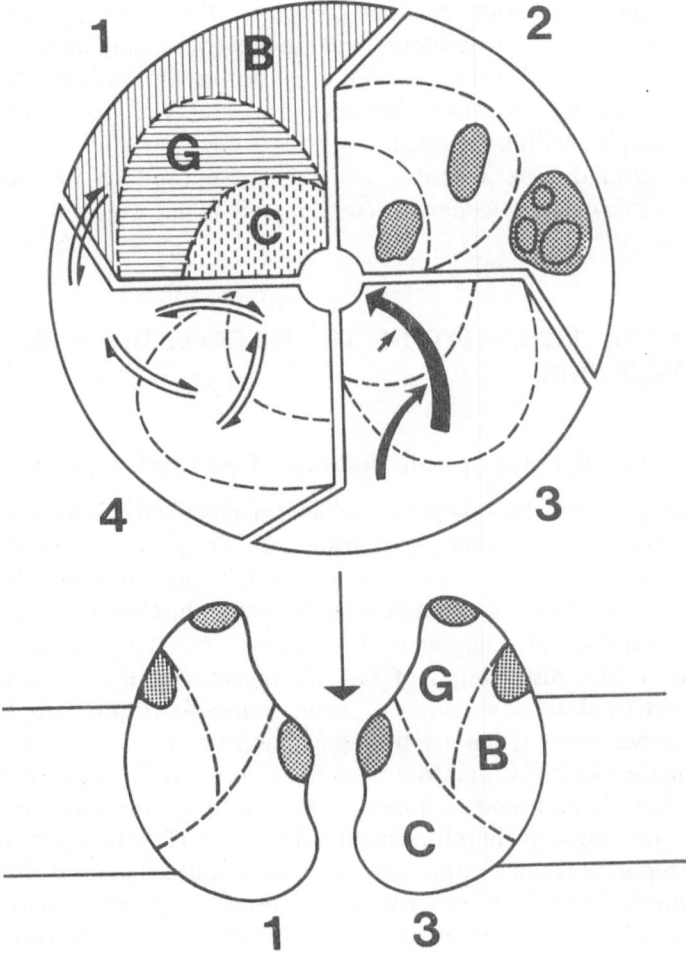

Figure 7 Hypothetical diagram of the GABA–benzodiazepine receptor-chloride channel complex and the effects of prototype ligands. The complex is seen from the extracellular site (above) and on a section through the cell membrane. The complex is shown to be composed of four identical monomers (for convenience). Each monomer contains 3 major anatomical and functional domains: the chloride-channel part (C), the GABA receptor (G) and the benzodiazepine receptor (B). Each domain carries a ligand binding site (shown on monomer 2), the chloride channel domain for barbiturates and several convulsants (e.g. picrotoxinin), the GABA receptor for GABA agonists and antagonists, and the benzodiazepine receptor for agonists, inverse agonists and antagonists. The main function of the complex is indicated on monomer 3: activation of the GABA receptors opens the chloride channel (large arrow), agonists of the benzodiazepine receptor and barbiturates allosterically facilitate chloride channel gating (small arrows). On monomer 4 is indicated that ligands to any of the 3 sites mutually affect the binding of the other ligands. Inverse agonists at the benzodiazepine receptor would reduce the GABA receptor–chloride channel coupling

31

According to this hypothetical model, the *physiological role of the benzodiazepine receptor* is to act as an allosteric modulatory site of the GABA receptor–chloride channel complex. It may be a receptor for benzodiazepines by pure accident, because it carries a domain accessible to benzodiazepines and other ligands (as do other proteins acting as benzodiazepine acceptors) and because of its ability to isomerize when it forms a complex with an agonist.

The benzodiazepine receptor has been proposed to be subject to regulation by *endogenous ligands* (see Haefely *el al.*, 1985).

FROM GABA POTENTIATION TO THERAPEUTIC EFFECTS OF BENZODIAZEPINES

Ubiquity of GABA and Specific Actions of Benzodiazepines

Benzodiazepines produce their various pharmacological effects by interacting with GABAergic inhibitory transmission. They enhance GABAergic transmission and, thus, in a way provide the CNS with a servomechanism for its most important system of internal brakes. It has been estimated that about one third of all synapses in the brain are GABAergic. Even more impressive is the distribution of GABA receptors: all central neurons investigated to date have, indeed, been found to respond to GABA. Moreover, wherever it has been studied, neurons responded to GABA applied on the cell body, dendrites as well as the axon. In addition, GABA receptors have been found on nonneuronal cells (e.g., the vascular smooth muscle). The question therefore inevitably arises: How is it possible that benzodiazepines produce rather specific somatic and behavioral effects and do not simply result in a uniform depression of neuronal activity? Even though no fully satisfactory answer can yet be offered, a few considerations should at least clarify some aspects of this issue.

Benzodiazepines do not act on all GABA receptor–effector complexes: Neuronal GABA receptors may be classified according to their location on a neuron into *synaptic receptors*, namely those present in the subsynaptic membrane of GABAergic synapses, and into *extrasynaptic receptors*, those present in membrane areas devoid of synapses. As examples, the primary sensory neurons from muscle spindles contain synaptic GABA receptors in the membrane areas of terminal *axo-axonal* GABAergic synapses as well as extrasynaptic receptors all along the axon and on the cell body, where GABAergic synapses are lacking. Another example are postganglionic sympathetic neurons, which have GABA receptors on the cell body/dendrites and on axon terminals. Yet all these receptors are extrasynaptic, since no GABAergic synapses exist on these neurons. A recent study by

Alger & Nicoll (1982a, 1982b) suggests that hippocampal pyramidal cells have synaptic GABA receptors on the soma and on dendrites, but also extrasynaptic receptors on dendrites. It appears that benzodiazepines do not enhance the effect of GABA on extrasynaptic receptors in the three cell types mentioned, and this might be a general rule for extrasynaptic receptors. The reason why extrasynaptic GABA receptors are unaffected by benzodiazepines is unknown. According to the model in Figure 7, these GABA receptor–chloride channel complexes could lack the benzodiazepine binding domain altogether or this domain may be inaccessible due to differences in the micro environment of the GABA receptor.

Another differentiation of the GABA receptors, which probably does not exactly parallel the differences in their location with respect to synaptic areas, has already been mentioned as the $GABA_A$ and $GABA_B$ types. It is based on differences in the specificity of the binding sites but probably also includes association with different effectors. It seems that GABA effects mediated by $GABA_B$ receptors are not enhanced by benzodiazepines.

Intensity of GABA potentiation by benzodiazepines: The maximal enhancement of the membrane effects of GABA by benzodiazepines is rather modest. In the study by Choi, Farb & Fischbach (1981) on chicken spinal cord neurons, the maximum shift to the left by chlordiazepoxide of the GABA dose–response curve for the induction of a chloride conductance was about twofold. Although this finding has to be expanded to other neurons and other benzodiazepines, it is consistent with the experience of most researchers that benzodiazepines are very potent (i.e., effective in low doses), but that the enhancement of GABA effects is smaller than that observed with barbiturates for example. This limited intensity of facilitation predicts that the enhancement will not be sufficient to enable GABA released into the synapse to completely block the excitability of target neurons.

The increase of GABA effects depends on the synaptic concentration of GABA: The modest parallel shift to the left of the GABA dose–response curve by benzodiazepines predicts that a functionally relevant increase of the GABA effect in a synapse will not occur in the presence of high, maximally effective synaptic concentrations of GABA (i.e., in synapses with high activity), and small or absent at very low synaptic GABA concentrations. Benzodiazepines should be most effective in those synapses where the synaptic GABA concentration fluctuates around the concentration producing a half-maximal saturation of the GABA receptors. Hence, the effect of benzodiazepines on GABAergic transmission will vary considerably from synapse to synapse, depending on the actual activities of the GABAergic neurons and the number of GABA receptors in the subsynaptic membrane area.

The potentiation of GABAergic transmission by benzodiazepines is self-limiting in certain neuronal circuits: Recurrent inhibitory circuits involving a GABAergic interneuron (see Figure 1, case d) are widely distributed in the CNS; they limit the maximal firing frequency of neurons and prevent firing in bursts of high-frequency discharges. When benzodiazepines reduce the firing rate of a neuron by enhancing the inhibitory effectiveness of GABAergic interneurons, the recurrent excitatory input to the interneuron is reduced. Thus, the effect of a benzodiazepine on the neuron in this situation is to stabilize the firing rate rather than to produce a progressive decrease in the firing rate.

Facilitation of firing rate by some GABAergic neurons: There are many synaptic connections between GABAergic neurons, particularly in the cerebellar cortex. Thus, some target neurons may, in fact, not decrease their firing rate under the influence of benzodiazepines, but rather increase their activity because of increased *disinhibition*.

Activity Changes in Neuronal Networks and Benzodiazepine Actions

To this point, focus has been on the well-established primary synaptic action of benzodiazepines – enhancement of GABAergic transmission – and speculation about the ways in which specific receptors for benzodiazepines may mediate GABA potentiation. A lot has been learned within a very short time about how benzodiazepines act on a molecular and synaptic level. A few factors were mentioned that may determine the effect of benzodiazepines on the level of single target neurons (e.g., the activity of a GABAergic synapse, the types of GABA receptors involved and the arrangement of target neurons within a network containing GABAergic cells).

This knowledge may be sufficient to explain in principle one outstanding effect of benzodiazepines, namely their *anticonvulsant* or *antiepileptic action*. Whatever the primary cause that leads to the generation of paroxysmal neuronal activity (Schwartzkroin & Wyler, 1980), the critical balance between inhibitory and excitatory synaptic activity is disturbed to begin with or as a consequence. Normal inhibitory mechanisms may temporarily prevent intrinsic bursting tendencies of epileptiform pacemaker neurons as well as the propagation of epileptiform activity from an epileptogenic focus to adjacent or distant structures. When these normal inhibitory mechanisms fail, enhancement of GABAergic transmissions will restore or enhance their control over hyperexcitation. Benzodiazepines have been shown to affect mainly propagation and generalization, while they are less effective in reducing the paroxysmal activity within a primary focus, probably because the GABAergic neurons within a focus are morphologically or functionally lesioned.

The *anxiolytic effect* of benzodiazepines are more difficult to explain. To do this, one needs to know the neuronal basis of anxiety, how the GABA potentiating effect of benzodiazepines affects the activity of a neuronal cell aggregate, and the output from it (such as the vertical columns or modules in the celebral cortex (Eccles, 1981)). Although this problem is very complex, it will eventually be unraveled. Gray (1982) postulated the existence of a 'behavioral inhibition system' that specifically responds to anxiogenic stimuli by producing behavioral inhibition and increases its activity in arousal and attention. The behavioral inhibition system in Gray's hypothesis includes parts of the limbic system which are rich in GABA, have a high density of benzodiazepine binding sites and are known to be sensitive to the action of benzodiazepines. Perhaps a deficient GABA system (in absolute or relative terms) with a resultant tonic hyperexcitability of the 'behavioral inhibition system' is a basis for trait anxiety, and a kind of epileptiform activity of the system is the neuronal basis of panic attacks. Anxiety is one form of emotional disturbance observed in temporal lobe epilepsy, and chemical convulsants (including inverse agonists of benzodiazepine receptors) induce states of anxiety in humans and behavioral changes in animals that are assumed to reflect fear or anxiety (Ninan et. al., 1982).

CONCLUSION

More is known about the mechanism of action of benzodiazepines than of any other psychotropic medications. Although it is known that anti-psychotics block dopamine, norepinephrine and serotonin receptors and that antidepressants probably enhance transmission of noradrenergic and/or serotoninergic neurons, the role of monoamines in schizophrenia or depression is still far from being understood. GABA, the primary neurotransmitter affected by benzodiazepines, is clearly an inhibitory neurotransmitter, and the mechanisms by which benzodiazepine receptors affect the GABA system are reasonably well understood. Soon these receptors will be isolated and become even more accessible to study.

Specific benzodiazepine receptor blockers are available and are undergoing clinical trials in anesthesiology (to shorten the duration of benzodiazepine anaesthesia or sedation) and in emergency medicine (in benzodiazepine overdosage). Inverse agonists of benzodiazepine receptors are a novel pharmacological principle not previously found with other pharmacological receptors. They are interesting probes for the study of molecular receptor mechanisms and may have mild vigilance increasing actions. Antagonists and inverse agonists support the feasibility of designing compounds with partial agonistic activity, which may well turn out to be the most significant progress in over two decades of efforts to improve on the first generation benzodiazepines.

Years of widespread use and misuse of benzodiazepines have led to a more appropriate therapeutic application of these drugs. The progress achieved in the understanding of the biological basis of benzodiazepine actions should further improve their rational use.

References

Albright JD, Moran DB, Wright WB, *et al*: Synthesis and anxiolytic activity of 6-(substituted-phenyl)-1,2,4-triazolo(4,3-b)pyridazines. *J Med Chem* 1981; 24:592-600.

Alger BE, Nicoll RA: Feedforward dendritic inhibition in rat hippocampal pyramidal cells studied in vitro. *J Physiol* 1982a;328:105-123.

Alger BE, Nicoll RA: Pharmacological evidence for two kinds of GABA receptor on rat hippocampal pyramidal cells studied in vitro. *J Physiol* 1982;328:125-141.

Blanchard JC, Boireau A, Garret C, *et al*: In vitro and in vivo inhibition by zopiclone of benzodiazepine binding to rodent brain receptors. *Life Sci* 1979;24:2417-2420.

Bonetti EP, Pieri L, Cumin R, *et al*: Benzodiazepine antagonist Ro 15-1788: Neurological and behavioral effects. *Psychopharmacology* 1982;78:8-18.

Bosmann HB, Case R, DiStefano P: Diazepam receptor characterization: Specific binding of a benzodiazepine to macromolecules in various areas of rat brain. *FEBS Lett* 1977;82:368-372.

Bowery NG, Hill DR, Hudson AL, *et al.*: Heterogeneity of mammalian GABA receptor, in Bowery NG (ed): *Actions and Interactions of GABA Benzodiazepines*. New York, Raven Press, 1987.

Braestrup C: Biochemical effects of anxiolytics, in Hoffmeister F, Stille G (eds): *Handbook of Experimental Pharmacology*. Vol. 55/III. Berlin, Springer, 1981.

Braestrup C, Nielsen M: Anxiety. *Lancet* 1982;2:1030-1034.

Braestrup C, Nielsen M: Benzodiazepine receptors, in Iversen LL, Iverson ID, and Snyder SH (eds): *Handbook of Psychopharmacology*. Vol. 17. New York, Plenum Press, 1983.

Braestrup C, Schmiechen R, Neef G, *et al*: Searching for endogenous benzodiazepine receptor ligands. *Trends Pharmacol Sci* 1980;424-427.

Braestrup C, Squires RF: Specific benzodiazepine receptors in rat brain characterized by high-affinity ^{3}H-diazepam binding. *Proc Natl Acad Sci* 1977;74:3805-3809.

Cerione RA, Sibley DB, Codina J, *et al.*: Reconstitution of a hormone-sensitive adenylate cyclase system. *J. Biol Chem.* 1984;259: 9979-9982.

Chang L-R, Bernard EA: The benzodiazepine/GABA receptor complex: Molecular size in brain synaptic membrane and in solution. *J Neurochem* 1982;39:1507-1518.

Choi DW, Farb DH, Fischbach GD: Chlordiazepoxide selectively potentiates GABA conductance of spinal cord and sensory neurons in cell cultures. *J Neurophysiol* 1981;45:621-631.

Cooper JR, Bloom FE, Roth RH: *The Biochemical Basis of Neuropharmacology*, New York, Oxford University Press, Fourth Edition, 1982.

Costa E, Guidotti A, Mao CC: Evidence for the involvement of GABA in the action of benzodiazepines: Studies on rat cerebellum, in Costa E, Greengard P (eds): *Mechanisms of Action of Benzodiazepines*. New York, Raven Press, 1975.

Costa E, Guidotti A, Toffano G: Molecular mechanisms mediating the action of diazepam on GABA receptors. *Br J Psychiatry* 1978;133:239-248.

Cumin R, Bonetti EP, Scherschlicht R, et al: Use of the specific benzodiazepine antagonist, Ro 15-1788, in studies of physiological dependence on benzodiazepines. *Experientia* 1982;38:833-834.

Czernik AJ, Petrack B, Kalinsky HJ, et al: CGS 8216: Receptor binding characteristics of a potent benzodiazepine antagonist. *Life Sci* 1982;30:363-372.

Dantzer R: Behavioral effects of benzodiazepines: A review. *Biobehav Rev* 1977;1:71-86.

Darragh A, Lambe R, Brick I, et al: Reversal of benzodiazepine-induced sedation by intravenous Ro 15-1788. *Lancet* 1981a;2:1042.

Darragh A, Lambe R, Brick I, et al: Antagonism of the central effects of 3-methyl-clonazepam. *Br J Clin Pharmacol* 1982a;14:871-872.

Darragh A, Lambe R, Kenny M, et al: Ro 15-1788 antagonizes the central effects of diazepam in man without altering diazepam bioavailability. *Br J Clin Pharmacol* 1982b;14:677-682.

Darragh A, Lambe R, Scully M, et al: Investigation in man of the efficacy of a benzodiazepine antagonist, Ro 15-1788. *Lancet* 1981b;2:8-10.

Eccles JC: The modular operation of the cerebral neocortex considered as the material basis of mental events. *Neuroscience* 1981;6:1839-1856.

File SE: Development and retention of tolerance to the sedative effects of chlordiazpoxide: Role of apparatus cues. *Eur J Pharmacol* 1982;81:637-643.

Geller J, Seifter J: The effects of meprobamate, barbiturates, d-amphetamine and promazine on experimentally induced conflict in the rat. *Psychopharmacologia* 1960;1:482-492.

Gray JA: *The Neuropsychology of Anxiety: An Enquiry into the Functions of the Septo-hippocampal System*. Oxford, Clarendon, 1982.

Griffiths RF, Ator NA: Benzodiazepine self-administration in animals and humans: A comprehensive literature review, in Szara SI, Ludord JP (eds): *Benzodiazepines: A review of Research Results, 1980*. NIDA Research Monograph 33. Rockville, Maryland, NIDA, 1981.

Haefely W: Synaptic pharmacology of barbiturates and benzodiazepines. *Agents Actions* 1977;7:353-359.

Haefely W: Behavioral and neuropharmacological aspects of drugs used in anxiety and related states, in Lipton MA, DiMascio A, Killam KF (eds): *Psychopharmacology: A Generation of Progress*. New York, Raven Press, 1978.

Haefely W: Biological basis of the therapeutic effects of benzodiazepines, in Priest RG, Vianna Filho U, Amrein R, et al (eds): *Benzodiazepines Today and Tomorrow*. Lancaster, England, MTP Press, 1980.

Haefely W: Antagonists of benzodiazepines. *L'Encéphale* 1983a;9:143 B-150 B.

Haefely W: Tranquillizers, in Grahame-Smith DG, Cowen PJ (eds): *Psychopharmacology 1*. Part 1: Preclinicel Psychopharmacology. Amsterdam, Excerpta Medica, 1983.

Haefely W: Antagonists of benzodiazepines: functional aspects, in Biggio G. Costa E (eds): *Benzodiazepine Recognition Site Ligands: Biochemistry and Pharmacology*. New York, Raven Press, 1983c.

Haefely W: Actions and interactions of benzodiazepine agonists and antagonists at GABAergic synapses, in Bowery NG (ed): *Actions and Interactions of GABA and Benzodiazepines*. New York, Raven Press, 1984a.

Haefely W: Pharmacological profile of two benzodiazepine partial agonists: Ro 16–6028 and Ro 17–1812. *Clin Neuropharmacol*. (1984); 7,suppl.1:S363–S364

Haefely W, Bonetti EP, Burkard WP, *et al*: Benzodiazepine antagonists, in Costa E (ed): *The Benzodiazepines: From Molecular Biology to Clinical Practice*. New York, Raven Press, 1983c.

Haefely W, Kulcsár A, Möhler H, *et al:* Possible involvement of GABA in the central actions of benzodiazepines, in Costa E, Greengard P (eds): *Mechanisms of Action of Benzodiazepines*. New York, Raven Press, 1975.

Haefely W, Kyburz E, Gerecke M, Möhler H: Recent advances in the molecular pharmacology of benzodiazepine receptors and in the structure–activity relationships of their agonists and antagonists, *Adv Drug Res*. (1985) (in press).

Haefely W, Pieri L, Polc P, *et al*: General pharmacology and neuropharmacology of benzodiazepine derivatives, in Hoffmeister F, Stille G (eds): *Handbook of Experimental Pharmacology* Vol. 55/II. Berlin, Springer, 1981.

Haefey W, Polc P: Electrophysiological studies on the interaction of anxiolytic drugs with GABAergic mechanisms, in Malick JB, Enna SJ, Yamamura HI (eds): *Anxiolytics: Neurochemical, Behavioral and Clinical Perspectives*. New York, Raven Press, 1983.

Haefely W, Polc P: Physiology of GABA enhancement by benzodiazepines and barbiturates, in Olsen RW and Venter JC (eds): *Benzodiazepine – GABA Receptors and Chloride Channels: Structural and Functional Properties*, New York, Alan R Liss, 1985

Haefely W, Polc P, Pieri L, *et al:* Neuropharmacology of benzodiazepines, in Costa E (ed): *The Benzodiazepines: From Molecular Biology to Clinical Practice*, New York, Raven Press, 1983a

Haefely W, Polc P, Schaffner R, *et al*: Facilitation of GABAergic transmission by drugs, in Krogsgaard-Larsen P, Scheel-Krüger J, Kofod H (eds): *GABA-Neurotransmitters*. Copenhagen, Munksgaard, 1978.

Hantraye P, Kaijima M, Prenant C, *et al.*: Central type benzodiazepine binding sites: a positive emission tomography study in the baboon's brain. *Neuroscience Letters* 1984;48:115-120

Hines LR: Toxicology and side-effects of anxiolytics, in Hoffmeister F, Stille G (eds): *Handbook of Experimental Pharmacology* Vol 55/II. Berlin, Springer, 1981.

Hunkeler W, Möhler H, Pieri L, *et al*: Selective antagonists of benzodiazepines. *Nature* 1981;290:514–516.

Hunt P, Husson J-M, Raynaud J-P: A radioreceptor assay for benzodiazepines. *J Pharm Pharmacol* 1979;31:448–451.

Jackson MB, Lecar H, Mathers DA, *et al*: Single channel currents activated by γ-aminobutyric acid, muscimol and (−) pentobarbital in cultured mouse spinal neurons. *J Neurosci* 1982;2:889–894.

Kilts CD, Commissaris RL, Rech RH: Comparison of anti-conflict drug effects in three experimental animal models of anxiety. *Psychopharmacology* 1981;74:290–296.

Klepner CA, Lippa AS, Benson DI, et al: Resolution of two biochemically and pharmacologically distinct benzodiazepine receptors. *Pharmacol Biochem Benav* 1979;11:457–462.

Laurent J-P, Mangold M, Haefely W: Reduction by two benzodiazepines and phenobarbitone of the multiunit activity in substantia nigra, hippocampus, nucleus locus coeruleus, and dorsal raphé nucleus of "encéphale isolé" rats. *Neuropharmacology* 1983, in press.

Little HJ: The effects of benzodiazepine agonists, inverse agonists and Ro 15–1788 on the responses of the superior cervical ganglion to GABA in vitro. *Br. J. Pharmacol* 1984;83:57–58.

Lukas SE, Griffiths RR: Precipitated withdrawal by a benzodiazepine receptor antagonist (Ro 15-1788) after 7 days of diazepam. *Science* 1982;217:1161–1163.

Lund J: Radioreceptor assay for benzodiazepines in biological fluids using a new drug and stable receptor preparation. *Scandinavian J Clin Lab Invest* 1981;41:275–280.

Martin WR, McNicholas LF, Cherian S: Diazepam and pentobarbital dependence in the rat. *Life Sci* 1982;31;721–730.

McNicholas LF, Martin WR: The effects of a benzodiazepine antagonist, Ro 15–1788. in diazepam dependent rats. *Life Sci* 1982;31:731–737.

Mennini T, Garattini S: Benzodiazepine receptors: Correlation with pharmacolog cal responses in living animals. *Life Sci* 1982;31:2025–2035.

Möhler H: Benzodiazepine receptors: Are there endogenous ligands in the brain? *Trends Pharmacol Sci* 1981;2:116–118.

Möhler H, Battersby MK, Richards JG: Benzodiazepine receptor protein identified and visualized in brain tissue by a photoaffinity label. *Proc Natl Acad Sci* 1980;77:1666–1670.

Möhler H, Burkard WP, Keller HH, et al: Benzodiazepine antagonist Ro 15–1788: Binding characteristics and interaction with drug-induced changes in dopamine turnover and cerebellar cAMP levels. *J Neurochem* 1981;37:714–722.

Möhler H, Okada T: Benzodiazepine receptors: Demonstration in the central nervous system. *Science* 1977;198:849–851.

Möhler H, Richards JG: Agonist and antagonist benzodiazepine receptor interaction in vitro. *Nature* 1981;294:763–764.

Möhler H, Wu J-Y, Richards JG: Benzodiazepine receptors: Autoradiographical and immunocytochemical evidence for their localization in regions of GABAergic synaptic contacts, in Costa E, DiChiara G, Gessa GL (eds): *GABA and Benzodiazepine Receptors*. New York, Raven Press, 1981.

Ninan PT, Insel TM, Cohen RM, et al: Benzodiazepine receptor-mediated experimental "anxiety" in primates. *Science* 1982;218:1332–1334.

Olsen RW: Drug interactions at the GABA receptor–ionophore complex. *Ann Rev Pharmacol Toxicol* 1982;22:245–277.

Phillis JW, Wu PH: Adenosine mediates sedative action of various centrally active drugs. *Med Hypotheses* 1982;9:361-367.

Polc P, Bonetti EP, Schaffner R, et al: A three-state model of the benzodiazepine receptor explains the interactions between the benzodiazepine antagonist Ro 15-1788, benzodiazepine tranquilizers, β-carbolines, and phenobarbitone. *Naunyn Schmiedebergs Arch Pharmacol* 1982;321:260–264.

Polc P, Haefely W: Benzodiazepines enhance the bicuculline-sensitive part of recurrent Renshaw inhibition in the cat spinal cord. *Neurosci Lett* 1982;28:193–197.

Polc P, Haefely W: Effects of two benzodiazepines, phenobarbitone and baclofen on synaptic transmission in the cat cuneate nucleus. *Naunyn Schmiedebergs Arch Pharmacol* 1976;294:121-131.

Polc P, Laurent J-P, Scherschlicht R, et al., Electrophysiological studies on the specific benzodiazepine antagonist Ro 15-1788. *Naunyn Schmiedebergs Arch Pharmacol* 1981;316:317–325.

Polc P, Möhler H, Haefely W: The effect of diazepam on spinal cord activities: Possible sites and mechanisms of action. *Naunyn Schmiedebergs Arch Pharmacol* 1974;284:319–337.

Popot, J-L Changeux, J-P: Nicotinic receptor of acetylcholine: structure of an oligomeric integral membrane protein. Physiol Rev 1984; 64: 1162-1239.

Richards JG, Möhler H, Haefely W: Benzodiazepine binding sites: Receptors or acceptors? *Trends Pharmacol Sci* 1982;3:233–235.

Rosenberg HC, Chiu TH: An antagonist-induced benzodiazepine abstinence syndrome. *Eur J Pharmacol* 1982;81:153–157.

Scherschlicht R, Marias J, Schneeberger J, et al: Model insomnia in animals, in Koella WP (ed): *Sleep 1980*. Basel, Karger, 1981.

Schmidt RF, Vogel ME, Zimmermann M: Die Wirkung von Diazepam auf die präsynaptische Hemmung und andere Rückenmarksreflexe. *Naunyn Schmiedebergs Arch Exp Pathol Pharmakol* 1967;258:69–82.

Schwartzkroin PA, Wyler AR: Mechanisms underlying epileptiform burst discharge. *Ann Neurol* 1980;7:95–107.

Sepinwall J, Cook L: Behavioral pharmacology of anti-anxiety drugs, in Iversen LL, Iversen SD, Snyder SH (eds): *Handbook of Psychopharmacology*. New York, Plenum Press, 1978, vol 13.

Sieghart W, Karobath M: Molecular heterogeneity of benzodiazepine receptors. *Nature* 1980;286:285-287.

Simon P, Soubrié P: Behavioral studies to differentiate anxiolytic and sedative activity of the tranquilizing drugs, in Boissier J-R (ed): *Modern Problems in Pharmacopsychiatry*. Basel, Karger, 1979, vol 14.

Skerritt JH, Willow M, Johnston GAR: Diazepam enhancement of low affinity GABA binding to rat brain membrane. *Neurosci Lett* 1980;18:323-327

Squires RF, Benson DI, Braestrup C, et al: Some properties of brain specific benzodiazepine receptors: New evidence for multiple receptors. *Pharmacol Biochem Behav* 1979;10:825-830.

Squires RF, Braestrup C: Benzodiazepine receptors in rat brain. *Nature* 1977;266:732.

Stephens DN, Shearman GT, Kehr W: Discriminative stimulus properties of β-carbolines characterized as agonists and inverse agonists at central benzodiazepine receptors. *Psychopharmacology*. 1984;233-239

Study RE, Barker JL: Diazepam and (–)-pentobarbital: Fluctuation analysis reveals different mechanisms for potentiation of γ–aminobutyric acid responses in cultured central neurons. *Proc Natl Acad Sci* 1981;78:7180–7184.

Tallman JF, Paul SM, Gallager DW: Receptors for the age of anxiety: Pharmacology of the benzodiazepines. *Science* 1980;207;274–281.

Thiébot M-H, Soubrié P: Behavioural pharmacology of the benzodiazepines, in Costa E, (ed): *Benzodiazepines – Molecular Biology to Clinical Practice*. New York, Raven Press, 1983.

Woods JH: Benzodiazepine dependence studies in animals: An overview. *Drug Dev Res Supp* 1982;1:77–81.

Yanagita T: Dependence-producing effects of anxiolytics, in Hoffmeister F, Stille G (eds): *Handbook of Experimental Pharmacology*. Berlin, Springer, 1981, vol 55/II.

Yokoyama N, Ritter B, Neubert AD: 2-Arylpyrazolo(4,3-c)quinolin-3-ones: Novel agonists, partial agonists and antagonists of benzodiazepines. *J Med Chem* 1982;25:337–339.

Young WS, Kuhar MJ: Radiohistochemical localization of benzodiazepine receptors in rat brain. *J Pharmacol Exp Ther* 1980;212:337-346.

2
Clinical Pharmacokinetics of the Benzodiazepines

David J. Greenblatt, MD
Richard I. Shader, MD

Studies of the pharmacologic and pharmacokinetic properties of the benzodiazepine derivatives during the last two decades has provided much important information relevant to the clinical actions of these drugs (Klotz *et al.*, 1980; Kanto & Klotz, 1982; Breimer *et al.*, 1980; Greenblatt *et al.*, 1982a, 1982b, 1983a, 1983b). This and related research also has taught us a great deal about the fate of foreign chemicals in general. The benzodiazepines are a class of drugs which are similar in structure, but vary in their physicochemical properties, patterns of distribution, and routes and rates of metabolism and clearance. This chapter summarizes the major pharmacological and pharmacokinetic properties of the benzodiazepine derivatives and the possible relation of these properties to their clinical actions.

PHYSICOCHEMICAL PROPERTIES

The benzodiazepines are a group of organic bases. Although some form water-soluble salts at acidic pH, at physiologic pH all benzodiazepine derivatives are moderately to highly lipid soluble substances (Greenblatt *et al.*, 1983c). There are wide differences among the benzodiazepines in their properties of lipid solubility (Figure 1), which in turn may influence some of their pharmacokinetic properties in vivo. For example, diazepam, midazolam, and desmethyldiazepam are very lipophilic benzodiazepines, causing them to have extensive tissue distribution in vivo, whereas less lipophilic compounds are less extensively distributed.

43

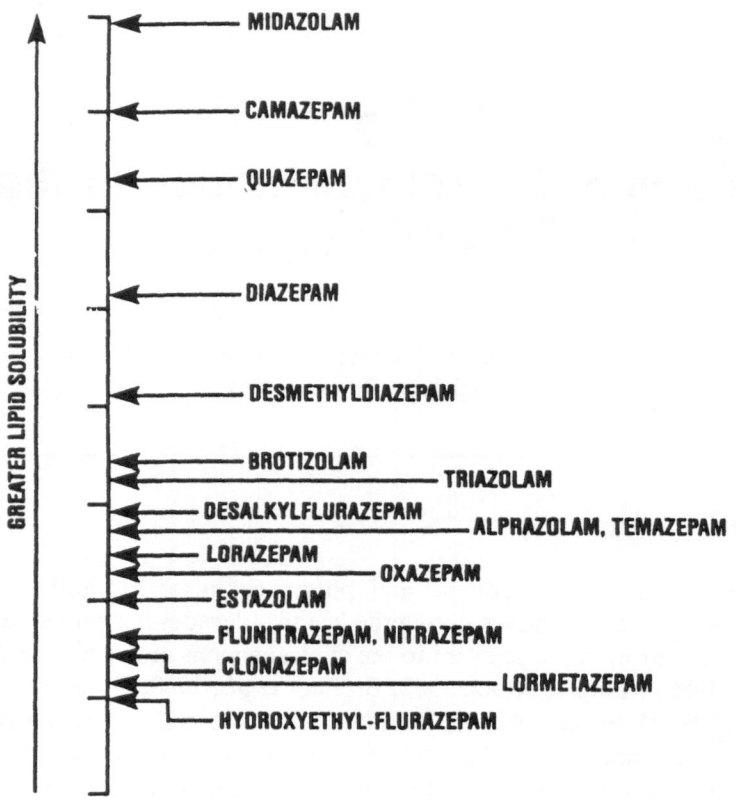

Figure 1. Relative lipid solubility of a number of benzodiazepines, based on the high-pressure liquid chromatographic (HPLC) retention procedure (Greenblatt *et al.*, 1983c). Compounds appearing higher on the list have greater relative lipid solubility.

Benzodiazepines also are extensively bound to plasma protein, but the extent of binding varies widely from drug to drug (Moschitto & Greenblatt, 1983). Of the commonly used benzodiazepine derivatives, diazepam is the most extensively protein-bound, whereas alprazolam is the least (Figure 2). Although the extent of protein binding as such does not influence clinical activity, it is an important pharmacokinetic variable which must be accounted for during studies of the distribution and clearance of benzodiazepines in vivo (Greenblatt *et al.*, 1982c). For example, since only the free drug is available for diffusion out of the vascular system, volume of distribution of free drug much more accurately describes the extent of drug distribution in vivo than does volume of distribution of total drug (Arendt *et al.*, 1983).

44

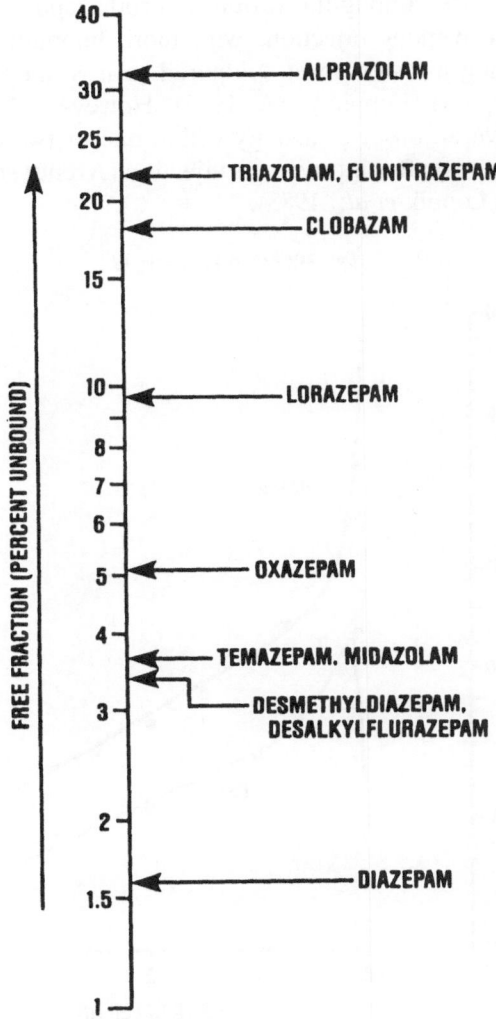

Figure 2.   Plasma protein binding of a number of benzodiazepines (Moschitto & Greenblatt, 1983).

ONSET OF ACTIVITY AFTER SINGLE DOSES

When benzodiazepines are injected directly into the vascular system, they rapidly reach their site of action in the brain (Figure 3). This is because all benzodiazepines, although they vary among themselves in lipid solubility, are lipophilic substances, and thereby easily traverse the blood-brain barrier to penetrate brain tissue (Arendt *et al.*, 1983). Some studies have indicated differences among the various benzodiazepines in their onset of action after intravenous injection, with more lipophilic drugs (such as diazepam) having a faster onset compared to less lipophilic compounds (such as lorazepam) (Leppik *et al.*, 1983). However all benzodiazepines nonetheless have an onset of activity within one or two circulation times (i.e., 30–60 seconds) after intravenous injection (Arendt *et al.*, 1983; Kanto & Klotz, 1982; Leppik *et al.*, 1983).

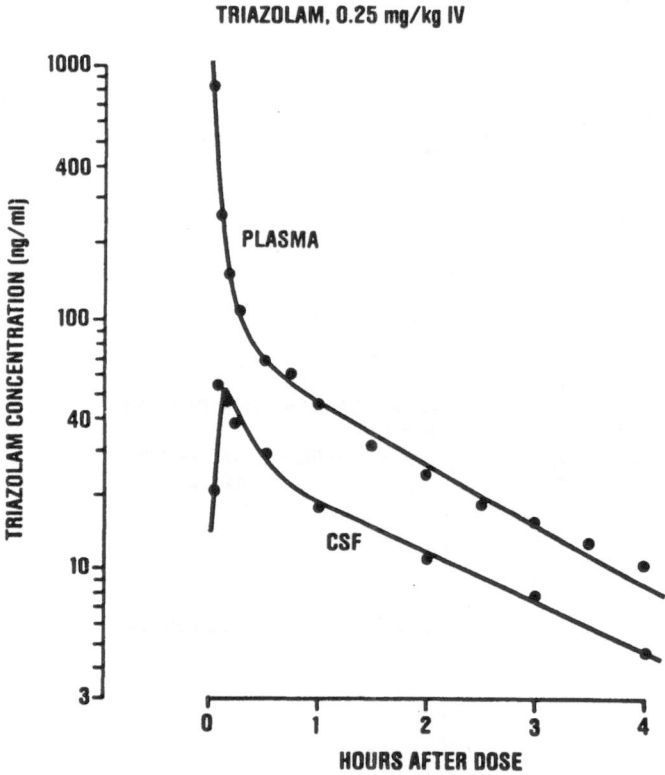

TRIAZOLAM, 0.25 mg/kg IV

Figure 3. Plasma and cisternal CSF concentrations of triazolam after a single intravenous dose of triazolam in an experimental study of anesthetized cats (Arendt *et al.*, 1983).

When benzodiazepines are given by extravascular routes of administration, such as by mouth or by intramuscular injection, the data strongly suggest that the rate of absorption from the gastrointestinal tract or the site of injection is the rate limiting step in onset of clinical activity. This is not surprising, since once they reach the blood, benzodiazepines rapidly enter brain tissue. These findings have important implications with regard to the onset of activity and clinical effects of benzodiazepines after oral dosage. Those benzodiazepines that are rapidly absorbed from the gastrointestinal tract have a prompt onset of clinical action, whereas those that are slowly

46

absorbed have a much slower onset of action (Shader *et al.*, 1984; Bliding, 1974). Table 1 ranks benzodiazepines in order of their absorption rate from the gastrointestinal tract after oral administration, based on studies in healthy volunteers of dosage forms used in the United States (Greenblatt *et al.*, 1983a). Diazepam, desmethyldiazepam (formed from its precursor clorazepate), and flurazepam (leading to its aldehyde and hydroxyethyl metabolites) are the most rapidly absorbed benzodiazepines, generally reaching peak concentrations in blood within one hour after dosage. In the treatment of insomnia, rapid onset of action after oral dosage is a desirable objective, to enhance efficacy in the treatment of sleep onset insomnia. During the treatment of anxiety, the benefits of rapid onset of action are less well defined. Many patients, for example, perceive the rapid onset of drug effects following administration of promptly absorbed benzo-diazepines as therapeutically beneficial, reflecting anxiolytic and calming effects of prompt onset. A few patients, on the other hand, perceive the very same pharmacokinetic property unfavorably, sensing some degree of drowsiness, loss of control, muscle relaxation, or feeling "spaced out" (Shader *et al.*, 1984). These perceptions, whether favorable or unfavorable, reflect the identical pharmacokinetic property of rapid drug absorption. It is not possible for a drug to have a fast onset of therapeutic action without the simultaneous possibility of causing unfavorable sensations in some patients. How a given patient perceives these effects will depend on his or her expectation, prior drug experience, and specific reason for drug adminis-tration.

Table 1 Absorption rates of orally administered benzodiazepines*

Drug	Time of peak plasma concentration (hours after dose)

Rapid
  Diazepam (conventional tablet)
  Desmethyldiazepam (from clorazepate)
  Flurazepam (leading to aldehyde and
    hydroxyethyl metabolites)
	less than 1.2 hours

Intermediate
  Triazolam
  Alprazolam
  Lorazepam
	1.2 to 2.0 hours

Slow
  Oxazepam
  Temazepam
	2.0 to 3.0 hours.

Ultra-slow
  Desmethyldiazepam (from prazepam)
  Diazepam (from slow-release diazepam)
	Longer than 3.0 hours

* Based on studies of young volunteers who ingested the medications in the fasting state. Dosage forms are those available in the United States.

Those benzodiazepines with slow rates of absorption from the gastrointestinal tract, such as oxazepam, temazepam, and prazepam, likewise must be evaluated in light of the specific clinical situation and the sensitivity of the individual patient. Slowly absorbed benzodiazepines might be of benefit for those anxious patients who wish to avoid the prompt onset of central effects following each dose. Prazepam, for example, is a reasonable choice of drug for highly drug-sensitive individuals who feel excessively drowsy or "spaced out" after taking rapidly absorbed benzodiazepines (Shader *et al.*, 1984). It is of interest that the hypnotic agent, temazepam, is slowly absorbed from the gastrointestinal tract when administered in the hard capsule dosage form currently available in the United States. This makes the drug relatively ineffective in the treatment of sleep latency insomnia (Bixler *et al.*, 1978).

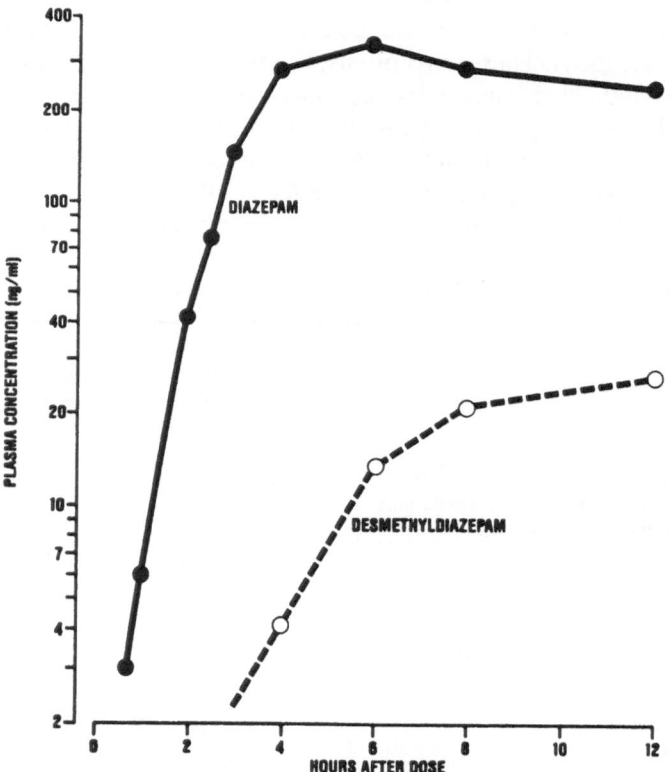

Figure 4 Plasma diazepam and desmethyldiazepam concentrations following a single 15-mg dose of slow-release diazepam (Valrelease) administered to a healthy volunteer.

All else being equal, the absorption of a given benzodiazepine is likely to be more rapid when taken on an empty stomach than when given concurrently with food (Greenblatt et al., 1978; Divoll et al., 1982). This is because the drug must be delivered to the site of absorption in the proximal small bowel before it can be absorbed into the systemic circulation. A promptly absorbed drug can be changed into a slowly absorbed drug simply by coadministration with food. Slowing of absorption will also occur if a drug is given concurrently with an aluminum-containing antacid such as Maalox (Greenblatt et al., 1976, 1978; Shader et al., 1978). The pharmaceutical preparation can also influence the rate of drug absorption. The formulation of diazepam, for example, into a sustained release preparation changes the rapidly absorbed conventional diazepam tablet into a slowly absorbed capsule (Gustafson et al., 1981; Locniskar et al., 1984).

DETERMINANTS OF THE DURATION OF ACTION

The duration of pharmacodynamic action of benzodiazepines is of considerable importance in clinical practice. As in the case of absorption rate, a long or short duration of action may be favorable or unfavorable, depending on the clinical circumstances. If a hypnotic agent has sedative actions that last longer than the length of time the patient wishes to stay asleep, the sedation produced during the waking hours may be unfavorable, and is sometimes termed "hangover". On the other hand, hypnotic drug action that is too short in duration may lead the patient to wake up early in the morning. Similar scenarios can occur in other clinical situations, as when benzodiazepines are used for the treatment of anxiety, for preoperative sedation, or for the treatment of acute seizure disorders.

Benzodiazepine actions may be terminated by at least three mechanisms. Two of these are pharmacokinetic, while the third involves a functional change in the receptor mediating drug action (Figure 5). In pharmacokinetic terms, benzodiazepine action may be terminated if the drug disappears from its receptor site, which can happen by one of two mechanisms. The first mechanism is by drug distribution, in which the drug egresses from its site of action in the brain and is taken up into peripheral storage sites, principally in adipose tissues. The second pharmacodynamic mechanism is biotransformation or clearance – the drug disappears from the receptor site as it is irreversibly biotransformed by the liver. The receptor or molecular mechanism for termination of drug action is independent of the above two pharmacokinetic events, and is sometimes termed "acute tolerance" or "acute adaptation". Acute tolerance operationally describes the observation that the receptors become less sensitive to drug effects as the duration of exposure to the drug becomes longer. Although the drug may have a constant concentration at the receptor site, its phar-

49

macodynamic effects are diminished as the receptor's intrinsic sensitivity to the drug decreases.

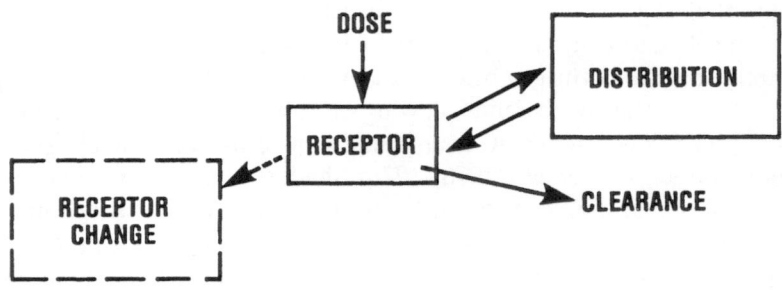

Figure 5. Possible mechanisms for termination of benzodiazepine action after single doses. The drug may be removed from its receptor site pharmacokinetically, either by reversible distribution or irreversible clearance. An alternative mechanism is adaptation or tolerance, in which the receptor changes functionally and becomes less sensitive to the effect of the drug.

Acute tolerance is operative as a terminator of action for essentially all benzodiazepines (Greenblatt *et al.*, 1983c). Although comparative studies of the degree to which various benzodiazepines produce tolerance are lacking, it is probable that all benzodiazepines are equally likely to produce acute tolerance. However, pharmacokinetic contributions to termination of drug action can be quite different among the various benzodiazepines. Current data suggest that distribution rather than clearance is the most important pharmacokinetic terminator of the action of benzodiazepines after single doses. The most lipophilic benzodiazepines, having the largest volumes of distribution in vivo, are those that have the shortest duration of action after a single dose. Midazolam and diazepam are by far the most lipid soluble benzodiazepines, and in experimental studies their duration of action is very short, consistent with their extensive volume of distribution (Arendt *et al.*, 1983). Drugs that are relatively less lipophilic and have smaller volumes of distribution have longer durations of action after single doses. Thus the extent of distribution, rather than the half-life of elimination, is the major determination of duration of action of benzodiazepines. In only a few cases does elimination or clearance contribute to terminating drug action in the first few hours after dosage. Midazolam is the most important example of such a drug. Not only does midazolam have a high degree of lipophilicity and a large volume of distribution in vivo, but it also has the highest metabolic clearance of any benzodiazepine (Greenblatt *et al.*, 1984a). Thus for midazolam, both clearance and distribution contribute to terminating drug action.

The dependence of single-dose pharmacodynamic action on drug distribution as opposed to elimination half-life explains why clinical "paradoxes" are not really paradoxical. Comparable intravenous doses of diazepam and lorazepam, for example, may have very different durations of action (George & Dundee, 1977; Conner *et al.*, 1978). All else being equal, lorazepam will have a longer duration of action after a single dose than will a clinically comparable dose of diazepam. This occurs even though the elimination half-life of lorazepam is much shorter than that of diazepam. As noted above, this is not really a paradox, since it reflects the relative volume of distribution of the drugs. An important general conclusion is that short half-life does not imply short duration of action, nor does long half-life imply long duration of action. A drug's half-life does not predict its duration of action.

CLINICAL CONSEQUENCES OF DRUG ACCUMULATION

Considerable misinformation appears in the literature on the clinical importance of drug accumulation or nonaccumulation during multiple dosage with benzodiazepines. The pharmacokinetic facts are clear, but the clinical relevance of these facts is not completely established.

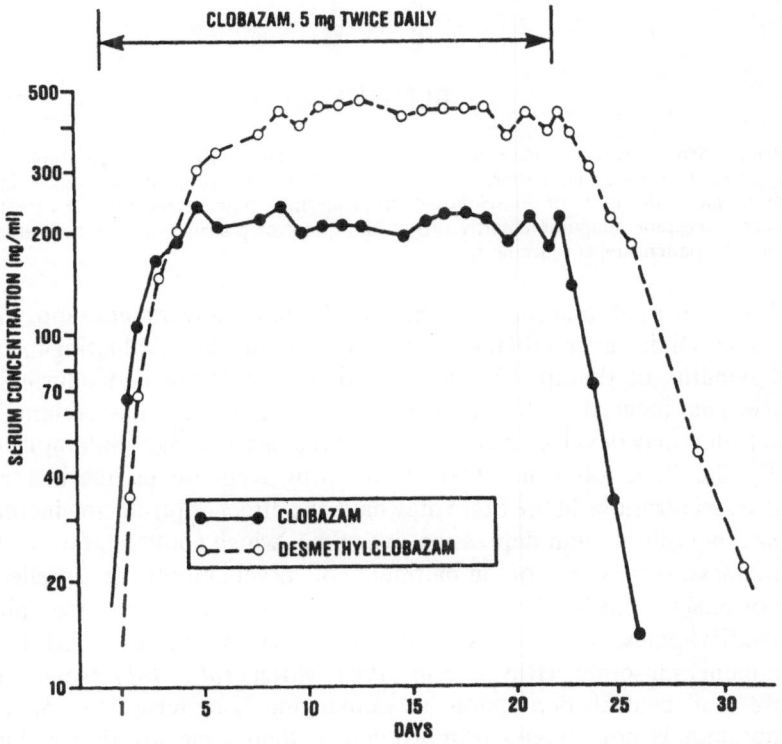

Figure 6. Serum concentrations of clobazam (a long half-life accumulating benzodiazepine) and its major pharmacologically active metabolite (desmethylclobazam) in a healthy volunteer who received 5 mg of clobazam twice daily for 3 weeks, then abruptly terminated treatment. (This case is reported with kind permission from Dr. Hermann R. Ochs.)

The extent of benzodiazepine accumulation during repeated dosage depends in large part on the drug's elimination half-life. Benzodiazepines with long values of elimination half-life will accumulate extensively and slowly during repeated dosage. Conversely, when treatment is terminated they will disappear from the body at an equally slow rate (Figure 6). Benzodiazepines with short values of elimination half-life will accumulate minimally during repeated dosage and will reach the steady-state condition shortly after initiation of therapy. Short half-life benzodiazepines likewise wash out very quickly after termination of multiple dose treatment.

FOR AN ACCUMULATING BENZODIAZEPINE:

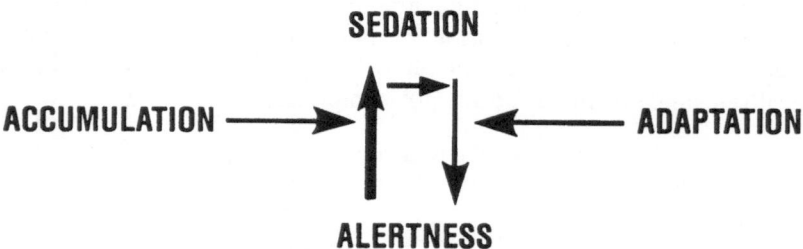

SEDATION

ACCUMULATION ⟶ **ADAPTATION**

ALERTNESS

Figure 7. Schematic representation of postulated clinical drug effects during multiple dosage with a long half-life accumulating benzodiazepine. Early in treatment, drug accumulation tends to move the level of consciousness from alertness toward sedation. As treatment proceeds, receptor adaptation partly offsets the effect of pharmacokinetic accumulation, moving the patient toward alertness.

Both types of pharmacokinetic profile have advantages and disadvantages; clinicians should take these into account when evaluating the risks and benefits of therapy. In the case of long half-life benzodiazepines, concern has focused on the cumulative sedative and performance-impairing effects that may develop over time during repeated dosage (Solomon *et al.*, 1979; Church & Johnson, 1979). As the drug accumulates, the increasing drug concentrations in the brain may have the effect of producing increased central nervous system depression over time, which could lead to daytime drowsiness, sedation, or impairment of psychomotor or intellectual performance. This has been demonstrated with a number of long half-life benzodiazepines, particularly when such compounds are used in the treatment of insomnia (Bliwise *et al.*, 1984; Mitler *et al.*, 1984). However the degree of central depression accompanying long-term use of these compounds is not directly proportional to their concentration in blood. Benzodiazepines are notorious for their capacity to produce adaptation or tolerance, analogous to the situation following single doses. Despite the continued drug buildup in blood and at the receptor site, central depression does not increase in parallel because the benzodiazepine receptor becomes tolerant to the nonspecific depressant effects of the drug. Drowsiness, sedation, or impairment of performance, may occur during the initial days or weeks of benzodiazepine treatment, but these effects tend to abate over time despite continued administration of the same dose and continued drug accumulation (Greenblatt *et al.*, 1977). Thus adaptation partially or completely offsets the tendency of accumulating benzodiazepines to produce cumulative sedative effects (Figure 7). After termination of treatment, long half-life benzodiazepines disappear from the body at a rate that is as slow as their rate of accumulation. This pattern of slow washout after termination of treatment appears to have clinical benefits, in that the "uncovering" of the receptor occurs at a similarly slow rate. This tends to minimize the likelihood of rapid recurrence of symptomatology and/or the development of withdrawal symptoms after treatment is terminated (Salzman *et al.*, 1983; Kales *et al.*, 1983).

Short half-life, nonaccumulating benzodiazepines likewise have some predictable benefits as well as disadvantages. During repeated dosage, the relative nonaccumulation of these compounds minimizes the likelihood of daytime sedative or performance-impairing effects, simply because there is not a continued buildup of drug over time (Bliwise *et al.*, 1984; Mitler *et al.*, 1984). Some studies, in fact, have suggested that some degree of receptor adaptation or tolerance may nonetheless occur, causing patients not only to avoid becoming drowsy but also to experience increased alertness during the daytime (Figure 8). After termination of treatment with short half-life benzodiazepines, the rapid disappearance of the drug from the blood and the brain rapidly uncovers the receptor and increases the likelihood that recurrence of symptoms or drug withdrawal will be of rapid onset (Kales *et al.*, 1983). This characteristic of short half-life benzodiazepines makes it essential that such drugs be tapered rather than abruptly discontinued at the termination of treatment.

FOR A NON-ACCUMULATING BENZODIAZEPINE:

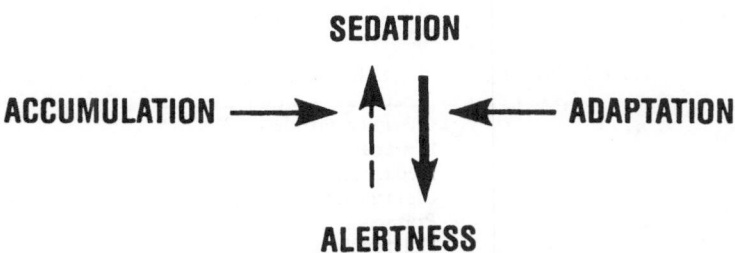

Figure 8. Schematic representation of postulated drug effects during multiple dosage with a short half-life non-accumulating benzodiazepine. Because the drug does not accumulate, there is no tendency toward increased sedation. However receptor adaptation still occurs, possibly leading to increased alertness.

The above discussion suggests that it would be helpful for clinicians to know the usual ranges of elimination half-life for the benzodiazepines in current clinical use. The values given in Figure 9 are only ranges for healthy young persons, and the half-life of a given benzodiazepine in a given patient may be difficult to predict with certainty. Many benzodiazepines in current clinical use are in fact metabolic precursors of desmethyldiazepam. Such drugs are either partially or entirely biotransformed into desmethyldiazepam prior to or shortly after reaching the systemic circulation (Table 2). Since desmethyldiazepam is a long half-life benzodiazepine, any drug that is transformed into desmethyldiazepam will behave as a long half-life accumulating compound.

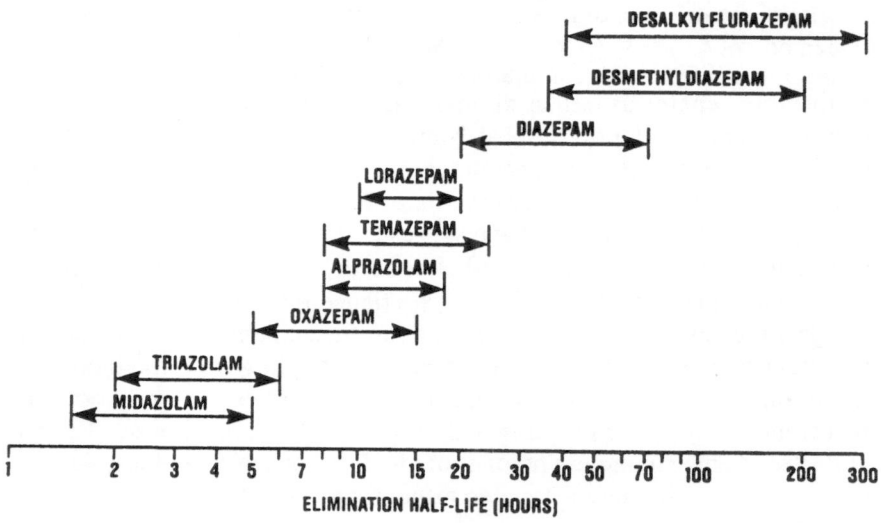

Figure 9. Ranges of half-life values for various benzodiazepines, based on studies of healthy young volunteers of normal body habitus.

Table 2 Precursors of desmethyldiazepam

Chlordiazepoxide
Diazepam
Medazepam
Clorazepate
Prazepam
Halazepam
Ketazolam
Oxazolam
Clazepam
Pinazepam

CLINICAL CONSEQUENCES OF DRUG OXIDATION VERSUS CONJUGATION

The clinical implications of the metabolic biotransformation pathways for the various benzodiazepine derivatives also is a subject of some controversy. The two major pathways for most currently available benzodiazepines involve hepatic biotransformation by one of two principal mechanisms: oxidation or conjugation (Greenblatt *et al.*, 1983a). Oxidative pathways produce relatively minor molecular modifications which may yield active pharmacologic intermediates. The two most common oxidative transformations are aliphatic hydroxylation and N-dealkylation. and many benzodiazepines are biotransformed by one of these pathways. Diazepam, for example, is oxidized by N-demethylation to yield the pharmacologically active compound desmethyldiazepam. This metabolite is in turn biotransformed by aliphatic hydroxylation, yielding oxazepam. The second principal biotransformation pathway of benzodiazepines is hepatic conjugation to glucuronic acid. Oxazepam, lorazepam, temazepam, and lormetazepam are metabolized by this mechanism (Greenblatt, 1981; Greenblatt *et al.*, 1983b). Unlike many products of oxidative biotransformation glucuronide conjugates are pharmacologically inactive and are excreted in the urine as such.

The pharmacokinetic differences between oxidation and conjugation are well established. Oxidation is termed a "susceptible" pathway, since oxidative activity can be impaired by a number of influences. These include: old age, liver disease such as cirrhosis or hepatitis, and coadministration of metabolic inhibitors such as cimetidine or estrogens. Conjugation, on the other hand, is a "nonsusceptible" pathway, since the same factors which can profoundly impair benzodiazepine oxidation may have little or no effect on conjugation (Greenblatt, 1981; Hoyumpa, 1978). In fact, even a disorder such as Gilbert's Syndrome, known to be associated with impaired bilirubin conjugation, apparently does not lead to impaired benzodiazepine conjugation (Shader *et al.*, 1981).

These pharmacokinetic differences have led many to conclude that benzodiazepines transformed by conjugation may be "preferable" for the treatment of the elderly patient, those with liver disease, or those also receiving inhibitors such as cimetidine. Oxidized benzodiazepines, on the other hand, may be "potentially hazardous" in the same group of patients. This argument has sound theoretical rationale, but at present is only incompletely supported by clinical findings.

During multiple dosage with a benzodiazepine (or any other drug), its steady-state concentration in serum or plasma will be determined as follows:

$$Css = \frac{\text{Dosing Rate}}{\text{Clearance}}$$

At any given dosing rate, C_{ss} will increase if some factor intervenes to reduce the drug's total metabolic clearance via hepatic biotransformation. However the increase in C_{ss} as a result of this impaired clearance cannot be assumed to be clinically important. Benzodiazepines have an inherently large therapeutic index – even a substantial increase in C_{ss} in a given patient does not necessarily lead to increased clinical effects or toxicity. Thus the clinical consequences of an alteration in benzodiazepine clearance (leading to an increased C_{ss}) due to a factor such as old age, cirrhosis, or administration of an inhibitor cannot be assumed until they have been proven. In one study, multiple dosage with diazepam in patients with cirrhosis led to increased steady-state concentrations of both diazepam and desmethyldiazepam compared to healthy controls with normal liver function. The increased steady-state levels did in fact lead to an increased perception of sedative effects (Ochs *et al.*, 1983). This suggests that the impaired clearance of diazepam in cirrhotic patients is of clinical importance and that the dosing rate of diazepam should be lower in cirrhosis relative to comparable patients with normal liver function. A second pharmacokinetic factor whose clinical importance has been evaluated is the interaction of diazepam and cimetidine. Coadministration of diazepam to cimetidine-treated patients leads to increased steady-state concentrations of diazepam and desmethyldiazepam. This interaction, on the other hand, is not of substantial clinical importance, since the change in steady-state concentrations apparently causes minimal if any alterations in therapeutic or potentially toxic drug effects (Greenblatt *et al.*, 1984b). Thus the clinical importance of altered benzodiazepine clearance in disease states or from drug interactions cannot be assumed until such consequences are established in controlled clinical trials.

COMMENT

In the last two decades much progress has been made in the understanding of the pharmacokinetics of benzodiazepines. The future of the discipline of clinical pharmacology lies in its capacity to link the pharmacokinetic profile of various benzodiazepines to the pharmacodynamic properties and to the nature of their interaction with the benzodiazepine receptor.

ACKNOWLEDGEMENTS

We are grateful for the collaboration and assistance of Darrell R. Abernethy, Marcia Divoll, Hermann R. Ochs, Rainer M. Arendt, and Jerold S. Harmatz.

Supported in part by Grant MH-34223 from the United States Public Health Service.

References

Arendt RM, Greenblatt DJ, deJong RH, et al: In vitro correlates of benzodiazepine cerebrospinal fluid uptake, pharmacodynamic action, and peripheral distribution. *J Pharm Exp Ther* 1983;227:95-106.

Bixler EO, Kales A, Soldatos CR, et al: Effectiveness of temazepam with shcrt-, intermediate-, and long-term use: sleep laboratory evaluation. *J Clin Pharmacol* 1978;18:110-118.

Bliding A: Effect of different rates of absorption of two benzodiazepines on subjective and objective parameters. *Europ J Clin Pharmacol* 1974;7:201-211.

Bliwise D, Seidel W, Greenblatt DJ, et al: Nighttime and daytime efficacy of flurazepam and oxazepam in chronic insomnia. *Am J Psychiatry* 1984;141:191-195.

Breimer DD, Jochemsen R, von Albert HH: Pharmacokinetics of benzodiazepines. *Arzneimittelforsch* 1980;30:875-881.

Church MW, Johnson LC: Mood and performance of poor sleepers during repeated use of flurazepam. *Psychopharmacology* 1979;61:309-316.

Conner JT, Katz RL, Bellville JW, et al: Diazepam and lorazepam for intravenous surgical premedication. *J Clin Pharmacol* 1978;18:285-292.

Divoll M, Greenblatt DJ, Ciraulo DA, et al: Clobazam kinetics: intra-subject variability, and effect of food on absorption. *J Clin Pharmacol* 1982;22:69-73.

George KA, Dundee JW: Relative amnesic actions of diazepam, flunitrazepam and lorazepam in man. *Br J Clin Pharmacol* 1977;4:45-50.

Greenblatt DJ: Clinical pharmacokinetics of oxazepam and lorazepam. *Clin Pharmacokin* 1981;6:88-105.

Greenblatt DJ, Abernethy DR, Morse DS, et al: Clinical importance of interaction of diazepam and cimetidine. *N Engl J Med* 1984b;310:1639-1643.

Greenblatt DJ, Abernethy DR, Locniskar A, et al: Effects of age, gender, and obesity on midazolam kinetics. *Anesthesiology* 1984a;61:27-35.

Greenblatt DJ, Allen MD, Shader RI: Toxicity of high-dose flurazepam in the elderly. *Clin Pharmacol Ther* 1977;21:355-361.

Greenblatt DJ, Allen MD, MacLaughlin DS, et al: Diazepam absorption: effect of antacids and food. *Clin Pharmacol Ther* 1978;24:600-609.

Greenblatt DJ, Arendt RM, Abernethy DR, et al: In vitro quantitation of benzodiazepine lipophilicity: relation to in vivo distribution. *Br J Anaesthes* 1983c;55:985-989.

Greenblatt DJ, Divoll M, Abernethy DR, et al: Benzodiazepine kinetics: implications for therapeutics and pharmacogeriatrics. *Drug Metab Rev* 1983a;14:251-292.

Greenblatt DJ, Divoll M, Abernethy DR, et al: Clinical pharmacokinetics of the newer benzodiazepines. *Clin Pharmacokin* 1983b;8:233-253.

Greenblatt DJ, Divoll M, Abernethy DR, et al: Benzodiazepine hypnotics: kinetic and therapeutic options. *Sleep* 1982b;5:s18-s27.

Greenblatt DJ, Sellers EM, Koch-Weser J: Importance of protein binding for the interpretation of serum or plasma drug concentrations. *J Clin Pharmacol* 1982c;22:259-263.

Greenblatt DJ, Shader RI, Abernethy DR, *et al*: Benzodiazepines and the challenges of the pharmacokinetic taxonomy, in Usdin E, Skolnick P, Tallman JF, *et al*. (eds): *Pharmacology of Benzodiazepines*. London, MacMillan Press, 1982a, pp 257-269.

Greenblatt DJ, Shader RI, Abernethy DR: Current status of benzodiazepines. *N Engl J Med* 1983c;309:354-358.

Greenblatt DJ, Shader RI, Harmatz JS, *et al*: Influence of magnesium and aluminum hydroxide mixture on chlordiazepoxide absorption. *Clin Pharmacol Ther* 1976;19:234-239.

Gustafson JH, Weissman L, Weinfeld RE, *et al*: Clinical bioavailability evaluation of a controlled release formulation of diazepam. *J Pharmacokin Biopharmaceut* 1981;9:679-691.

Hoyumpa AM: Disposition and elimination of minor tranquilizers in the aged and in patients with liver disease. *SA Med J* 1978;71(supplement):23-28.

Kales A, Soldatos CR, Bixler EO, *et al*: Rebound insomnia and rebound anxiety: a review. *Pharmacology* 1983;26:121-137.

Kanto J, Klotz U. Intravenous benzodiazepines as anesthetic agents: pharmacokinetic and clinical consequences. *Acta Anaesth Scand* 1982;26:554-569.

Klotz U, Kangas L, Kanto J: Clinical pharmacokinetics of benzodiazeines. *Prog Pharmacol* 1980;3(No.3):1-72.

Leppik IE, Derivan AT, Homan RW, *et al*: Double-blind study of lorazepam and diazepam in status epilepticus. *J Am Med Assoc* 1983;249:1452-1454.

Locniskar A, Greenblatt DJ, Zinny MA, *et al*: Absolute bioavailability and effect of food and antacid on diazepam absorption from a slow-release preparation. *J Clin Pharmacol* 1984;24:255-263.

Mitler MM, Seidel WF, van den Hoed J, *et al*: Comparative hypnotic effects of flurazepam, triazolam, and placebo: a long-term simultaneous nighttime and daytime study. *J Clin Psychopharm* 1984;4:2-13.

Moschitto LF, Greenblatt DJ: Concentration-independent plasma protein binding of benzodiazepines. *J Pharm Pharmacol* 1983;35:179-180.

Ochs HR, Greenblatt DJ, Eckardt B, *et al*: Repeated diazepam dosing in cirrhotic patients: cumulation and sedation. *Clin Pharmacol Ther* 1983;33:471-476.

Salzman C, Shader RI, Greenblatt DJ, *et al*: Long versus short half-life benzodiazepines in the elderly: kinetics and clinical effects of diazepam and oxazepam. *Arch Gen Psychiatry* 1983;40:293-297.

Shader RI, Divoll M, Greenblatt DJ: Kinetics of oxazepam and lorazepam in two subjects with Gilberts Syndrome. *J Clin Psychopharm* 1981;1:400-402.

Shader RI, Georgotas A, Greenblatt DJ, *et al*: Impaired absorption of desmethyldiazepam from clorazepate by magnesium aluminum hydroxide. *Clin Pharmacol Ther* 1978;24:308-315.

Shader RI, Pary RJ, Harmatz JS, *et al*: Plasma concentrations and clinical effects after single oral doses of prazepam, clorazepate, and diazepam. *J Clin Psychiatry* 1984;45:411-413.

Solomon F, White CC, Parron DL, *et al*: Sleeping pills, insomnia and medical practice. *N Engl J Med* 1979;300:803-808.

3
Pharmacokinetic Considerations in the Treatment of Chronic Anxiety

Ute Weiershausen, PharmD

The scientific background for more rational clinical use of the benzodiazepines established in recent years is mainly based on extensive investigations into the metabolic, pharmacokinetic and receptor binding features of these compounds. Since the profiles of clinical action of benzodiazepines show close relation to certain characteristics of invasion and elimination kinetics, a sound knowledge of these data is a prerequisite to safe and effective benzodiazepine medication prescription. Also, there is a substantial pharmacokinetic influence on the abuse potential of these drugs. Thus attention must be paid to the three aspects of the compound's behaviour in the organism: the plasma invasion rate, the plasma level curve following multiple dosing, and the plasma elimination rate (Weiershausen, 1981).

Benzodiazepines are mainly lipophilic compounds and are therefore rapidly absorbed. Those derivatives, however, with the most rapid absorption produce such steep rises in plasma levels that peak plasma levels occur within half an hour after drug intake ($t_{max} < 1$ h). Peak plasma levels of a second group are recorded after 2 hours ($t_{max} = 2$ h) while plasma levels of a third group rise continuously to reach peak levels after 4-6 hours ($t_{max} = 4$-6 h) (Figure 1). A classification of benzodiazepines according to their plasma invasion (or absorption) kinetics (Weiershausen 1981; Cooper, 1982; Greenblatt *et al.*, 1983) is of particular interest in view of the compounds' phase of initial drug action.

Bliding (1974) was the first who, on the basis of controlled clinical studies, related the speed of plasma invasion of benzodiazepines to the induction of subjective perceptible drug effects which he supposes to bear a special risk of abuse. From additional, albeit rare clinical data recorded in the literature, it is suggested that, with derivatives of the rapidly invading type, phenomena like rush, euphoria, amnesia, induction of sleepiness, or decreases of vigilance in the initial phase of drug action occur more commonly than with derivatives released less readily into the circulation. Further, because drug addicts want to experience a discernible drug effect, psychotropic drugs with a rapid onset of action are preferred for abuse by these individuals. The phenomena may affect the patient if extremely rapidly-absorbed derivatives also display high specific receptor-binding activity. Since a smoother, more delayed onset of action militates against perceptible drug effects, more slowly-released compounds should be preferred unless a rapid onset of effects is needed (e.g., sleep induction, or treatment of acute anxiety attacks).

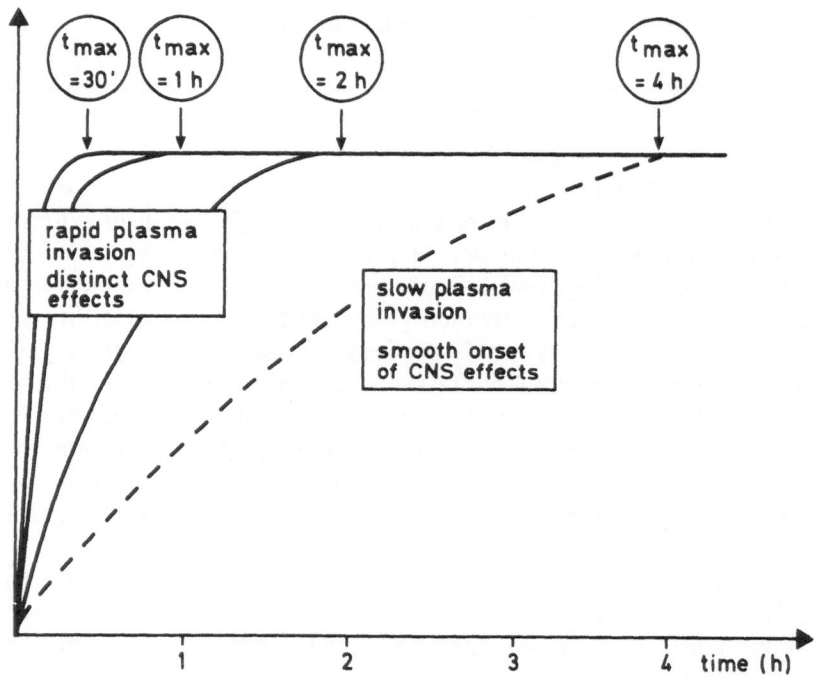

Figure 1 Plasma invasion characteristics of common benzodiazepines (t_{max} = time of peak plasma level).

The induction of perceptible psychotropic effects in the drugs' invasion phase as a function of plasma level changes over time is particularly a matter of interest in multiple dosing. Repeated, short-lived, marked CNS effects (e.g. sedation) occurring in the course of benzodiazepine daytime tranquillization in patients who need antianxiety effects, can cause distress, preventing these substances from fully developing a psychoregulative function. They are expected also to influence the abuse potential of the drug (Bliding, 1974). Thus, major fluctuations in effect between single doses should be avoided. In order to achieve a continuous plateau of effects, efforts are therefore made to build up plasma concentrations with as little fluctuation as possible. Due to the benzodiazepines' high therapeutic index, accumulation can be used to build up steady-state plasma levels in an effective non-toxic concentration range. Compounds with a long half-life are most suitable for this purpose. Benzodiazepines may be classified in derivatives with a short ($t_{1/2}$ = 5–6 h), intermediate ($t_{1/2}$ = 10–25 h), and long ($t_{1/2}$ = 50–80 h) half-life (Kales, 1979; Vollmer, 1981; Greenblatt *et al.*, 1983). Derivatives with a long half-life reach a state of equilibrium after several days of treatment. The plasma level curves of these compounds are characterized by only slight fluctuation between individual doses, even when the drug is administered only once a day (Figure 2). This can be an advantage in treatment of chronic anxiety requiring continuous drug administration to prevent recurrent cycles of symptoms, conditions which could result in operant conditioning of the patient to drug intake.

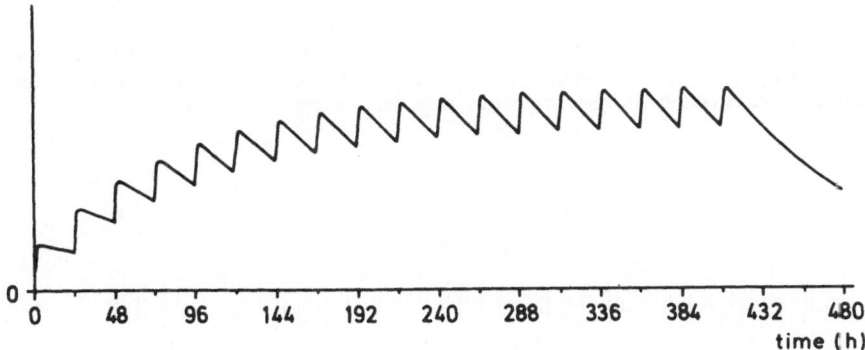

Figure 2   Plasma level curve following multiple dosing of a benzodiazepine with slow plasma invasion (t_{max} = 1 h) and short half-life ($t_{1/2}$ = 4.5 h). Dose schedule: one tablet b.i.d. (From Weiershausen, U: *Fortschr. Med.*, 1981, reproduced with permission)

A plasma level plateau of the kind produced by benzodiazepines with long half-lives cannot be obtained by means of compounds with short or intermediate half-lives, which can well be visualized by computer-simulated plasma level curves, kindly produced by Dr. E. U. Köelle, Freiburg, FR Germany. In the case of benzodiazepines with a short half-life, plasma levels drop almost to zero between individual doses (Figure 3). Even when the daily dose of such compounds is divided into several single doses, significant fluctuations in plasma levels occur (Figure 4). Therefore, benzodiazepine derivatives with half-lives causing major fluctuations of effects between individual doses cannot be considered the drugs of choice for daytime tranquillization. A factor also to be borne in mind with respect to multiple benzodiazepine dosing is the possible presence of more than one active substance in the plasma. Even in the presence of an active metabolite with a long half-life, a single dose can produce distinct CNS effects when considerable quantities of an active parent compound invade the plasma rapidly at the same time.

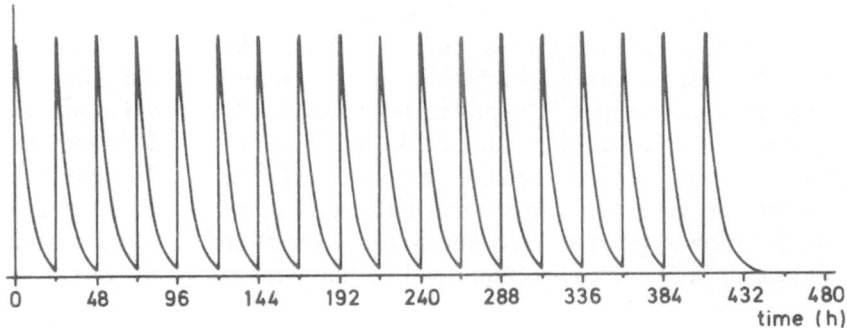

Figure 3 Plasma level curve following multiple dosing of a benzodiazepine with rapid plasma invasion (t_{max} = 1 h) and short half-life ($t_{1/2}$ = 4.5 h). Dose schedule: two tablets once a day. (From: Weiershausen, U: *Fortschr. Med., 1981,* reproduced with permission)

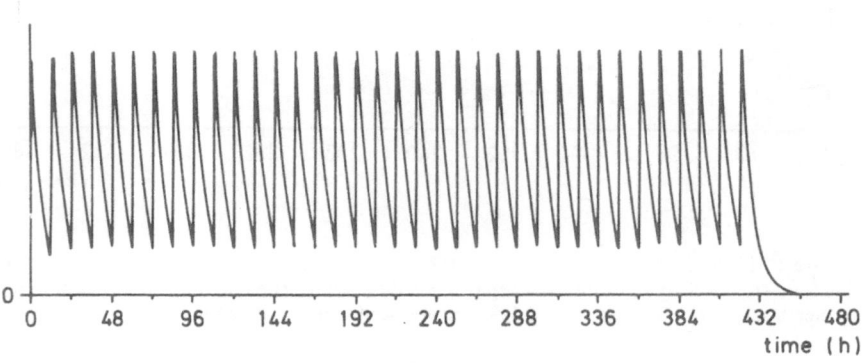

Figure 4 Plasma level curve following multiple dosing of a benzodiazepine with rapid plasma invasion (t_{max} = 1 h) and short half-life ($t_{1/2}$ = 4.5 h). Dose schedule: one tablet b.i.d. (From Weiershausen, U: *Fortschr. Med.*, 1981, reproduced with permission)

A further factor which has to be carefully considered with any kind of benzodiazepine medication is the avoidance of so-called rebound phenomena on discontinuance of therapy, well known of the barbiturates and commented on in detail elsewhere in this book. Marked rebound effects are assigned a pacemaker function for abuse of the substance concerned because they act as a strong stimulus to continue treatment as a means of overcoming rebound symptoms. On the basis of clinical observations it was concluded that rebound effects are induced by benzodiazepine derivatives with short and intermediate half-lives, whereas compounds with a long half-life may not produce rebound phenomena (Kales, *et al.*, 1979). In a critical review of their studies (1983) the authors take into consideration that increased follow-up periods after drug withdrawal could have revealed some degree of rebound phenomena also with benzodiazepines with long half-lives. Additional clinical studies seem to indicate that rebound effects may occur with these derivatives, however less markedly and more delayed. In such instances it appears especially difficult to draw a clear distinction between a substance-related rebound and a recurrence of the original symptoms. Computer-simulated plasma level curves demonstrate that after discontinuance of therapy, the plasma level of a compound with a short half-life drops abruptly to zero within 24 hours in contrast to a gradual decrease over a period of 10 days in the case of a compound with a long half-life (Figure 5). From Figure 5 it is also apparent that gradual dose reduction of a compound with an intermediate half-life may produce a decrease in plasma level resembling the elimination curve of the compound with a long half-life. The slow decline in plasma level reduces risk of rebound phenomena of benzodiazepine derivatives with a long half-life: a desirable property for daytime tranquillisation.

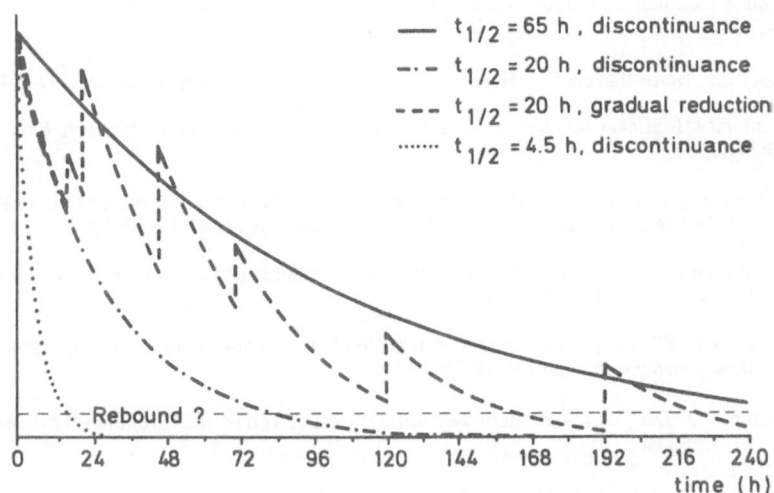

Figure 5 Time of plasma clearance (h) of benzodiazepines with different half-lives ($t_{1/2}$) following discontinuance and gradual dose reduction, respectively. (From: Weiershausen, U: *Fortschr. Med.*, 1981, reproduced with permission)

SUMMARY

Benzodiazepine daytime tranquillisers should provide a smooth onset of action, minimal perceptible CNS effects in the initial phase of drug action, a continuous plateau of psychotropic action with multiple dosing, a gentle subsidence of effects upon discontinuance of therapy, a once-a-day dose schedule, and as low an abuse potential as possible. Of the benzodiazepines presently available on the market these features seem best provided by derivatives with slow plasma invasion and elimination kinetics, e.g. benzodiazepines with a slow absorption and long half-life. The balanced profile of action of this type of drug in multiple dosing provides the preconditions for effective daytime tranquillisation. Since these compounds prepare the patients during the day for a restful night, they may also help to restore a physiological wake/sleep pattern. Benzodiazepines of this type are most appropriate for the treatment of chronic anxiety, especially since they may induce drug abuse less frequently than compounds with rapid invasion and elimination characteristics (Schöenhöefer, 1980). Patients must be monitored, however, on a regular basis in order to assess whether dosage escalation is occurring, and periodically given a trial of stopping the benzodiazepine to see if benzodiazepine therapy is still needed.

References

Bliding A: Effects of different rates of absorption of two benzodiazepines on subjective and objective parameters: significance for clinical use and risk of abuse. *Eur J Clin Pharmacol* 1974;7:201-211.

Cooper AJ: Benzodiazepines: Towards more logical use. *Scott Med J* 1982;27:297-394.

Greenblatt DJ, Shader RJ, Abernethy DR: Current status of benzodiazepines. *N Engl J Med* 1983;309:354-358

Kales A, Scharf MB, Kales JD, *et al*: Rebound insomnia: a potential hazard following withdrawal of certain benzodiazepines. *J Am Med Assoc* 1979;241:1692-1695.

Kales A, Soldatos CR, Bixler EO, *et al*: Rebound insomnia and rebound anxiety: A review. *Pharmacology* 1983; 26: 121-137.

Schöenhöefer PS: Pharmakodynamische faktoren bei der entwicklung von drogenabhängigkeit. *Therapiewoche* 1980;30:1167-1176.

Vollmer K-O: Zur pharmakokinetischen differenzierung von benzodiazepinen. *Fortschr Med* 1981; 21: 829-834.

Weiershausen U: Zur klinischen relevanz pharmakokinetischer unterschiede bei benzodiazepinen. *Fortschr Med* 1981; 23: 919-924.

II. Therapeutic Application

4
An International Overview

John Marks, MD

During the almost 25 years since the introduction of Librium^R, the first benzodiazepine, benzodiazepines have become among the most widely used pharmaceutical substances in the history of medicine. These compounds have been of interest to me since they were first discovered, and I was responsible for some of the early clinical studies with Librium^R (Marks 1960a, 1960b). There is now a large number of benzodiazepines and some are antagonists rather than agonists to specific benzodiazepine receptors in the central nervous system (Braestrup & Squires, 1977; Moehler & Okada, 1977).

Despite their therapeutic success, the benzodiazepines have not been without their critics. Misgivings have been voiced about the extent of their use (Cooperstock, 1976), their adverse effects (Tyrer et al., 1981), and particularly the sociological ramifications of the use of tranquilizers in general (Koumjian, 1981).

It is important, however, to assess drugs' adverse effects not in isolation, but in relation to their effectiveness, their use in therapeutics, and the availability of alternatives. This review highlights those aspects of such an assessment in which there are international implications.

INDICATIONS

There is broad international acceptance of the main clinical indications for the benzodiazepines: anxiety, psychosomatic disorders, insomnia. The therapeutic application of benzodiazepines in the treatment of these disorders are considered in more detail in Chapters 6 and 7. It is also accepted that the benzodiazepines have no place in the treatment of depression, but may be useful adjuvant therapy for any severe anxiety associated with the depression.

The exact indications for which the benzodiazepines are prescribed shows variation from one nation to another. This probably depends on the extent to which the patients present with psychological or physical manifestations of their anxiety. In some countries, e.g., Italy, Spain, France, they are prescribed mainly for anxiety states presenting as such and for insomnia, but in others the major prescribing is for physical disorders in which physicians believe that anxiety is a significant aspect in the genesis of the disorder, e.g., U.S.A., United Kingdom. The most frequently prescribed benzodiazepine also varies from one country to another.

Other internationally accepted indications include muscle spasticity, use in status epilepticus, and anaesthetic uses. In anaesthesia, an appropriate benzodiazepine may be used both as an amnesiac sedative preoperatively and during minor operations.

Most of these medical indications are common to all countries, both industrially developed and the developing Third World countries. Although benzodiazepines are often presented as being of use only in the "decadent west", the availability of the benzodiazepines in the Third World is just as important, if not more so, though often for different indications. For example, in the treatment of tetanus which is still common in many Third World countries, particularly in the neonatal form, diazepam has produced a dramatic reduction in the mortality rate. Other important indications for benzodiazepines in Third World countries include cerebral malaria and the treatment of major psychosis.

One cannot review the clinical uses of the benzodiazepines internationally without also stressing that the remarkable safety record of these drugs in overdosage is accepted in nearly all countries.

DOSAGE

An interesting feature with many drugs is the variation in dosage that exists internationally. This is also true for the benzodiazepines (Yamashita & Asano: personal communication, 1982). Whether there are rational explanations for the differences, based perhaps on different rates of metabolism, is not known. From the practical viewpoint, it is important to be aware of these dosage differences and to interpret cross national and cross cultural clinical results with caution.

Even within Europe there are substantial differences in the dosage at which benzodiazepine hypnotics are prescribed, particularly to the elderly. This may explain why a greater frequency of some side effects is reported in some countries than in others.

INTERNATIONAL AVAILABILITY OF DIFFERENT MEMBERS OF THE SERIES

The U.S. Food and Drugs Administration has, over the years, retarded the introduction of drugs into the United States of America, sometimes with beneficial effects (e.g., thalidomide), sometimes to the detriment of patient care. Other countries, e.g., Japan, United Kingdom, Germany, have introduced new benzodiazepines more rapidly than the U.S. Moreover, varying patent laws and their varying interpretation by the courts have meant that the number of copies of the original drugs has varied between countries. One of the difficulties for those treating international travellers, or those concerned with international therapeutics, is the availability of different medicines in different countries and the different trade names under which they may be prescribed. In a rapidly growing series like the benzodiazepines, the list of all the available preparations is constantly changing. Table 1 therefore only indicates the commercial availability of representatives of the series in selected countries. It demonstrates the wide variation that exists in benzodiazepines that may be prescribed internationally and may be met by those treating the increasing numbers of international travellers.

INTERNATIONAL VIEWS ON PHARMACOKINETICS AND PHARMACODYNAMICS

The pharmacokinetics of different members of the benzodiazepines differ markedly, particularly in respect of the metabolic pathway, receptor affinity, lipid solubility, and elimination half-life. Based upon the elimination half-life, the group was broadly divided into the so-called short and long half-life members (Breimer, Jochemsen & von Albert, 1980) and different therapeutic indications were proposed for each. Skilled clinical application requires consideration of other factors as well as elimination half-life.

First, in common with all orally administered drugs there are three phases of the pharmacokinetic history of a drug: the absorption, the distribution, and the elimination (by metabolism, conjugation or direct excretion). The rapidity of onset of initial effects and the length of action of each dose of benzodiazepine depends more on the absorption and distribution phase than on the elimination half-life. However it is the elimination figure (beta half-life) that is quoted, and this can give a false picture. The elimination half-life and the metabolic pathway define the degree of accumulation of varying components with different pharmacological intensities of effect that occurs with different dosage schedules. It also defines the rate at which the substance will disappear from the blood when the last dose is given (Nicholson & Marks, 1983).

Table 1. Representatives of the benzodiazepine series that are commercially available in various countries.

Generic name	USA	UK	Germany	Italy	Japan	France
Alprazolam	Yes	Yes	Yes	—	—	Yes
Bromazepam	—	Yes	Yes	Yes	Yes	Yes
Camazepam	—	—	Yes	Yes	—	—
Chlordiazepoxide	Yes	Yes	Yes	Yes	Yes	Yes
Clobazam	—	Yes	Yes	Yes	—	Yes
Clonazepam	Yes	Yes	Yes	Yes	Yes	Yes
Clorazepic acid	Yes	Yes	Yes	Yes	Yes	Yes
Clotiazepam	—	—	Yes	—	Yes	—
Cloxazolam	—	—	—	—	Yes	—
Delorazepam	—	—	—	Yes	—	—
Diazepam	Yes	Yes	Yes	Yes	Yes	Yes
Estazolam	—	—	—	Yes	Yes	Yes
Ethyl loflazepate	—	—	—	—	—	Yes
Fludiazepam	—	—	—	—	Yes	—
Flunitrazepam	—	Yes	Yes	Yes	Yes	Yes
Flurazepam	Yes	Yes	Yes	Yes	Yes	—
Flutazolam	—	—	—	—	Yes	—
Halazepam	Yes	—	—	—	—	—
Haloxazolam	—	—	—	—	Yes	—
Ketazolam	—	Yes	Yes	—	—	—
Loprazolam	—	Yes	—	—	—	—
Lorazepam	Yes	Yes	Yes	Yes	Yes	Yes
Lormetazepam	—	Yes	Yes	Yes	—	—
Medazepam	—	Yes	Yes	Yes	Yes	Yes
Midazolam	—	Yes	—	—	—	—
Nimetazepam	—	—	—	—	Yes	—
Nitrazepam	—	Yes	Yes	Yes	Yes	Yes
Nordiazepam	—	—	—	Yes	—	—
Oxazepam	Yes	Yes	Yes	Yes	Yes	Yes
Oxazolam	—	—	Yes	—	Yes	—
Pinazepam	—	—	—	Yes	—	—
Prazepam	Yes	Yes	Yes	Yes	Yes	Yes
Temazepam	Yes	Yes	Yes	Yes	—	Yes
Tetrazepam	—	—	Yes	—	—	Yes
Tofisopam	—	—	—	—	—	Yes
Triazolam	Yes	Yes	Yes	Yes	Yes	Yes

Second, current pharmacokinetics is based largely on *blood* level determinations. While these appear to represent brain levels in general, the distribution in different parts of the brain and of the dynamics of the interaction between the substance and the receptor may be variable. *Hence current pharmacokinetics may not correspond to brain receptor dynamics.* Thus, because of receptor binding, the length of pharmacological action does not always match the pharmacokinetic predictions. In some countries, e.g., United Kingdom, Germany, pharmacokinetics have been exerting a powerful effect on academic therapeutics and some of the differences in the use and dosage of drugs from one country to another can be explained on this basis. It is now becoming more widely accepted that it is important to determine the clinical activity and time relationships rather than the blood levels.

A recent development is the introduction of benzodiazepines with variations in the heterocyclic ring. It is still too early to assess their merits. The traditional series had nitrogen atoms at position 1 and 4, while some newer members have been developed with the nitrogen at positions 1,5 and 3,4. It is claimed that a 1,5 benzodiazepine retains the anxiolytic effect while eliminating the psychomotor impairment of the originals (Lader, 1980). Whether this will stand the test of extensive study (Feely, Calvert & Gibson, 1982) is uncertain.

EXTENT OF INTERNATIONAL USE

Following their introduction, the use of the benzodiazepines increased rapidly and some people believe too markedly. I estimated in 1978 that there was a compound increase of use of about 2% per year over their first 15 years in the United Kingdom. A significant part of this growth replaced the dangerous barbiturates.

In most countries, the number of prescriptions peaked during the mid 1970s. In many countries, the level of use has declined since then. The extent of use is of current wide interest. Hence it is important to define the ways in which the level of use of a therapeutic substance can be represented. The first of these is by sales in monetary terms. This is inaccurate nationally and internationally, since it takes no account of price differences and need not be considered further.

The second and most commonly used method is based on prescription audits. This technique compiles the number of prescriptions written by practitioners representative of physicians in a given country. A prescription can be for a short or long period even in the same patient, let alone from one practice to another or one country to another. Caution is necessary over the interpretation of the findings (Marks, 1983b).

The peak of tranquilizer prescriptions in the United States was reached in 1975 (Rickels, 1983). Nearly all West European countries also showed a peak during the 1970s (Boethius & Westerholm, 1976). In the United Kingdom, the rise continued for longer than in many countries, but the level has now started to decline (Figure 1).

The third method adopted by the World Health Organisation expresses the level of use in terms of "defined daily doses" (D.D.D.) per year per 1000 population (Bergman, 1981; Stika et al., 1981; Lunde et al., 1979). This method is particularly valuable when comparisons are to be made from one country to another and when the members of a therapeutic class that are being used change significantly with time. However, even with D.D.D. figures, international comparisons may not be reliable because patient audits show that the average dose used in different countries may vary markedly from the D.D.D.

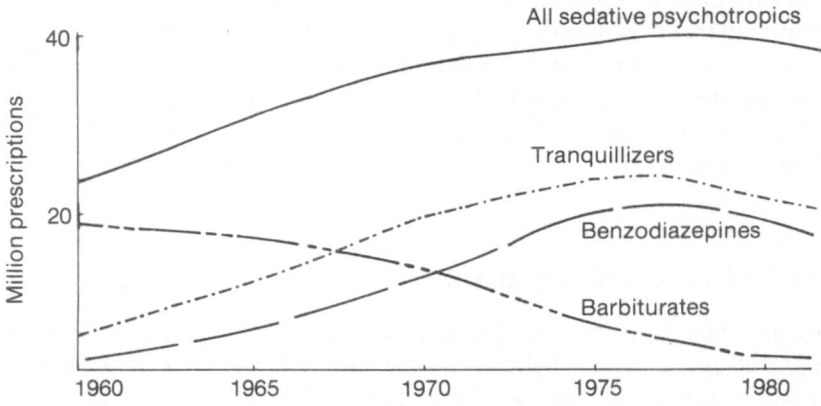

Figure 1. Level of prescription of sedative psychotropic substances in the United Kingdom (1960-1979). Based on various Government statistics.

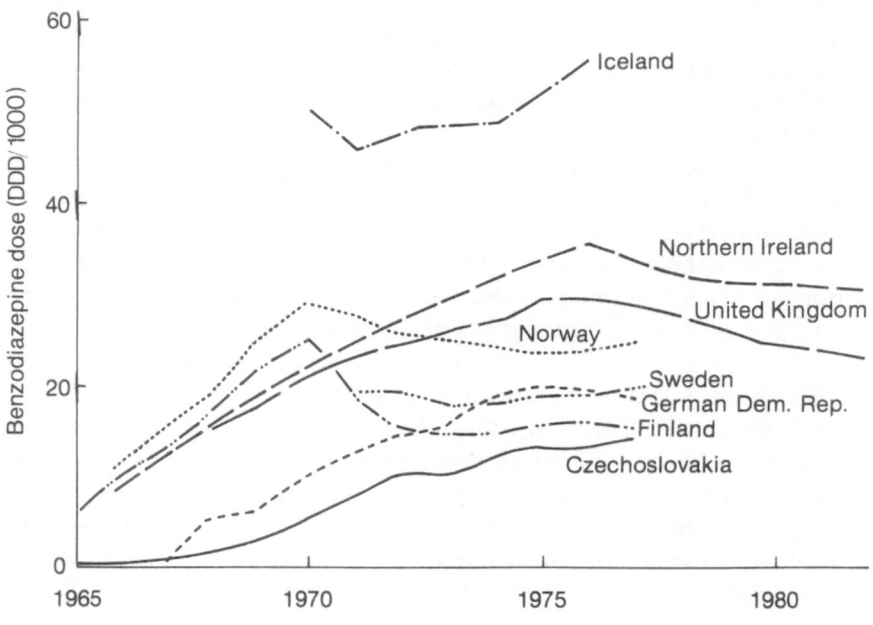

Figure 2. Level of benzodiazepine use (expressed in terms of D.D.D. per 1000 adult population in various European countries. Based on Blaha & Brickman, 1983 and my own calculations.

The figures for the consumption of benzodiazepines during the 1970s for several west European countries, expressed in terms of the D.D.D., are shown in Figure 2. No equivalent yearly D.D.D. figures appear to be available for the United States but I have calculated that the 1981 figure is 21.8 and the 1983 figure 18.8, which is relatively low in the international order. With the possible exception of Iceland, the consumption of the benzodiazepines is reasonably uniform from one country to another. Decreasing levels of use are occurring in most countries.

But even with D.D.D. figures, any information on the extent of use must be viewed with caution until all the factors involved have been studied. For example, the pattern of drugs used as anxiolytics and sedatives differs even between close neighbours like Norway and Sweden (Table 2). Moreover, any conclusions about the level of drug *use* based solely on sales volume or prescriptions takes no account of the evidence from the U.S.A. (and which is also true for the U.K.) that patients actually consume far less tranquilizers than are prescribed (Marks, 1981). Until the proportion consumed in other countries is known, the amount actually *consumed* in different countries cannot be known with certainty.

Table 2. Comparison of the use of psychotropic drug classes in Norway and Sweden expressed in D.D.D. terms.

	NORWAY			SWEDEN		
	1971	*1976*	*% change*	*1971*	*1976*	*% change*
Anxiolytics	27.4	23.4	−14.6%	19.2	18.7	−2.4%
Hypnotics	34.2	35.3	+3.2%	49.6	40.7	−18.0%
Neuroleptics	9.8	8.4	−14.3%	11.2	15.1	+34.8%
Total	71.4	67.1	−6.0%	80.0	74.5	−6.9%

The fourth method for expressing the level of use is by defining the proportion of the population that is receiving the drug. This may be the proportion that have used the drug over a defined period (often the last year) or the point prevalence of use. The former clearly gives significantly higher figures than the latter depending upon the length of the period over which the incidence is determined. Errors of interpretation can thus occur.

Studies reported early in the 1970s (Balter, Levine & Manheimer, 1974; Parry *et al.*, 1973) found a level of new use of tranquilo-sedatives of approximately 15% over the year, of which benzodiazepines represented about 60%. The studies of Balter and colleagues (1974) showed that there was a fairly uniform use of tranquilizers and sedatives in several countries in Europe. Between 10 and 17% of the population had used these drugs during the previous year with a regular use between 3 and 8%. Mellinger and

Balter (1981) have produced 1979 figures for the United States. These comparative figures, over a gap of almost a decade, also confirm the decline in the level of use.

Taken together, the data suggest that currently about one in ten of the adult population of most industrially developed countries receives a prescription for a tranquilizer during the course of the current year and that about 50% of these will be receiving a benzodiazepine. The point prevalence is about 2%.

The favoured benzodiazepines and the exact form in which they are prescribed will vary from one country to another. In Spain, for example, a significant proportion receive fixed combinations including the benzodiazepines (LaPorte et al., 1981), whereas combinations would be the exception in Anglo-Saxon and Nordic countries. Various studies indicate that about twice as many women as men are prescribed tranquilizers and that the elderly are higher users than the young (Lader, 1980; Marks, 1980).

JUSTIFICATION FOR THE LEVEL OF INTERNATIONAL USE

Various recent studies have shown an annual level of significant psychiatric morbidity in the population of industrially developed countries of about 30% with a point prevalence of about 15%. Morbid anxiety accounts for the major share (Marks, 1980). According to various studies by psychiatrists (Marks, 1980), only about half this morbidity is recognised by medical practitioners. Hence the current level of prescription compounds to help relieve anxiety (annual level about 10%) is low rather than high compared with this level of morbidity.

In Third World countries, studies have suggested a similar frequency of psychiatric morbidity (Harding, et al., 1980; Harding & Chrusciel, 1975). In Hong Kong, the incidence of neuroses among Chinese new patients has now risen to some 30–40% (from a previous figure of some 10%), bringing it into line with many Western nations (W.H. Lo: personal communication, 1981).

The mere finding that the proportion who received a group of drugs corresponds to the proportion with a disorder requiring treatment does not indicate that the correct patients are being treated. However, there is evidence of valid use in the case of the tranquilizers. In a careful study in over 1000 people in Pennsylvania, U.S.A., Hesbacher et al., (1976) found a very good "illness–treatment fit;" i.e., 99.1% of patients diagnosed as having no emotional disorders had never received tranquilizers, while of those diagnosed as suffering from emotional illness, over half had never had any treatment with psychoactive drugs. A study by Uhlenhuth, Balter and Lipman (1978) showed that the level of tranquilizer use correlated well with the level of anxiety (Figure 3). In a U.S. National Institute of Mental Health sponsored study of medication use and psychic distress, virtually all the regular users of psychotherapeutic drugs reported psychic distress or life crises. On the other hand, of those reporting both a high level of emotional distress and life crises, only 35% of the women and 21% of the men had used any psychoactive medication at any time in the previous year (Mellinger, *et al.*, 1978). Unfortunately, no comparable studies appear to be available outside the United States, though there is no reason to believe that they would reach a different conclusion.

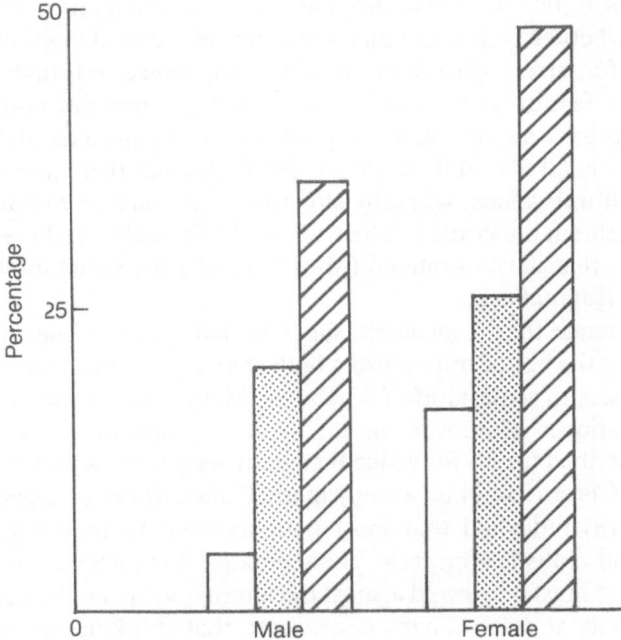

Figure 3. Correlation of tranquilizer use with the level of anxiety (based on Uhlenhuth, Balter & Lipman, 1978).

The finding that in most developed countries women are twice as likely as men to be treated with tranquilizers (Bass, 1981) has also been subjected to critical examination recently. Women report more symptoms of both physical and mental illness and use practitioner and hospital services at higher rates than do men (Roskies, 1978). Moreover, women are more willing to talk about their emotional problems (Verbrugge, 1978). In the National Institute of Mental Health study (Mellinger *et al.*, 1978) about 30% of the women were rated "high" on a psychic distress index compared with only 20% men.

There is, moreover, evidence that the level of prescription of tranquilizers for women who report with emotional problems is higher (Bass & Baskerville, 1981; McCranie, 1978; Manheimer, Davidson & Balter, 1973).

This is also true for those who are treated by female doctors (Hasday & Karch, 1981; McCranie, 1978). Hence there is justification for the argument that the level of use in women is not too high, but that the level in men is too low. With increased appropriate prescription of benzodiazepines, some cases of alcoholism, evolving from self-medication of emotional distress, might be prevented. Also, work absenteeism, resulting from significant emotional factors, might be reduced.

However, before deciding that the prescribing practices of physicians are reasonable as far as benzodiazepines are concerned, it is important to ascertain whether benzodiazepine use is not reducing the search for social solutions for stress disorders. It has been suggested that this is an undesirable feature of the use of the benzodiazepines (Koumjian, 1981). Sociologists have also claimed that people are being prescribed drugs which they do not need (Twaddle & Sweet, 1970) and that there may be a recent shift in cultural values, whereby stoicism in the face of discomfort is no longer a fashionable virtue (Cohen, 1976). Unfortunately, there have been few studies that have examined (Marks, 1983b) the social implications of the use of tranquilizers.

The evidence that is available suggests that there are beneficial social effects from the use of tranquilizers both at work (Proctor, 1981) and in the circumstances of general life (Whybrow, Matlins & Greenberg: personal communication). Moreover, in the United Kingdom, tranquilizers are rarely prescribed for ills for which there is an easy social solution (Williams, Murray & Clare 1982), and a study in the United States (Tessler, Stokes & Pietras 1978) indicated that most patients want to reduce their use, a sensible and realistic approach. The sociological implications of the use of tranquilizers must be viewed against the alternative means by which society deals with its stresses. There is evidence that drinking alcohol may be practised as a form of self-medication alternative to taking prescription tranquilizers, at least as far as males are concerned (Mellinger, 1978). In this respect, it is salutory to note that in Finland, allegedly as the result of publicity and altered prescribing procedures, there was a decline in the use of psychotropic drugs. Coinciding with this, there was a rise in the consumption of alcohol, suggesting that the overall result was the substitution of alcohol use for tranquilizers (Idanpaan-Heikkila, 1979) (Figure 4).

Hence there is currently no valid evidence of undesirable sociological consequences from the current level of tranquilizer prescriptions although further and more extensive studies are desirable.

The concept that their administration retards social solutions would be more telling if it could be demonstrated that withholding benzodiazepines encouraged social solutions. As Mellinger (1978) has pointed out, those in distress who are refused treatment seek solace elsewhere in less appropriate form, e.g., use of alcohol, and he notes that "society often does not provide a great deal in the way of viable alternatives that are much better".

Viewed overall, we may conclude that current tranquilizer use is medically and socially valuable: that "benzodiazepines are far more beneficial than harmful" (Greenblatt & Shader, 1981). As Morrison (1974) put it: "Rational responsible use of psychotropic drugs to relieve even ill defined psychological disorders should not be considered as a craven surrender to human weakness. There is nothing really noble about needless suffering".

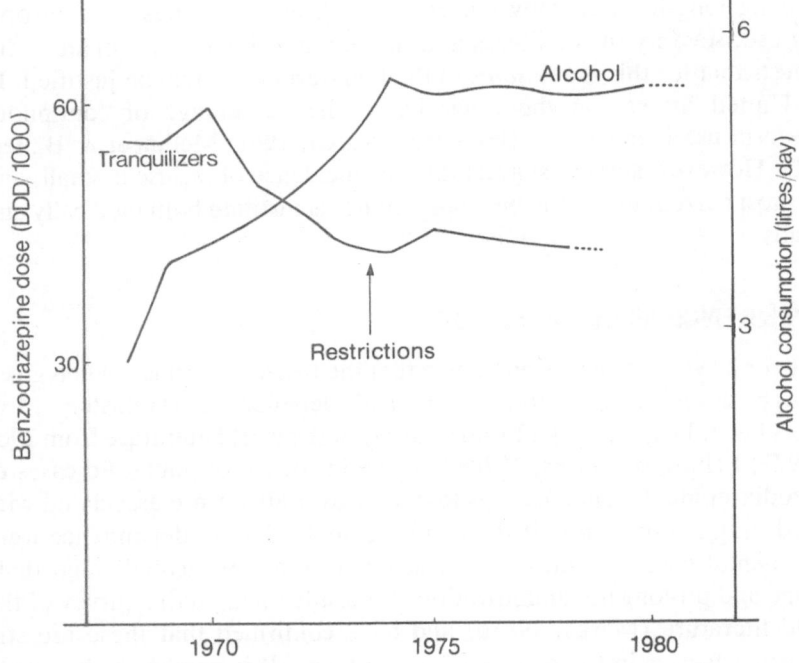

Figure 4. Comparison of psychotropic drug use and alcohol consumption in Finland.

MISUSE

Within this level of justified use, is there any misuse? The answer is "yes". First, benzodiazepines are not always prescribed appropriately. Some of the poor results of benzodiazepine prescription are due to failure to recognise and treat appropriately the depressive component of a co-existing anxiety/depression.

Second, there may be inappropriate use of tranquilizers as the sole means of therapy. Psychoactive medication is only one component of total therapy, and its use does not preclude the need to provide all appropriate forms of treatment.

Third, benzodiazepines can be used for too long a period. It is essential that these drugs should be withdrawn as soon as they are no longer required for therapeutic purposes (Marks, 1981). The amount of long-term use differs from one country to another. For example, there is evidence of inappropriate long-term prescribing in the United Kingdom (Marks, 1983b). Thus, in one prospective study of therapeutic outcome in a group of patients treated with psychotropic drugs in general practice, about 20% were still receiving the drugs at the end of a six month period of therapy (Williams, Murray & Clare, 1982). The likelihood that they would be receiving long-term therapy correlated with age, previous psychotropic drug use, severity of the illness and the number of social problems. This suggests that for this group *some* of the long-term use could be justified. In the United States, on the other hand, the percentage of continuous long-term use is much less (Hasday & Karch, 1981; Mellinger & Balter, 1981). However, surveys suggest that the incidence of misuse is small, and that most current use of the benzodiazepines is justified both medically and socially.

DEPENDENCE IN CLINICAL USE

For over 20 years, it has been known that the benzodiazepines, when given in high doses, could produce physical dependence (Hollister, Motzenbecker & Degan, 1961). From a survey of the world literature from 1960 to 1977, I showed (Marks, 1978) that the incidence of published cases of benzodiazepine dependence was low, that over 80% were associated with mixed drug abuse, and that the main factors leading to dependence were coincidental consumption of other sedative drugs or alcohol, high daily dosage and prolonged administration. I recently updated this survey of the world literature (Marks, 1983b) and have confirmed that these are still important factors in the genesis of dependence. It is now clear, however, that dependence can also develop at normal therapeutic dose levels (Petursson & Lader, 1981; Tyrer, Rutherford & Huggett, 1981) and this finding needs to be put into clinical perspective.

As with most, if not all, sedative compounds, dependence can be physical, psychological or both. Physical dependence is only demonstrated at the time of abrupt or rapid withdrawal of the substance. During maintained administration, there are no clinical signs that indicate the existence of physical dependence. Abrupt withdrawal leads to a reaction similar to that encountered upon withdrawal of alcohol, barbiturates or sedatives. The interval after withdrawal at which the reactions appear depends on the elimination half-life of the compound concerned. For compounds with long elimination half-life, the maximum effects occur about 5 to 8 days after withdrawal.

Although these manifestations occur in patients who are physically dependent, the phenomenon is not necessarily pathognomonic of physical dependence (Table 3).

Table 3. Effects of sudden withdrawal of tranquilo–sedative substances.

1. No problems

2. "Crutch" phenomenon

3. Rebound anxiety/insomnia

4. Pseudo-dependence

5. Later return of chronic anxiety state

6. True psychological dependence

7. True physical dependence

Psychological dependence, a craving for the drug, is very difficult to quantify for the benzodiazepines. The traditional drug-seeking pattern through different doctors which is classical of psychological dependence is unusual for the benzodiazepines due to the low incidence of tolerance and wide medical availability of these substances.

For these reasons, it is probably more logical and helpful to refer to "withdrawal reactions" rather than to "dependence" associated with the benzodiazepines. These, whatever the cause, can give rise to patient discomfort and an unnecessary continuation of therapy beyond that which is required for the treatment of the original disorder.

The best indication of the incidence of withdrawal problems is seen in studies in which *therapeutic doses* of benzodiazepines are suddenly stopped. I have recently undertaken an appraisal of 8 such studies (Marks, 1983b). Below 4 months, the incidence of dependence is virtually nil unless alcohol, other sedatives or narcotics are also being taken. Up to about one year's continuous use, the incidence of significant withdrawal phenomena is estimated to be less than 5%. Over one year of continuous use, the incidence appears to rise steeply and may reach substantial levels (Tyrer, Rutherford & Huggett, 1981). Dependence is more likely to occur in individuals with a particular personality – the so-called "dependence-prone" individuals (Hollister, 1977; Smith & Wesson, 1983).

The higher the unit dose the shorter is the exposure for reaching a risk level, but the single most important factor in the genesis of withdrawal reactions appears to be the length of administration. All benzodiazepines that have been available commercially for some time are implicated (Marks, 1983b).

It appears from several publications that the short and rapidly acting compound lorazepam may have a higher dependence risk than some other members of the series (Tyrer, Rutherford & Huggett, 1981; Lapierre, 1981; Marks, 1983b). Not only can dependence occur at an earlier stage (under 3 months) and the incidence be greater, but due to the rapid elimination of the active substance, reactions occur sooner after withdrawal and are more intense.

Dependence during therapeutic use is primarily a disorder of developed countries. In the Third World, it is rare for any psychotropic drug to be given for more than a brief period, mainly because the patient cannot afford the costs. Hence dependence from therapeutic use in the Third World is rare.

The estimated incidences of abrupt withdrawal effects given above are based on *uninterrupted* administration. However, few patients take benzodiazepines on a continuous basis. Either on the advice of their doctors, or at the patient's own instigation, the majority now use benzodiazepines episodically "as needed", only taking a dose when the level of distress justifies the use (Hollister, 1977; Bowden & Fisher, 1980; Ayd, 1981; Marks, 1981). The majority of the patients use doses below those that are prescribed for them (Tessler, Stokes & Pietras, 1978). With this pattern of discontinuous and low dose use, the incidence of dependence with recommended therapeutic doses of benzodiazepines is still regarded as low, certainly lower than that estimated in the recent studies (Marks, 1983b).

Although the dependence risk is low, a certain number of patients experience considerable difficulty in discontinuing the benzodiazepine. However, the pattern of use is unusual for a "drug of dependence" (e.g., the low level of tolerance) and an alternative hypothesis for the difficulty would have attractions.

There is a possible additional cause for the problem. Caffeinism, intoxication with high levels of intake of coffee or tea, is a disorder which has been recognised relatively recently. Its manifestations closely resemble chronic anxiety (Greden, 1974; Gilbert, 1976). Caffeinism has been found to be associated with increased cigarette smoking (Friedman, Siegelaub & Seltzer, 1974). Some recent studies (Downing & Rickels, 1981; Greden, Proctor & Vistor, 1981) have shown that there is an interrelationship between tranquilo-sedatives and coffee intake. The level of use of tranquilo-sedatives is high in those persons who consume more than 750 mg caffeine per day (Downing & Rickels, 1981). There is evidence too that caffeine is a competitive inhibitor of diazepam binding at the brain "benzodiazepine" receptors (Tallman, Paul & Skolnick, 1980).

This raises the interesting hypothesis that some people who chronically use benzodiazepines are suffering from caffeinism and that symptoms which emerge on discontinuation of the benzodiazepine are due to caffeine rather than benzodiazepine dependence. The anxiety state which they experience on cessation of the benzodiazepine therapy is the consequence of the anxiety mimicking effect of the high caffeine intake converted to a vicious circle by the sedative effect of the benzodiazepines. If this hypothesis is established, then this particular group of patients can be relieved of the problems of long-term use of benzodiazepines by reducing or eliminating their intake of caffeine.

The relationship between dependence in therapeutic use, misuse and abuse is considered in greater detail in Chapter 13.

MINIMISING THE DEPENDENCE PROBLEM IN CLINICAL PRACTICE

First, it is important to achieve good selection of patients. Not all patients with anxiety or insomnia require pharmacological treatment. Other methods of treatment may be equally or even more effective and these should be tried. It is important to realise that a proportion of inappropriate long-term use of this group of drugs seems to stem from the failure to recognise and treat a masked depression.

Second, patients who have been, or are, dependent on other drugs (narcotics, alcohol or barbiturates) develop dependence more readily. In such patients any sedative, including the benzodiazepines, should be used with great caution.

Third, the lowest effective dose should be given for the shortest period. If that period exceeds 3 months, there should be careful review of the therapeutic need. Long-term benzodiazepine therapy is justified if there is continued distress which does not respond to other forms of therapy.

Some anxious patients can only live in the community with the help of anxiolytics and may need long-term therapy. In such patients, the dose should be as low as possible and the patient advised to reduce or discontinue dosage for brief or long periods if the level of distress makes this possible. When long-term treatment is discontinued, it should be done slowly by small increments, e.g., a quarter of the dose at weekly intervals.

Fourth, in a patient who is dependent, the greatest chance of successfully withdrawing therapy exists when the physician is supportive to the patient over the period during and after which the drug is being gradually withdrawn.

INTERNATIONAL LEGISLATION

In most countries, the benzodiazepines have been placed in a category which requires a doctor's prescription and dispensing either by the doctor or a qualified pharmacist. It is widely accepted that this legislation is appropriate for this class of drugs.

It has been argued that since the benzodiazepines are safer than the socially acceptable alternative tranquilizers – e.g., alcohol and tobacco –

they should, logically, be equally available. Nevertheless most people accept that the current level of legislative control for the benzodiazepines is correct and that the removal of this class of drugs from prescription control is not currently justified.

The United Nations Convention on Psychotropic Substances (1971) imposes international control on those psychotropic drugs where there is a problem which requires *international* control and where the social danger resulting from dependence and abuse outweighs the therapeutic benefit of the drug being more easily available to the community. The controls imposed by the least stringent schedules are intended to allow ready medical availability. However it is found in practice that in Third World countries, drugs in even less stringent schedules often disappear from the medical scene but can still be bought illicitly in the black market.

After discussion and consideration which has lasted many years, all the benzodiazepines have just been included (1984) in Schedule IV (the least stringent schedule) of the Convention (United Nations 1971). International control is considered in Chapter 19.

SUMMARY AND CONCLUSIONS

This paper reviews the main current international issues relating to benzodiazepine use. On the basis of the information that is currently available, the following conclusions may be drawn:

1. The benzodiazepines are still accepted as the drugs of choice for morbid anxiety, insomnia and several disorders that involve muscle spasms. Internationally, other indications that are rarely encountered in the United States are important, e.g., neonatal tetanus.

2. In most countries, the level of use of benzodiazepines has now stabilized or is declining. There is considerable uniformity of use between developed countries.

3. The incidence of illnesses for which the use of benzodiazepines is justified correlates well with the level of use. In the developing countries, recent surveys have indicated that there is a similar level of psychiatric morbidity. Moreover, there is a close correlation between the level of psychiatric distress and the use of benzodiazepines.

4. There is no evidence that the use of benzodiazepines leads to a reduced determination to seek a social solution to the problems that produce distress in the community.

5. The benzodiazepines should be used prudently, with careful selection of patients, dosage should be as low and brief as therapeutically reasonable, with adequate followup. Particular care should be taken when treating patients with known predisposition to dependence (e.g., those currently abusing alcohol or other drugs).

6. A "withdrawal phenomenon" can occur on abrupt withdrawal after prolonged administration at therapeutic doses.

7. With continuous therapeutic doses there is no evidence of dependence to 4 months, but with more prolonged use, at higher dose levels, with high intake of alcohol or previous dependence to barbiturates, the incidence of dependence is higher. The level of dependence may rise to a substantial figure after more than one year of continuous administration.

8. The majority of the patients require only a short course of the benzodiazepine. Therapy should not be continued beyond 3 months without a clear appraisal being made of the need for long-term therapy.

9. A proportion of patients with chronic anxiety can only live in society without distress when they are under treatment with benzodiazepines. In such patients, long-term use is justified for there is no evidence of significant social, moral or mental deterioration with their use. Intermittent use of benzodiazepines to cover periods of distress has much to commend it in such patients. It is essential to discontinue therapy gradually.

References

Ayd F: Diazepam – the question of long-term therapy and withdrawal reactions. *Drug Ther* 1981;Special Supplement.

Balter MB, Levine J, Manheimer DI: Cross-national study of the extent of anti-anxiety/sedative drug use. *N Engl J Med* 1974;290:769-774.

Bass MJ: Do physicians overprescribe for women with emotional problems? *Can Med Assoc J* 1981;125:1211.

Bass MJ, Baskerville JC: Prescribing of minor tranquilizers for emotional problems in family practice. *Can Med Assoc J* 1981;125:1225-1226.

Bergman U: Studies on patterns and prevalence of psychiatric drug use – data from the Nordic countries, in Tognoni G, *et al.* (eds): *Epidemiological Impact of Psychotropic Drugs.* Elsevier, North-Holland, Biomedical Press, 1981.

Blaha D, Brickmann J-V: Benzodiazepines in the treatment of anxiety (Angst): European experience, in Costa E (ed): *The Benzodiazepines: From Molecular Biology to Clinical Practice.* New York, Raven Press, 1983, pp 311-324.

Boethius G, Westerholm B: Is the use of hypnotics, sedatives and minor tranquilizers really a major health problem? *Acta Med Scand* 1976;199:507-512.

Bowden CL, Fisher JG: Safety and efficacy of long-term diazepam therapy. *South Med J* 1980;73:1581-1584.

Braestrup C, Squires RF: Brain specific benzodiazepine receptors in rat characterized by high affinity ^{3}H-diazepam binding. *Proc Natl Acad Sci* 1977;74:3805-3809.

Breimer DD, Jochemsen R, Von Albert HH: Pharmacokinetics of benzodiazepines: short-acting versus long-acting. *Arzneimittelforsch* 1980;30:875-881.

Cohen S: Valium: its use and abuse. *Drug Abuse Alcohol Newslt* 1976;5:

Cooperstock R: Psychotropic drug use among women. *Can Med Assoc J* 1976;115:760-763.

Downing RW, Rickels K: Coffee consumption, cigarette smoking and reporting of drowsiness in anxious patients treated with benzodiazepines or placebo. *Acta Psychiat Scand* 1981;64:398-408.

Feely M, Calvert R, Gibson J: Clobazam in catamenial epilepsy. *Lancet* 1982;2:71-73.

Friedman GD, Siegelaub AB, Seltzer CC: Cigarettes, alcohol, coffee and peptic ulcer. *N Engl J Med* 1974;290:469-473.

Gilbert RM: Caffeine as a drug of abuse, in Gibbin RG, Israel Y, *et al.* (eds): *Research Advances in Alcohol and Drug Problems.* New York, John Wiley & Sons, 1976.

Greden JF: Anxiety or caffeinism: a diagnostic dilemma. *Amer J Psychiatry* 1974;131:1089-1094.

Greden JF, Procter A, Victor B: Caffeinism associated with greater use of other psychotropic agents. *Compr Psychiatry* 1981;22:565-571.

Greenblatt DJ, Shader RI: Clinical use of the benzodiazepines. *Ration Drug Ther* 1981;15:1-6.

Harding JW, Chrusciel TL: The use of psychotropic drugs in developing countries. *Bull WHO* 1975;52:359-367.

Harding JW, De Arango MV, Baltazar J, *et al*: Mental disorders in primary health care: a study of their frequency and diagnosis in four developing countries. *Psychol Med* 1980;10:231-241.

Hasday JD, Karch FE: Benzodiazepine prescribing in a family medical center. *J Am Med Assoc* 1981;246:1321-1325.

Hesbacher P, Stepansky P, Stepansky E, *et al*: Psychotropic drug use in family practice. *Pharmakopsychiatrie Neuro-psychopharmakologie* 1976;9:50-60.

Hollister LE: Valium: a discussion of current issues. *Psychosomatics* 1977;18:44-58.

Hollister LE, Motzenbecker FP, Degan RO: Withdrawal reactions from chlordiazepoxide (Librium). *Psychopharmacologia* 1961;2:63-68.

Idanpaan-Heikkila J: *Studies in Drug Utilisation.* WHO Regional Publications European Series No.8. Copenhagen, WHO, 1979.

Koumjian K: The use of Valium as a form of social control. *Soc Sci Med* 1981;15E:245-249.

Lader MH: The present status of benzodiazepines in psychiatry and medicine. *Arzneimittelforsch* 1980;30:910-912.

Lapierre YD: Benzodiazepine withdrawal. *Can J Psychiatry* 1981;26:93-95.

Laporte J-R, Capella D, Gisbert R, *et al*: The utilization of sedative-hypnotic drugs in Spain, in Tognoni G, *et al*. (eds): *Epidemiological impact of psychotropic drugs*. Elsevier, North Holland, Biomedical Press, 1981.

Lunde PK, Baksaas I, Halse M, *et al*: Studies in Drug Utilisation. WHO Regional Publications European Series No.8. Copenhagen, WHO, 1979.

Manheimer DI, Davidson ST, Balter MB: Popular attitudes and beliefs about tranquilizers. *Am J Psychiatry* 1973;130:1246-1253.

Marks J: Methaminodiazepoxide (Librium) - a new psychotropic drug. *Chemother Rev* 1960a;1:141-143.

Marks J: Tranquillizing drugs. *Med Press* 1960b;244:426-430.

Marks J: *The Benzodiazepines: Use, Overuse, Misuse, Abuse?* Lancaster, MTP Press, 1978.

Marks J: The benzodiazepines – use and abuse. *Arzneimittelforsch* 1980;30:898-901.

Marks J: Diazepam – the question of long-term therapy and withdrawal reactions. *Drug Ther* (Special Supplement) 1981.

Marks J: Measurement of the benefits of benzodiazepines, in Teeling-Smith G (ed): *Measuring the Social Benefits of Medicine*. London, Office of Health Economics, 1983a.

Marks J: Benzodiazepines – for good or evil. *Neuropsychobiology* 1983b;10:115-126.

McCranie EW: Alleged sex-role stereotyping in the assessment of women's physical complaints: a study of general practitioners. *Soc Sci Med* 1978;12:111-115.

Mellinger GD: Use of licit drugs and other coping alternatives: some personal observations on the hazards of living, in Lettier DJ (ed): *Drugs and Suicide – When Other Coping Strategies Fail*. Beverly Hills, CA, Sage Publications, 1978.

Mellinger GD, Balter MB: Prevalence and patterns of use of psychotherapeutic drugs: results from a 1979 national survey of American adults. Read before the International Seminar on the Epidemiological Impact of Psychotropic Drugs, Milan, June 24-26, 1981.

Mellinger GD, Balter MB, Manheimer DI, *et al*: Psychic distress, life crisis and the use of psychotherapeutic medications. *Arch Gen Psychiatry* 1978;35:1045-1052.

Moehler H, Okada T: Benzodiazepine receptor: demonstration in the central nervous system. *Science* 1977;198:849-851.

Moehler H, Okada T, Ulrich J, *et al*: Biochemical identification of the site of action of benzodiazepines in human brain by ^{3}H-diazepam binding. *Life Sci* 1978;22:985-996.

Morrison AA: Regulatory control of the Canadian Government over the manufacture, distribution and prescribing of psychotropic drugs, in Cooperstock R (ed): *Social Aspects of Psychotropic Drugs*. Toronto, Alcohol and Drug Addiction Foundation, 1974, pp 9-19.

Nicholson AN, Marks J: *Insomnia: A Guide for Medical Practitioners*. Lancaster, MTP Press, 1983.

Parry HJ, Balter MB, Mellinger GD, et al: National patterns of psychotherapeutic drug use. *Arch Gen Psychiatry* 1973;28:869-784.

Petursson H. Lader MH: Withdrawal from long-term benzodiazepine treatment. *Br Med J* 1981:283:643-645.

Proctor RC: Prescription medication in the workplace. *NC Med J* 1981;42:545-547.

Rickels K: Benzodiazepines in the treatment of anxiety: North American experience, in Costa E (ed): *The Benzodiazepines: From Molecular Biology to Clinical Practice.* New York, Raven Press. 1983, pp 295-310.

Roskies E: Sex, culture and illness – an overview. *Soc Sci Med* 1978;12B:139-144.

Smith DE, Wesson DR: Benzodiazepine dependency syndromes. *J Psychoactive Drugs* 1983;15:85-96.

Stika L, Kubat K, Elis J, et al: Studies on patterns and prevalence of psychotropic drug use (data from Czechoslovakia), in Tognoni G, et al. (eds): *Epidemiological Impact of Psychotropic Drugs.* Elsevier, North Holland, Biomedical Press, 1981.

Tallman JF, Paul SM, Skolnick P: Receptors for the age of anxiety: pharmacology of the benzodiazepines. *Science* 1980;207:274-276.

Tessler R, Stokes R, Pietras M: Consumer response to Valium: a survey of attitudes and patterns of use. *Drug Ther* 1978;8:179-186.

Twaddle AC, Sweet RH: Characteristics and experiences of patients with preventable hospital admission. *Soc Sci Med* 1970;4:141-145.

Tyrer P, Rutherford D, Huggett T: Benzodiazepine withdrawal symptoms and propranolol. *Lancet* 1981;1:520-522.

Uhlenheth EH, Balter MB, Lipman RS: Minor tranquillizers: clinical correlates of use in an urban population. *Arch Gen Psychiatry* 1978;35:650-655.

United Nations Convention on Psychotropic Substances, 1971. New York, United Nations, 1971.

Verbrugge LM: Complaints and diagnoses: sex differences in the vocabulary and attribution of illness. Read at the American Public Health Association Meeting, Los Angeles, 1978.

Williams P, Murray J, Clare A: A longitudinal study of psychotropic drug prescription. *Psychol Med* 1982;12:201-206.

5
Principles of Therapeutic Applications of Benzodiazepines

Leo E. Hollister, MD

In the more than two decades that benzodiazepines have been available to physicians throughout the world, they have become one of the most widely used group of drugs in all of medical history. The popularity seems to be well deserved, based upon the many uses to which these drugs have been put. Although many of the current indications for the use of benzodiazepines have in the past been accomplished with other drugs, most notably the barbiturates, the consensus presently is that the benzodiazepines are not only more effective, but are safer drugs than those which predated them.

Several thousand benzodiazepines or homologs have been synthesized. Perhaps as many as 100 have been marketed in various parts of the world or are in various stages of clinical development. The majority are marketed as antianxiety drugs or as hypnotics. Some of those drugs marketed either as antianxiety or hypnotic drugs are shown in Figures 1 and 2. The listing is by no means complete.

Most clinical indications of these drugs derive from three principal pharmacologic actions: sedative–hypnotic, muscle relaxant and anticonvulsant. The principal indications for benzodiazepines are shown in Table 1. Perhaps the widest application is in the treatment of anxiety and insomnia – classic uses for sedative–hypnotic drugs of this type. Their use in the control of seizures is more limited. Intravenously administered diazepam is a well-recognized treatment for status epilepticus, but must very quickly be followed by loading doses of longer-acting anticonvulsants, such as phentoin. Diazepam has been the most widely used benzodiazepine as a muscle relaxant and is beneficial and safe for many individuals. Treating alcohol withdrawal with drugs that are cross-tolerant to alcohol is an established tradition. The benzodiazepines meet this requirement, and

87

which benzodiazepine to use for this purpose is a matter of individual choice. Diazepam has a potential advantage over the others in that it can be administered intravenously to obtain very rapid control of disturbed behavior. Finally, intravenously administered diazepam has been frequently used as an induction agent for anesthesia or as an anesthetic for short operations.

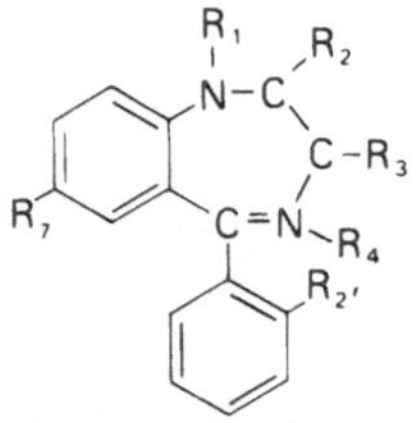

Anxiolytic Benzodiazepines

Benzodiazepine nucleus and
points of chemical substitution

alprazolam
$R_2 = =N-N-CH(CH_3)-R_1$; $R_7 = Cl$

bromazepam
$R_2 = O$; $R_7 = Br$ 2-pyridine side-chain

camazepam
$R_1 = CH_3$; $R_2 = O$; $R_3 = -OCON(CH_3)_2$; $R_7 = Cl$

chlordiazepoxide
$R_2 = NCH_3$; $R_7 = Cl$

clobazam
$R_1 = CH_3$; $R_2 = O$; $R_7 = Cl$ 1,5 benzodiazepine

clonazepam
$R_2 = O$; $R_{2'} = Cl$; $R_7 = NO_2$

clorazepate
$R_2 = OH, O^-$; $R_3 = COO^-$; $R_7 = Cl$

diazepam
$R_1 = CH_3$; $R_2 = O$; $R_7 = Cl$

halazepam
$R_1 = CH_2CF_3$; $R_2 = O$; $R_7 = Cl$

ketazolam
$R_1 = CH_3$; $R_2 = O$; $R_4 =$

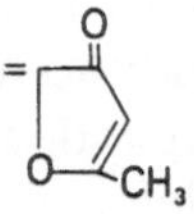

lorazepam
$R_2 = O$; $R_3 = OH$; $R_7 = Cl$; $R_{2'} = Cl$

medazepam
$R_1 = CH_3$; $R_7 = Cl$ dihydro diazepine ring

oxazepam
$R_3 = OH$; $R_7 = Cl$

prazepam
$R_1 = CH_2-CH_2-CH_2$; $R_2 = O$; $R_7 = Cl$

Figure 1. Structural relationships between benzodiazepines marketed as antianxiety drugs and those marketed as hypnotics.

Hypnotic Benzodiazepines

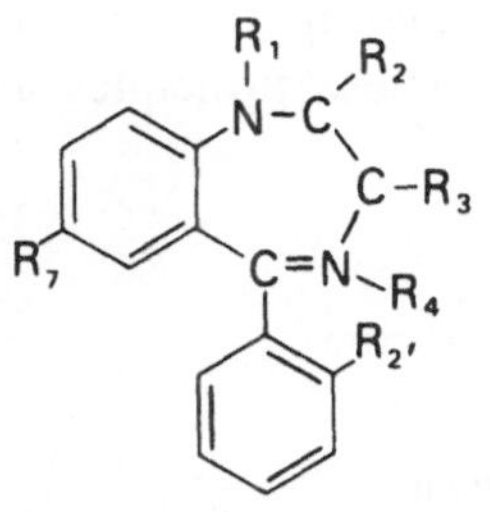

Benzodiazepine nucleus and points of chemical substitution

flunitrazepam
$R_2=0; R_7=NO_2$

flurazepam
$R_1=CH_2CH_2N(C_2H_5)_2; R_2=0; R_{2'}=F; R_7=Cl$

lormetazepam
$R_1=CH_3; R_2=0; R_3=OH; R_{2'}=Cl; R_7=Cl$

nitrazepam
$R_2=0; R_7=NO_2; R_{2'}=F$

temazepam
R_1 $CH_3; R_3$ $OH; R_7$ Cl

triazolam
R_2 $N-N-CH(CH_3)-R_1; R_7$ $Cl; R_{2'}$ Cl

Figure 2.

Table 1

Anxiety, nervousness, panics
Sleeplessness, insomnia
Repeated seizures, status epilepticus
Withdrawal from alcohol
Muscle relaxation in true spasticity
Intravenous anesthetic or induction agent

Virtually all of these indications have in the past been met by one or another type of barbiturate. Benzodiazepines are now considered to be both more effective and safer. One safety factor is that of not inducing drug-metabolizing enzymes that could cause pharmacokinetic interactions with other drugs. Another is that when taken by themselves in overdose, they are remarkably unlikely to kill, thereby nullifying this misuse of sedative–hypnotic drugs.

The benzodiazepines may be among the most widely used class of drugs in medical history. For most of the more than two decades since its introduction, diazepam has been the most widely prescribed drug in the U.S. In 1981, it had regained first place after having been displaced temporarily by cimetidine. Flurazepam was the tenth most widely prescribed drug. Several others, including some benzodiazepines in combination with other agents, were in the top 100 most widely prescribed drugs. Similar patterns of use have been documented in other countries as well.

This widespread clinical use of these drugs has engendered some concerns. Are they being over-used, either for trivial conditions or those which might be managed as well or better by other methods? Are physicians inadvertently making many patients dependent on these drugs either by prescribing too large a dose or by prescribing for too long a period of time? We shall try to examine these and other issues in considering the principles to be used in the proper use of benzodiazepines. These principles are summarized in Table 2.

Table 2

Use benzodiazepines only when indicated
Use non-drug methods when feasible
Drug treatment should be brief and intermittent
Doses should be titrated individually
Efficacy should be assessed early
Avoid classical sedative-hypnotics in drug abuses
Gradually discontinue drugs after chronic treatment

PRINCIPLE 1: USE BENZODIAZEPINES ONLY FOR GOOD INDICATIONS

Benzodiazepines should be used only for those indications for which they have proven benefit. In the case of anxiety, when to use drug therapy is often a matter of judgment. Many cases of anxiety are clearly related to life experiences that may be temporary and are relieved by the mere passage of time. The major reasons for using drugs to treat anxiety would be the degree of discomfort and disability that anxiety produces in the individual patient. Some patients are more stoic than others and can endure anxiety with less discomfort and less disability. Relief of disabling or discomforting symptoms is paramount in all of medical practice. Some physicians have taken the moral position that anxiety should be borne so as to develop character. Oddly, physicians who have little difficulty using analgesics to provide relief of physical pain may be troubled about using drugs for the relief of psychic pain. This inconsistency of attitude is not congruent with good medical practice.

Prior to the use of these drugs for treating sleep disturbances, one should try to determine the cause of the problem. For instance, sleep disturbed by depression may be better treated with antidepressants than with benzodiazepines. Daytime sleepiness associated with sleep apnea syndrome might not be remedied by hypnotics, and their use in this situation might be dangerous. Not only should one determine the possible causes of insomnia but one should also assess its severity. Many patients who complain of insomnia are found in sleep laboratory studies to sleep for adequate periods of time. The perceived impairment of performance that they attribute to sleeplessness may be unreal or due to some other causes. Even when insomnia is real, it may not be of a degree that requires treatment with drugs. Sometimes deliberate avoidance of daytime naps or re-adjusting one's daily schedule to a different time for bed and arising may be all that is needed. The main indication for using these drugs as hypnotics is the degree of discomfort and disability produced by insomnia.

PRINCIPLE 2: USE NONDRUG METHODS WHEN FEASIBLE

A variety of nondrug methods may be used for managing patients with anxiety. These include various types of psychotherapy and various manipulations of the environment, the traditional treatment of the past. Recently, use of such maneuvers as biofeedback, muscle relaxation training, autogenic training and different kinds of massage has becme popular. Except for psychotherapy and environmental manipulation, the value of which has been proven in traditional medical practice, the efficacy of the other forms of nondrug treatment is still questionable. Nonetheless, for many patients these may be acceptable alternatives. The simplest and cheapest nondrug treatments are meditation, which costs only time, and exercise, which costs only calories. Some patients are unwilling to accept psychotherapy or cannot afford it. In this case, less expensive nondrug alternatives might be tried. No matter which nondrug alternative is tried, it can be used successfully with concomitant drug treatment.

Some nondrug approaches to managing insomnia have already been mentioned. As with anxiety, daily exercise and meditation may be cheap and effective alternatives. The avoidance of drugs that may aggravate insomnia, such as alcohol (which may cause early awakening, possibly because of "mini-withdrawal"), caffeine-containing beverages, and nasal decongestants or other preparations with sympathomimetic drugs, is another approach. Although the benefits are more likely to be psychological than due to any pharmacological effects, some patients may sleep better if they take a glass of milk and some crackers before going to bed.

PRINCIPLE 3: DRUG TREATMENT SHOULD BE PROPOSED AS INTERMITTENT AND BRIEF

The principle is extraordinarily important in assuring that patients do not get overtreated with drugs. Many episodes of anxiety are transitory, and even patients with chronic anxiety have fluctuations in their course, when anxiety becomes unbearable on some occasions while at other times it is not. Generally speaking, a course of treatment extending two or three weeks should be adequate to determine the efficacy of treatment. It should also provide enough relief of symptoms to allow a determination whether treatment should be extended or withdrawn.

From what is known of the pharmacokinetics of these drugs, steady-state plasma concentrations will be attained within a week or two with most of the commonly used drugs. Assuming that doses have been properly titrated, the drug should be fully effective by that time. Almost everyone who will improve with these drugs will show some degree of improvement within the first week or two. Maximal improvement, however, may not occur until after several weeks of treatment. Thus, it seems reasonable to think of initial short courses of treatment for most patients. If anxiety is relieved at the end of that time, one can propose to the patient that the drug be discontinued and used again when symptoms return. The arguments for doing so are, first, that effective treatment is available for future use, and second, to avoid possible tolerance and/or dependence that might follow sustained treatment. Most patients these days are so frightened of the possibility of becoming dependent on these drugs that this argument is quite convincing. Furthermore, the knowledge that an effective treatment is available for future use sustains the patient over succeeding episodes of anxiety.

It is equally important to establish limits on the use of these drugs as hypnotics. It does not seem to be reasonable to allow patients to take a hypnotic every night, except in unusual circumstances (such as severe emotional trauma or grief) where several days of consecutive treatment may be justified. Rather, one should negotiate with the patient at the onset of treatment for an intermittent dosage schedule. Patients should be assured that poor sleep, though it may make one feel poorly the next day, is not a life-threatening disorder. Thus, a couple of nights of poor sleep is tolerable and probably does not lead to as much impairment as may be subjectively felt. Therefore, hypnotics need not be used after a single night of poor sleep. By avoiding napping during the day, the normal corrective influences of the body should allow patients to sleep well the following night. Only if poor sleep occurs on two consecutive nights should patients take the hypnotic.

This rule of "at least two bad nights" should be tolerable for most patients and effectively reduces the amount of hypnotic that needs to be prescribed. By not taking the hypnotic on consecutive nights, the patient may also be able to detect rebound insomnia or anxiety that may follow the use of short-acting hypnotics. On the other hand, if a long-acting hypnotic is used, some carry-over to the second night often is experienced. Such an understanding about dosage should be reached at the outset of treatment. The total amount of hypnotic prescribed should be no more than that necessary to follow such a program during the period between visits.

PRINCIPLE 4: TITRATE DOSES

Some patients respond to the same dose of a drug quite differently from others. Many factors influence the individual patient's response to drugs.

One of the principal lessons learned from pharmacokinetic studies is that patients differ greatly either in peak plasma concentrations from single doses of a drug or steady-state plasma concentrations after repeated doses. Such differences among patients are generally in the order of several-fold. Consequently, it is of the utmost importance to titrate the dose of the drug to the individual patient's response.

One of the major effects of initial doses of benzodiazepines is sedation. Sedation is clearly appreciated by the patient with anxiety and is easily quantified. It is best tested, not with the first dose of the drug being in the morning, but rather at a time when the consequences will be minimal if oversedation occurs. Accordingly, it is wise to establish what this author calls the "minimally effective hypnotic dose". The definition of this dose is (a) that it is a dose which, if taken two or three hours before usual bedtime, will make one turn in earlier, (b) that the night's sleep will be good by whatever criteria the patient uses to make this determination and (c) that the patient will awake with a mild degree of hangover. The advantage of using this method for determining the proper dose for the patient is that very little harm can be done by having the patient sedated during the evening and night hours, and quite possibly some major benefit may occur by alleviating sleep problems.

The technique for doing this kind of dose titration is extremely simple. One starts out with a low dose of the drug the first night, instructing the patient to take it 2 or 3 hours before normal bedtime. If the criteria for the minimally effective hypnotic dose are not met on the first night, twice the dose is given the second night, four times this dose the third night and eight times the dose on the fourth night. To give an example, if one were to crack a 10 mg tablet of diazepam twice, one would have dose units of 2 to 3 milligrams (one-quarter tablet); once, 5 milligrams (one-half tablet); and whole, 10 milligrams (a full tablet). The patient, therefore, could take the one-quarter tablet the first night, the half-tablet the second night, the full tablet the third night and, if necessary, 2 tablets the fourth night. Thus, within a period of 4 nights, one could explore an eight-fold range of doses. Actually, most patients, if they are drug naive and are not cross-tolerant because of excessive alcohol use, will find the minimally effective hypnotic dose to be 10 milligrams or less. This dose then becomes the basic daily dose for the patient in the case of long-acting drugs. If the patient requires additional doses during the day, they may be taken as needed, usually one-half to one-third of the nighttime dose.

The advantages of abandoning the traditional equally divided dose schedule throughout the day are many. First, one can exploit the hypnotic effects, as most, if not all, patients with severe anxiety have some concurrent disturbance of sleep. Second, one avoids using more drug than is actually needed by having reckoned the patient's response. Third, one allows the patient to determine when additional drug is needed in a fashion similar to the determination made by anginal patients when they need additional nitroglycerine. Such flexibility makes much more sense in treating a fluctuating symptom than a fixed dose schedule. It also tends to minimize oversedation during the daytime hours.

This approach is best when used with long-acting benzodiazepines rather than with short-acting drugs (see Table 3 for this classification of benzodiazepines). Shorter-acting drugs may be required in regular divided doses, although not necessarily equally divided. One could increase the evening dose and decrease the daytime dose.

Table 3 Classification of benzodiazepines by plasma half-life

Very short	
triazolam	2 – 6 hours
Short	
alprazolam	6 – 20 hours
lorazepam	9 – 22 hours
oxazepam	6 – 24 hours
temazepam	5 – 20 hours
Intermediate	
chlordiazepoxide	7 – 46 hours
diazepam	14 – 90 hours
Long	
clorazepate	30 – 200 hours
halazepam	30 – 200 hours
prazepam	30 – 200 hours
Very long	
flurazepam	90 – 200 hours

The same principles apply when dosing with hypnotic benzodiazepines. Many of the patients requiring these drugs are elderly, in whom smaller doses are more appropriate. In any case, the smallest possible dose unit should be used initially. For many patients, this dose may be quite adequate, especially if the aim of treatment is to help initiate sleep. A considerable amount of placebo effect is attendant with the use of hypnotics, so one may wish to turn it to therapeutic advantage. If the smallest possible dose is not adequate, it is easy to titrate doses upward until one finds the effective dose for a particular patient. A dose that is too large initially may be quite satisfactory, but one will thereafter be overtreating the patient.

PRINCIPLE 5: ASSESS EFFICACY EARLY ON

The patient's response to the drug should be closely monitored. If the patient has shown little or no response after two or three weeks of treatment with an adequate dose of drug, it is unlikely that they will ever respond. Of course, if the dose has been pegged too low, it may be necessary to augment it before giving up. One should always be suspicious that the patient whose anxiety fails to be alleviated, at least in part, during the early phases of treatment, may have a more severe disorder. Anxiety is a prominent part of all depressive syndromes, being both as frequent and severe as depression itself. A misdiagnosis may have been made and the wrong drug chosen. Another possibility is that the patient with anxiety that does not improve with these drugs is alcoholic. Cross-tolerance may require much higher doses than usual, or concomitant use of alcohol may aggravate anxiety. Most serious of all is the possibility that the patient may be schizophrenic. Anxiety is a prominent symptom in the incipient stages of schizophrenia; the characteristic thought disorder of schizophrenia may not be apparent at this time. Therefore, any failure of the patient to respond early during treatment with benzodiazepines should be a clue for the consideration of other diagnosis.

Failure to respond to an adequate dose of hypnotic benzodiazepines also suggests some degree of cross-tolerance. If this is not the case, one should suspect also that some more serious emotional disorder, most likely depression, is the cause of the difficulty.

PRINCIPLE 6: AVOID BENZODIAZEPINES IN PATIENTS WITH A KNOWN RECORD OF DRUG ABUSE

Of special concern in this regard is the patient who is abusing alcohol. This patient may show disturbances of sleep and daytime anxiety during periods of "mini-withdrawal". When alcoholic patients are placed on benzodiazepines, these drugs may be used as substitutes. The vast majority of patients who have abused benzodiazepines have also abused alcohol. Much less common would be the abuse of other social–recreational drugs, but these should also be considered. With such drug abusing patients, one would prefer to use drugs that may be sedatives, but are less attractive in large doses. In this situation, sedative antihistamines (e.g., hydroxyzine) or tricyclic antidepressants (e.g., doxepin, amitriptyline) are useful. These drugs are not well tolerated because of their noxious side effects, which mitigate potential abuse by the alcoholic.

PRINCIPLE 7: GRADUALLY DISCONTINUE THE DRUG AFTER CHRONIC TREATMENT

Chronic treatment with benzodiazepines, even with therapeutic doses, seems to lead to some change in benzodiazepine receptors. "Receptor rebound" may follow abrupt discontinuation of the drug. This situation is somewhat analogous to that of propranolol. After continued use of the beta-adreno-receptor blocking drug, propranolol, supersensitivity of receptors develops. Rebound exacerbations of either angina pectoris, hypertension or cardiac arrhythmias have been well documented. The mechanism of therapeutic dose withdrawal reactions from benzodiazepines may be similar, but it is not entirely clear. This phenomenon has been only recently discovered, and still seems to be fairly uncommon. The principal determinant is not so much the dose of the drug as the duration of constant exposure to it. Accordingly, exposure to therapeutic doses of benzodiazepines of 3 months or more may put the patient at risk, albeit slight, of experiencing such a withdrawal reaction. The wisest thing to do would be gradually discontinue treatment in any patient who has had this degree of exposure. The longer the duration of exposure, the slower the rate of discontinuation. For instance, if a dose of 20 mg/day has been taken for 12 months, one might wish to reduce by 5 mg decrements each week for 2 weeks, then by 2 mg decrements for the succeeding 5 weeks. It is impossible to predict in any given patient what will be acceptable. The main point is that initially one can use larger decrements, but as the total dose declines, decrements should be progressively smaller.

The symptoms of therapeutic dose withdrawal are often confounded with the return of the original symptoms of anxiety, and consequently lead to the erroneous notion that the drug is continually needed. Although it is said that the symptoms of anxiety tend to be progressive and also recur more slowly than those of the withdrawal syndrome, these distinctions are not always clear.

Any return of symptoms of anxiety during the period of discontinuation probably indicates a continuing need for the drug. The frequency with which this phenomenon occurs is still uncertain. At the moment there are no adequate prospective studies to provide firm information on this matter. Although the risk is small, it is definite, and therefore this policy of gradual discontinuation should be adopted for all patients chronically treated with benzodiazepines.

CONCLUSION

One hopes that by following the general principles of treatment outlined above that benzodiazepines may be used effectively and safely in the many patients who require these drugs. Following these principles may cause less drug to be used, but not necessarily in fewer patients. Above all, one wants to avoid overtreating the patient who really needs the drug, either by giving too large a dose or by giving the dose for too long a period of time. With these reservations, the benzodiazepines can be safely and effectively used by virtually any physician.

6
Benzodiazepines in Emotional Disorders

Karl Rickels, MD

The efficacy of the benzodiazepines in the symptomatic treatment of non-psychotic anxiety has been well established. Hundreds of studies, many of them conducted under stringent double-blind conditions, have consistently shown that the benzodiazepines produce significantly more improvement than placebo in both somatic and emotional manifestations of anxiety (Lader, 1980; Rickels, 1978; Greenblatt & Shader 1974). In fact, comparing the clinical efficacy of the benzodiazepines with that of the barbiturates, meprobamate and placebo, one finds again and again the same rank order of efficacy, with benzodiazepines producing the most and placebo the least amount of improvement (Rickels, 1978; Cohen et al., 1976; Lader, Bond & James, 1974). Yet, by far, not every patient improves with benzodiazepines, and moderate to marked improvement is obtained only in about 65 to 75 percent of benzodiazepine-treated patients. In addition, as this author's research group demonstrated years ago, even patients reporting moderate improvement, representing about 40 percent of patients treated with benzodiazepines, by far do not reach "normative" anxiety levels (Rickels, 1978). An excellent review of the current status of benzodiazepines was recently provided by Greenblatt, Shader & Abernethy (1983).

Eight benzodiazepines are presently available in the United States as anxiolytics (Table 1). Five of them have long half-lives and include: chlordiazepoxide, the first benzodiazepine introduced into medicine; diazepam, the most frequently prescribed benzodiazepine; and clorazepate, prazepam and halazepam, pharmacologically inactive pro-drugs of the major active metabolite of diazepam, namely desmethyl-diazepam. The remaining three benzodiazepines have short to intermediately long half-lives. Two of them, oxazepam and lorazepam, have no active metabolites, and the recently introduced triazolo-benzodiazepine, alprazolam, has several active but clinically insignificant metabolites. In equipotent dosages, alprazolam appears to be less sedating than other benzodiazepines (Rickels *et al.*, 1983; Aden & Thein, 1980; Dawson, Tue & Brogden, 1984) and, most interestingly, it also seems to possess antidepressant properties (Rickels, 1982; Feighner *et al.*, 1981; Rickels *et al.*, 1984).

Table 1 Benzodiazepines marketed as anxiolytics in the United States

Drugs	*Dosage* (mg)	*Half-life* (hrs.)	*Active metabolites*
Moderately long-acting			
Diazepam	4–40	26–53	N-desmethyldiazepam
Chlordiazepoxide	15–100	8–28	Several
Long acting			
Clorazepate	7.5–60	30–100	N-desmethyldiazepam
Prazepam	10–60	30–100	N-desmethyldiazepam
Halazepam	20–160	30–100	N-desmethyldiazepam
Short-intermediate acting			
Oxazepam	30–120	5–15	None
Lorazepam	1–8	10–20	None
Alprazolam	0.5–4.0	12–15	Not clinically important

Several clinically effective benzodiazepines are available in many countries other than the United States (Tochemson & Breimes, 1984). Three of them have a long half-life (Table 2), as for example medazepam, a pro-drug of desmethyldiazepam, ketazolam whose major metabolite is also desmethyldiazepam, and the 1,5 benzodiazepine clobazam, which is supposedly less sedating that other benzodiazepines (Nicholson, 1981; John *et al.*, 1983), and bromazepam which has an intermediately long half-life and no major active metabolites. Ketazolam (Nair *et al.*, 1982; Rickels *et al.*, 1980) and clobazam (Jacobson *et al.*, 1983; Rickels *et al.*, 1981; Hindmarsh & Stonier, 1981) were extensively studied in the U.S. Bromazepam was studied already many years ago in the U.S. (Mahler & Holms, 1975; Rickels *et al.*, 1973) and more recently in Canada (Fontaine *et al.*, 1983; Lapierre *et al.*, 1978), and Scandinavia (Fynbroe *et al.*, 1981).

Table 2 Some benzodiazepines not marketed in the U.S.

Drug	*Active metabolites*	*Half-life*
Ketazolam	Desmethyldiazepam	Long
Medazepam	Desmethyldiazepam	Long
Clobazam	Desmethyldiazepam	Long
Bromazepam	3-Hydroxy bromazepam ?	Intermediate

PHARMACOKINETICS AND PHARMACOLOGICAL ACTION

All benzodiazepine derivatives have similar pharmacological properties. They reduce anxiety and tension, produce sedation and sleep, and possess varying degrees of anticonvulsant and muscle relaxing properties. The most common side effects arise from their central nervous system (CNS) depressant effect. Sedative side effects are commonly seen in early phases of treatment and are usually dose related. Interestingly, while some tolerance to the sedative effects of the benzodiazepines develops initially, this usually is not true for the anxiolytic effect. The benzodiazepines are extremely safe and, unless combined with alcohol or other CNS depressant drugs taken in excessive dosages, overdosing is not lethal. Some of the literature related to toxicity and drug overuse has recently been reviewed (Rickels, 1981).

While all benzodiazepines should be given sparingly if at all during pregnancy, any possible relationship between oral cleft and diazepam use during pregnancy has never been demonstrated (Rosenberg et al., 1983).

The clinical relevance of BZ drug interactions with cimetidine, propranolol and oral contraceptives are still far from established, as patients and physicians easily adjust treatment regimen to cope with increased or impaired drug clearance (Abernethy et al., 1984).

Benzodiazepines as a group possess more pharmacological and clinical similarities than dissimilarities, and in general they cannot be differentiated from each other in terms of overall clinical efficacy, all produce significantly more clinical improvement than placebo (Lader, 1980; Rickels, 1978, 1980; Greenblatt & Shader, 1974). However, the benzodiazepines do differ both in terms of pharmacokinetics and pharmacodynamics.

Diazepam and its pro-drugs, prazepam and clorazepate, are in some ways quite similar, having a long duration of action and a relatively sedating component as they share the active metabolite desmethyldiazepam (Greenblatt, 1980). Yet, even here, drug differences are seen. The clinical effects produced by diazepam, for example, are caused not only by desmethyldiazepam, but also by diazepam, itself an active drug. And while clorazepate has a fairly fast onset of action, prazepam does not.

Diazepam, the most lipophilic of the benzodiazepines, has the fastest onset of action of any benzodiazepine and is, therefore, one of the preferred benzodiazepines for acute or p.r.n. (as required) dosing. The main active ingredient is diazepam itself when given acutely. It enters the brain swiftly and also disappears relatively swiftly from the plasma, being distributed rapidly throughout all body tissues. Therefore, diazepam, given in an acute dose, disappears more quickly from the plasma than its long half-life would lead one to expect, and pattern of distribution, not plasma half-life, determines diazepam's acute effects. During chronic treatment, however, once distribution is complete, the elimination phase, which has a long half-life, now becomes the dominant factor. Thus, the wide use of diazepam as an anxiolytic can probably be explained in part by its fast onset of action when used acutely or p.r.n., its possession of two major components rather than one, its relatively long half-life such that during chronic use compliance may be less of a problem, and its muscle relaxant properties.

Oxazepam and lorazepam, two benzodiazepines with a relatively short duration of action (i.e., shorter half-lives), have to be taken more regularly and thus compliance may become a problem at times. Since both compounds have no active metabolites and are glucuronized into inactive compounds, they are considered to represent safer drugs for the treatment of the elderly or of patients with serious liver impairment (Greenblatt & Shader, 1980; Hoyumpa, 1978). Yet, even long-acting benzodiazepines with active metabolites can be managed quite effectively in the elderly or in persons with liver impairment by prescribing the drug in smaller dosages and by increasing the interval between dosings. Thus, anxiety can be appropriately managed even in the elderly with both short- and long-half-life benzodiazepines (Bandera et al., 1984).

It is interesting that the length of drug half-life has no clear-cut relationship to onset of action and is of relatively little importance for a patient's response during p.r.n. dosing. What is important for onset of action is speed of absorption as well as rate and extent of distribution (Greenblatt, 1980). While, for example, the long-half-life benzodiazepine, diazepam, is very quickly absorbed, the short-half-life, less lipophilic benzodiazepines, oxazepam and lorazepam, are absorbed more slowly.

Length of drug plasma half-life may be relevant in determining the time course of return of symptoms after the benzodiazepine is abruptly discontinued. One may expect that the shorter the half-life the sooner the original symptoms may return, and the longer the half-life the longer it will take for original symptoms to return (de Figueiredo et al., 1981; Ponciano et al., 1981). Half-life may also play a role in determining the incidence and intensity of withdrawal reactions when a benzodiazepine, prescribed in therapeutic doses, is stopped abruptly after many months of treatment (Tyrer, Rutherford & Huggett, 1981).

Pharmacodynamic differences exist between benzodiazepines. Some benzodiazepines, such as diazepam, have more muscle relaxant and sedative properties, while others possess more anticonvulsant effects, such as clonazepam, a benzodiazepine marketed in the United States only as an anticonvulsant. Another example is alprazolam which seems to possess more antidepressant properties than other anxiolytics and which is presently being intensively studied for the treatment of panic disorder with or without agoraphobia.

There also have been claims, particularly in the American literature, that some benzodiazepines increase aggression, while others, such as oxazepam, do not (Salzman et al., 1974; DiMascio, Shader & Harmatz, 1969). Much of this work has been conducted with normals or has been reported anecdotally. In a review of the benzodiazepines, Lader (1980) came to the conclusion that the reports that claim these drugs produce aggression or hostility are inconsistent, contradictory and often anecdotal. This author also could not confirm any consistent aggression-enhancing properties (Downing & Rickels, 1981; Rickels & Downing, 1974). It is true, however, that such responses may occur occasionally as paradoxical reactions, just as with other sedative drugs or alcohol. Such paradoxical responses are probably related to an interaction between some disinhibiting drug effect and patient personality. Thus, in the majority of anxious patients, benzodiazepines decrease rather than increase hostility and aggression.

INDICATIONS FOR BENZODIAZEPINE USE

Research conducted over many years has shown that non-psychotic anxious patients respond best to anxiolytics if they suffer from high levels of emotional and somatic symptoms of anxiety and from low levels of depression and interpersonal problems (Rickels, 1978). Benzodiazepines are usually not very effective in clear-cut depressions (Schatzberg & Cole, 1978), in anxiety associated with schizophrenia or borderline personalities, in agitation associated with chronic brain syndrome, and in phobic, obsessive-compulsive disorders. Many social phobias, which frequently improve with behavior therapy or with imipramine or MAO inhibitors, do however also respond at least to some degree to treatment with benzodiazepines. Panic disorder with or without agoraphobia or with other phobic avoidance behavior is claimed to respond better to alprazolam (Sheehan, 1982) than to other benzodiazepines and is similar in its efficacy to imipramine (Zitrin et al., 1983). Much of this research is confounding patients suffering from pure panic disorder with patients suffering from panic attacks and agoraphobia, and much more systematic research needs to be done for this particular indication. It should be stressed, however, that other benzodiazepines are not ineffective in the treatment of panic disorder (Rickels, unpublished data; Noyes et al., 1984). Noyes et al. reported diazepam to be significantly more effective than propranolol in alleviating symptoms of patients who suffered from panic disorder with or without agoraphobia. Indications for benzodiazepine use, employing *DSM-III Diagnostic Criteria* (American Psychiatric Association, 1980), are given in Table 3. In addition, many nonpsychotic anxiety reactions not clearly diagnosable according to *DSM-III*, such as anxiety in patients who have been told of the need for a coronary bypass operation, anxiety in cancer patients or anxiety present with or triggered by many physical illnesses are disorders where benzodiazepines might be profitably used.

While the benzodiazepines are presently the drugs of choice for the treatment of transient, acute and chronic anxiety, they are also effective hypnotics. Benzodiazepines, especially marketed in the U.S. for the treatment of insomnia are flurazepam with its long half-life metabolite desalkyl flurazepam and its very short half-life metabolite hydroxyethyl flurazepam, temazepam, a diazepam metabolite with an intermediate half-life, and triazolam, a triazolo benzodiazepine with a very short half-life. Other benzodiazepines used almost exclusively for the indication of insomnia outside of the U.S.A. are nitrazepam, flunitrazepam and more recently also midazolam and brotizolam (Rickels, 1982; Rickels, 1983).

Table 3

*DSM-III major indications
for benzodiazepine use*

Generalized anxiety disorder
Atypical anxiety disorder
Panic disorder
Anticipatory anxiety
Post-traumatic anxiety
Adjustment disorder with anxious mood
Somatization disorders

One of the most significant predictors of six-week treatment outcome has been identified by this author's group (Rickels, 1980) as the patient's initial response to a benzodiazepine (diazepam in this case) during the first week of treatment ($p<.001$). Of patients who were unimproved or who felt worse after one week on diazepam treatment, only 20 percent were markedly improved after six weeks of treatment. In fact, if a patient does not show at least some improvement within a few weeks of initiating benzodiazepine treatment, the physician would be wise to reassess his/her earlier diagnosis. S/he may have overlooked a depression or missed a personality problem, such as borderline personality. In the former case, a shift to a tricyclic antidepressant, and in the latter case, a shift to a low dosage of neuroleptic medication would probably represent a more appropriate treatment regimen than benzodiazepines. Finally, if a patient fails to improve with benzodiazepines, and if a reassessment of the diagnosis confirms the original anxiety diagnosis, one may consider measuring benzodiazepine plasma levels. Plasma levels of benzodiazepines do correlate strongly with daily dosage, but only weakly with clinical improvement (Rickels, 1980; Rickels *et al.*, 1984). Determination of benzodiazepine plasma levels may help the physician if compliance appears to be a problem. It may also help to identify the occasional fast or slow drug metabolizers (i.e., patients with excessive side effects on low benzodiazepine dosages or unimproved patients with a lack of side effects on high daily dosages).

LONG-TERM BENZODIAZEPINE TREATMENT AND DEPENDENCE

Maximal improvement with benzodiazepines is usually obtained within the first six weeks of treatment and, as a rule, no measurable additional improvement occurs after that time, even when daily dosage is increased within therapeutic range. In other words, increase of daily dosage as well as prolonged drug treatment does not produce additional improvement in patients resistant to benzodiazepine treatment (Rickels, Case & Downing, 1982). At the same time, tolerance to the anxiolytic effect of the benzodiazepine does not seem to be a significant problem even with long-term treatment (Rickels *et al.*, 1983; Greenblatt *et al.*, 1981; Hollister *et al.*, 1981).

Whether a shift to other benzodiazepines would be helpful in patients experiencing little or no improvement is questionable. One may speculate that *state anxiety* is more susceptible to anxiolytic drug therapy than *trait anxiety*. Thus, either a patient is happy with the level of anxiety reduction obtained, or should consider other therapeutic modalities and/or changes in life situation.

Since high relapse rates occur within six months after discontinuation of acute benzodiazepine treatment in chronically anxious patients (Rickels, Case & Diamond, 1980), chronic benzodiazepine treatment of several months duration, and possibly even years, appears to be an appropriate treatment regimen for a significant subgroup of chronically anxious patients frequently also suffering from panic symptoms and general dysphoria. There also may exist an indication for the chronic use of benzodiazepines in postcoronary patients or in patients with angina pectoris, to mention only a few chronic disease states in which these drugs may have beneficial effects (Dowling, 1980; Wheatley, 1980; Rickels, 1978).

If a protracted treatment course is warranted for chronically anxious patients, it is generally considered prudent to use the lowest daily dose that produces beneficial effects. Since anxiety frequently waxes and wanes, p.r.n. dosing or intermittent use should be considered whenever possible. Even chronically anxious patients should not be indiscriminantly treated with benzodiazepines for extended periods of time without assessing the need for such continuous treatment at regular time intervals. Also, a variety of nondrug therapies ranging from simple support to analytic psychotherapy should be considered as treatment options by patient and physician. In fact, medication is seldom given in a therapeutic vacuum. Balmer *et al.* (1981) employed diazepam in combination with psychotherapy for a 6-month period and found cautious use, beneficial effects, and no decrease of motivation for psychotherapy.

Dependence, both psychological and physical, may develop with benzodiazepines, as with other drugs in this general class, when medication is prescribed for prolonged periods of time. In fact, withdrawal responses to abrupt discontinuation of treatment are not unique for the benzodiazepines, but have also been reported for tricyclic antidepressants (Charney *et al.*, 1982) and for such antihypertensive drugs as propranolol, clonidine and methyldopa, to mention only a few (Rangno & Langlois, 1982; Garbus *et al.*, 1979).

Very high dosages of benzodiazepines, given over prolonged periods of time, are usually necessary before serious withdrawal reactions, including convulsions, are observed (Allgulander, 1978; Hollister, Motzenbecker & Degan, 1961). However, it appears that the majority of patients on long-term benzodiazepine medication do not use more than medically accepted dosages, even when treated for years (Greenblatt *et al.*, 1981; Hollister *et al.*, 1981; Bowden & Fisher, 1980; Winokur *et al.*, 1980). Despite the widespread use of benzodiazepines, it has not been easy to demonstrate tolerance or physical dependence to these drugs when used in therapeutic doses (Marks, 1978). Occasionally, case reports of withdrawal responses to abrupt discontinuation of benzodiazepines, primarily diazepam as the most frequently used benzodiazepine, have appeared in the literature, but even here, frequently excessive dosages were taken over extensive periods of time. Literature concerning benzodiazepine dependence has been reviewed by Rickels (1981), Greenblatt & Shader (1978) and Marks (1978). Since these 3 reviews, several case reports of lorazepam withdrawal have appeared in the literature (De la Fuente *et al.*, 1980; Einerson, 1980; Howe, 1980; Stewart, Salem & Springer, 1980).

More recently, two British studies (Petursson & Lader, 1981; Tyrer, Rutherford & Huggert, 1981) and one American study (Rickels *et al.*, 1983) reported some withdrawal responses, but no convulsive or psychotic reactions after abrupt discontinuation of therapeutic doses of diazepam, lorazepam and clobazam in patients treated from 6 months to 10 years. Two American studies by Laughren *et al.* (1982) and Bowden and Fisher (1980) could not confirm the occurrence of clear-cut withdrawal responses after the abrupt discontinuation of therapeutic doses of diazepam taken for years. In most cases, benzodiazepine withdrawal reactions can be effectively prevented by tapering off drug intake slowly, usually by an eighth to a quarter the daily dose every 1 to 2 weeks (Winokur *et al.*, 1980; Smith, 1979).

CONCLUSION

The time has come to consider benefit/risk and cost/benefit ratios when discussing the use of benzodiazepines for the treatment of anxiety. If benzodiazepines are not provided and if expensive nondrug interventions such as various psychotherapies are not acceptable, not affordable, or not helpful for the patient, what alternative coping options are available? Is the excessive intake of alcohol, over-eating, smoking of cigarettes or marijuana, sniffing of cocaine, or the use of other illicit drugs more acceptable than the use of benzodiazepines to cope with anxiety (Rickels,

1981)? In the author's opinion, such alternative coping mechanisms are certainly less appealing from the Public Health point of view than the use of benzodiazepines. On the contrary, benzodiazepines prescribed cautiously and judiciously by a caring physician lending an empathetic ear and offering practical advice represent an important medical option for the treatment of anxiety. While abuse as well as physical and psychological dependence certainly do occur, their incidence when considering the wide use of these drugs is minimal. While the majority of anxious patients can probably be treated for relatively short periods of time with benzodiazepines, a minority of chronically anxious patients may well need prolonged treatment. Such treatment should be under the careful supervision of an experienced physician. In fact, the prudent use of benzodiazepines demands the same skills that are required for the use of any other type of medication. In many instances, a combination of medication and psychotherapy appears to be the treatment of choice, with medication being given for more immediate, and psychotherapy offered for more prolonged and extended, benefits. Intermittent chronic treatment is preferred to uninterrupted chronic treatment. P.R.N. usage should be attempted whenever possible. Compared to most other psychiatric therapies, including several types of psychotherapy, the benefit/risk as well as cost/benefit ratios appear to greatly favor the use of benzodiazepines in the treatment of a significant number of anxious patients.

References

Abernethy DR, Greenblatt DJ, Ochs HR, *et al*: Benzodiazepine drug-drug interactions commonly occurring in clinical practice. *Curr Med Res Opin* 1984;8:Supp4,80.

Aden GC, Thein SG: Alprazolam compared to diazepam and placebo in the treatment of anxiety. *J Clin Psychiatry* 1980;41:245-248.

Allgulander C: Dependence on sedative and hypnotic drugs: A comparative clinical and social study. *Acta Psychiatr Scand* 1978;270.

American Psychiatric Association, Taskforce on Nomenclature and Statistics: *Diagnostic and Statistical Manual of Mental Disorders* (DSM-III), ed 3. Washington, DC, American Psychiatric Association, 1980.

Balmer R, Battegay R, von Marschall R: Long-term treatment with diazepam: investigation of consumption habits and the interaction between psychotherapy and psychopharmacotherapy: a prospective study. *Int Pharmacopsychiatry* 1981;16:221-234.

Bandera R, Bollini P, Garattini S: Long-acting and short-acting benzodiazepines in the elderly: kinetic differences and clinical relevance. *Curr Med Res Opin* 1984;8:Supp4,94

Bowden CL, Fisher JG: Safety and efficacy of long-term diazepam therapy. *South Med J* 1980;73:1581-1584.

Charney DS, Heninger GR, Sternberg DE, *et al*: Abrupt discontinuation of tricyclic antidepressant drugs: Evidence for noradrenergic hyperactivity. *Br J Psychiatry* 1982;141:377-386.

Cohen J, Gomez E, Hoell NL, *et al*: Diazepam and phenobarbital in the treatment of anxiety: A controlled multicenter study using physician and patient rating scales. *Curr Ther Res* 1976;20:184-193.

Dawson GW, Jue SG & Brogden RN: Alprazolam: a review of its pharmacodynamic properties and efficacy in the treatment of anxiety and depression. *Drugs* 1984;27:132-147.

de Figueiredo R, Franchini A, Martinho A, *et al*: Differences in the effect of two benzodiazepines in the treatment of anxious outpatients. *Int Pharmacopsychiatry* 1981;16:57-65.

De la Fuente JR, Rosenbaum AH, Martin HR, *et al*: Lorazepam-related withdrawal seizures. *Mayo Clin Proc* 1980;55:190-192.

DiMascio A, Shader RI, Harmatz J: Psychotropic drugs and induced hostility. *Psychosomatics* 1969;10:46-47.

Dowling JT: Relief of anxiety and pain in cardiac patients. *Drugs* 1980;19:437-442.

Downing RW, Rickels K: Hostility conflict and the effect of chlordiazepoxide on change in hostility level. *Comp Psychiatry* 1981;22:362-367.

Einarson TR: Lorazepam withdrawal seizures. *Lancet* 1980;1:151.

Feighner JP, Aden GC, Fabre LF, *et al*: Comparison of alprazolam, imipramine, and placebo in the treatment of depression. *J Am Med Assoc* 1983;249:3057-3064.

Fontaine R, Annable L, Chouinard G, *et al*: Bromazepam and diazepam in generalized anxiety: a placebo-controlled study with measurement of drug plasma concentrations. *J Clin Psychopharmacol* 1983;3:80-87.

Fynboe C, Christensen N, Halberg T, *et al*: Bromazepam (Lexotan[R]) and chlorprothixene (Taractan[R]) in acute psychoneurotic anxiety: a randomized double-blind comparison in general practice concerning the effect and risk of treatment resumption. *Curr Ther Res* 1981;30:1014-1023.

Garbus SB, Weber MA, Priest RT, *et al*: The abrupt discontinuation of antihypertensive treatment. *J Clin Pharmacol* 1979;19:476-486.

Greenblatt DJ: Pharmacokinetic comparisons. *Psychosomatics* 1980;21S:9-14.

Greenblatt DJ, Laughren TP, Allen MD, *et al*: Plasma diazepam and desmethyldiazepam concentrations during long-term diazepam therapy. *Br J Clin Pharmacol* 1981;11:35-40.

Greenblatt DJ, Shader RI: Effects of age and other drugs on benzodiazepine kinetics. *Drug Res* 1980;30:886-890.

Greenblatt DJ, Shader RI: Dependence, tolerance and addiction to benzodiazepines: Clinical and pharmacokinetic considerations. *Drug Metab Rev* 1978;8:13-28.

Greenblatt DJ, Shader RI: *Benzodiazepines in Clinical Practice*. New York, Raven Press, 1974.

Greenblatt DJ, Shader RI, Abernethy DR: Current status of benzodiazepines *N Engl J Med* 1983;309:354-358;410-416.

Hollister LE, Conley FK, Britt RH, et al: Long-term use of diazepam. J Am Med Assoc 1981;246:1568-1570.

Hollister LE, Motzenbecker FP, Degan RO: Withdrawal reactions from chlordiazepoxide (Librium[R]). Psychopharmacologia 1961;2:63-68.

Howe JG: Lorazepam withdrawal seizures. Br Med J 1980;281:1163-1164.

Hoyumpa AM: Disposition and elimination of minor tranquilizers in the aged and in patients with liver disease. South Med J 1978;71:23-28.

International Symposium on Clobazam. 13-15 April 1981. Proceedings. London/New York, Royal Society of Medicine International Congress and Symposium Series (No. 43), 1981.

Jacobson AF, Goldstein BJ, Dominguez RA, et al: A placebo-controlled, double-blind comparison of clobazam and diazepam in the treatment of anxiety. J Clin Psychiatry 1983;44:296-300.

Jochemsen R, Breimer DD: Pharmacokinetics of benzodiazepines: metabolic pathways and plasma level profiles. Curr Med Res Opin 1984;8:Supp4,60.

John J, Roy A, Verghese A: Clobazam and diazepam as anxiolytics and their effect on motor co-ordination. Curr Ther Res 1983;33:990-996.

Lader M: The present status of the benzodiazepines in psychiatry and medicine. Drug Res 1980;30:910-913.

Lader MH, Bond AJ, James DC: Clinical comparison of anxiolytic drug therapy. Psychol Med 1974;4:381-387.

Lader M, Petursson H: Rational use of anxiolytic/sedative drugs. Drugs 1983;25:514-528.

Lapierre YD, Oyewumi LK, Ghadirian A, et al: A placebo-controlled study of bromazepam and diazepam in anxiety neurosis. Curr Ther Res 1978;23:475-484.

Laughren TP, Battey Y, Greenblatt DJ, et al: A controlled trial of diazepam withdrawal in chronically anxious outpatients. Acta Psychiatr Scand 1982;65:171-179.

Marks J: The Benzodiazepines: Use, Overuse, Misuse, Abuse. Lancaster, England, MTP Press, 1978.

Nair NPV, Singh AN, Lapierre Y, et al: Ketazolam in the treatment of anxiety: a standard- and placebo-controlled study. Curr Ther Res 1982;31:679-691.

Nicholson AN: Studies on the effects of 1,4- and 1,5-benzodiazepines on sleep in man. Royal Society of Medicine International Congress and Symposium Series 1981;43:67-71.

Noyes R, Anderson DJ, Clancy J, et al: Diazepam and propranolol in panic disorder and agoraphobia. Arch Gen Psychiatry 1984;41:287-292.

Petursson H, Lader MH: Withdrawal from long-term benzodiazepine treatment. Br Med J 1981;283:643-645.

Ponciano E, Relvas J, Mendes F, et al: Clinical effects and sedative activity of bromazepam and clobazam in the treatment of anxious outpatients. Royal Society of Medicine International Congress and Symposium Series 1981;43:125-131.

Rangno RE, Langlois S: Comparison of withdrawal phenomena after propranolol, metoprolol and pindolol. *Br J Clin Pharmacol* 1982;13S:345-351.

Rickels K: Clinical trials of hypnotics. *J Clin Psychopharmacol* 1983;3:133-139.

Rickels K: The significance of pharmacokinetics in practical application in sleep disturbances, in Hippius H (ed): *Benzodiazepine in der Behandlung von Schlafstorungen.* München, Germany, Upjohn GmBH, 1982, pp 41-47.

Rickels K: Are benzodiazepines overused and abused? *Br J Clin Pharmacol* 1981;11S:71-83.

Rickels K: Clinical comparisons, in "Benzodiazepines 1980: Current Update". *Psychosomatics* 1980;21S:15-20.

Rickels K: Use of antianxiety agents in anxious outpatients. *Psychopharmacology* 1978;58:1-17.

Rickels K, Brown AS, Cohen D, *et al*: Clobazam and diazepam in anxiety. *Clin Pharmacol Ther* 1981;30:95-100.

Rickels K, Case WG, Diamond L: Relapse after short-term drug therapy in neurotic outpatients. *Int Pharmacopsychiatry* 1980;15:186-192.

Rickels K, Case DG, Downing RW: Issues in long-term treatment with diazepam therapy. *Psychopharmacol Bull* 1982;18:38-41.

Rickels K, Case WG, Downing RW, *et al*: Long-term diazepam therapy and clinical outcome. *J Am Med Assoc* 1983;250:767-771.

Rickels K, Cohen D, Csanalosi I, *et al*: Alprazolam and imipramine in depressed outpatients: a controlled study. *Curr Ther Res* 1982;32:157-164.

Rickels K, Csanalosi I, Greisman P, *et al*: A controlled clinical trial of alprazolam for the treatment of anxiety. *Am J Psychiatry* 1983;140:82-85.

Rickels K, Csanalosi I, Greisman P, *et al*: Ketazolam and diazepam in anxiety: a controlled study. *J Clin Pharmacol* 1980;20:581-589.

Rickels K, Downing RW: Chlordiazepoxide and hostility in anxious outpatients. *Am J Psychiatry* 1974;131:442-444.

Rickels K, Feighner JP, Smith WT: A double-blind comparison of alprazolam, amitriptyline, doxepin and placebo in the treatment of major depression. *Arch Gen Psychiatry* In press.

Rickels K, Pereira-Ogan J, Chung HR, *et al*: Bromazepam and phenobarbital in anxiety: a controlled study. *Curr Ther Res* 1973;15:679-690.

Rosenberg L, Mitchell AA, Parsells JL, *et al*: Lack of relation of oral clefts to diazepam use during pregnancy. *N Engl J Med* 1983;309:1282-1285.

Salzman C, Kochansky GE, Shader RI, *et al*: Chlordiazepoxide-induced hostility in a small group setting. *Arch Gen Psychiatry* 1974;31:401-405.

Schatzberg AF, Cole JO: Benzodiazepines in depressive disorders. *Arch Gen Psychiatry* 1978;35:1359-1365.

Sheehan DV: Panic attacks and phobias. *N Engl J Med* 1982;307:156-158.

Smith DE: Importance of gradual dosage reduction following low-dose benzodiazepine therapy. *Newsletter*, California Society for the Treatment of Alcoholism and Other Drug Dependencies 1979;6:1-3.

Sonne LM, Holm P: A comparison between bromazepam (Ro5-3350, Lexotan[R]) and diazepam (Valium[R]) in anxiety neurosis. *Int Pharmacopsychiatry* 1975;10:125-128.

Stewart RB, Salem RB, Springer PK: A case report of lorazepam withdrawal. *Am J Psychiatry* 1980;137:1113-1114.

Tyrer P, Rutherford D, Huggett T: Benzodiazepine withdrawal symptoms and propranolol. *Lancet* 1981;1:520-522.

Wheatley D: Coronary heart disease: Treating the anxiety component. *Prog Neuropsychopharmacol* 1980;4:537-544.

Winokur A, Rickels K, Greenblatt DJ, *et al*: Withdrawal reaction from long-term administration of diazepam. *Arch Gen Psychiatry* 1980;37:101-105.

Zitrin CM, Klein DF, Woerner MG: Treatment of agoraphobia with group exposure in vivo and imipramine. *Arch Gen Psychiatry* 1980;37:63-72.

7

Anxiety

Donald R. Wesson, MD

Patients' presentations of anxiety are ubiquitous to medical practice. Some patients specifically complain of anxiety to their physicians; other patients present with pathophysiological consequences of anxiety (e.g., tachycardia, tension headaches, or duodenal ulcers). For good reasons, physicians' first choice of medication for treatment of anxiety is a benzodiazepine. Compared with their sedative-hypnotic predecessors, benzodiazepines have definite advantages: lower lethality, even when taken in massive overdose; they do not activate microsomal liver enzymes; and they have lower abuse potential.

Many physicians (particularly biologically-oriented psychiatrists) view anxiety as a primary biological disorder. There is strong empirical evidence to support this view for at least one type of anxiety disorder: panic attacks. Two lines of research suggest a biological basis for panic attacks. First, intravenous infusions of sodium lactate will induce acute panic attacks in subjects with anxiety neurosis, but not in normal controls. Second, an asymmetry of cerebral blood flow in the a region of the parahippocampal gyrus has been described by one group of investigators (Reiman, Raichle *et al.*, 1984).

Other forms of anxiety may also have a biological basis. The presence of a benzodiazepine receptor in the central nervous system naturally raises the question about the natural ligand for the receptor. Although the receptor site binds benzodiazepines, they cannot be the natural ligand since benzodiazepines do not naturally occur. It is reasonable to assume that the receptor has a natural function, and a benzodiazepine receptor-mediated model of anxiety has been proposed (Insel, Ninan *et al.*, 1984).

Psychodynamically-oriented psychotherapists believe that anxiety is produced by preconscious recognition of unacceptable thoughts, wishes, or impulses. Consequently, anxiety is formulated as a secondary symptom of unconscious conflict, and psychotherapeutic treatment of anxiety is directed toward understanding and resolving the *conflict*. Psychotherapists are generally opposed to their patients taking anti-anxiety medications because of the concern that reducing anxiety would remove the drive for conflict resolution. Although their concern has validity, there are some patients in whom anxiety is too high for productive work in psychotherapy. By reducing the patient's anxiety to tolerable levels with a benzodiazepine or other sedative-hypnotic, the physician may assist the patient in their psychotherapeutic work.

Many people believe that anti-anxiety medications are overprescribed. Underlying their judgment that physicians overprescribe anti-anxiety medications is the, usually unstated, belief that anxiety is a normal part of everyone's life and that medication treatment for anxiety is tantamount to promoting pharmacological solutions to everyday problems in living. Physicians who prescribe anti-anxiety medication are viewed as having been unduly influenced by pharmaceutical companies' advertising promoting pills for all human ills.

Physicians are often advised to use benzodiazepines only for severe, disabling anxiety, however patients often come to physicians specifically to obtain psychotropic medication treatment of anxiety regardless of whether their day-to-day functioning is impaired. Patients view their symptoms of anxiety as intrusive, unnecessary and purposeless, and they want their physician to help them in extinguishing their symptoms. Such patients will respond to the physician's refusal to prescribe anti-anxiety medications by viewing the physician as unreasonable, uncaring, or not taking their complaints seriously. The physician will then either acquiesce to the patient's request or attempt to educate the patient about anxiety, pharmacological treatment, and alternative ways of learning to control or accept anxiety.

A rational approach to the treatment of anxiety follows from an understanding that anxiety is the final common pathway for different intrapsychic and biochemical processes. Physicians have a unique role in diagnosing physiological causes of anxiety (e.g., hypoglycemia, hyperthyroidism, stimulant toxicity, alcohol or other drug withdrawal) while maintaining sensitivity to issues of psychological causality.

The prevalence of anxiety among alcoholics is higher than non- alcoholics for several reasons. Some anxious people are predisposed to excessive drinking because they perceive alcohol as anxiolytic. Thus some people drink in an effort to self-medicate anxiety. In one study of patients admitted to hospitals for alcohol detoxification, 23% met American Psychiatric Association's Diagnostic and Statistical Manual (DSM-III, 1980) diagnostic criteria for one or more anxiety disorders (Weiss & Rosenberg, 1985). Establishing causality of anxiety in an alcoholic is often nebulous because alcohol can often be a cause of anxiety. A short-term abstinence syndrome (rebound from the sedation) occurs in the 8-12 hours following intoxication, and with longer periods of abstinence from alcohol, the classical alcohol abstinence syndrome, which always includes anxiety as a prominent symptom, may occur.

As with alcohol, other sedative-hypnotics can produce anxiety either as a paradoxical response, during rebound from the sedation, or as a withdrawal phenomena.

Although benzodiazepines are generally effective in treating anxiety, benzodiazepines can also be a *cause* of anxiety. With chronic daily use of benzodiazepines, physical dependency may develop. When the benzodiazepine is suddenly stopped, a withdrawal syndrome, which includes anxiety, may occur. The frequency with which this happens may be more common than generally diagnosed. Rickels *et al.* (1983), in a study of chronically anxious outpatients treated with diazepam (15-40 mg/day), reports that 43% of patients treated for 8 months or more demonstrated clear withdrawal reactions when the benzodiazepine was stopped. Even a marked decrease in dose, or the substitution of a short-acting benzodiazepine for a long-acting one, may precipitate withdrawal symptoms (Conell & Berlin, 1983). The physical dependency syndromes of benzodiazepines are presented in detail in Chapter 17.

Given current standards of prescription for benzodiazepines, even careful and experienced physicians are likely to treat a few patients who develop physical dependency on benzodiazepines. Although development of physical dependency should be of concern, physical dependency should be viewed as an undesirable side effect and should not dissuade physicians from prescribing benzodiazepines for patients who will benefit from them. Physicians can, however, use treatment strategies that minimize the possiblity of dependence. Of primary importance is the length of time the patient takes them continuously. The prescription of benzodiazepines should generally be for a short duration, and the physician should always give consideration to mobilization of non-pharmacological treatment (e.g., individual or group psychotherapy, biofeedback and relaxation training) in addition to, or as an alternative to, anxiolytic medication treatment.

CLINICAL ASSESSMENT OF ANXIETY

Clinical assessment of anxiety may be based on history from the patient, measurements of physiological signs of anxiety, or the behavioral correlates of anxiety. Each of these will be considered in more detail.

A patient's report of "anxiety" needs to be carefully explored as patients may use the term to describe a variety of unpleasant subjective states. For example, patients may equate worry, or rumination, with anxiety. The subjective state of anxiety is apprehension, fear, or terror, often associated

113

with feelings of impending doom. If the patient's anxiety is triggered by specific environmental stimuli, the term "phobia" is more appropriate.

Physiological correlates of anxiety are generally mediated through the sympathetic nervous system (e.g., increased heart rate, blood pressure, peripheral vasoconstriction and sweating of the palms). Some patients report a feeling of shortness of breath and in response, hyperventilate. If the patient's blood gases are measured during hyperventilation, oxygen saturation of the blood is normal, however the carbon dioxide content is decreased. It is the decrease in carbon dioxide that produces secondary symptoms: paresthesias and muscle spasms.

Some people experience anxiety with gastro-intestinal symptoms. The gastro-intestinal tract can respond to anxiety in a variety of ways including painful cramping, the urge to defecate, a feeling that the stomach is "tied up in knots", or acute abdominal pain.

Tension, an increased musculo-skeletal tone, may result from anxiety.

Behavioral correlates of anxiety include purposeless motor movements, facial grimace, or rigid body movements.

Patients show great individual differences in how anxiety is manifested. For example, some patients deny the subjective experience of anxiety while showing a physiological response pattern typical of anxiety. If patients manifest anxiety as increased muscle tone, particularly of the facial and neck muscles, musculo-skeletal complaints or tension headaches may occur, and these patients may complain of pain without recognizing that anxiety is the cause.

ACUTE ANXIETY STATES

Although acute anxiety may be superimposed on a chronic anxiety state, acute anxiety is episodic and more intense. During an acute attack, patients feel helpless, unable to control themselves, and often fear dying or "going crazy". Phobias are a type of acute anxiety in which the anxiety attacks are triggered by specific phobic stimulus or situations.

Panic disorder is a discrete type of acute anxiety. In panic disorder, acute recurrent panic attacks occur unpredictably and are unrelated to environmental or psychological precipitants (Shader, Goodman, Gever, 1982). The acute attacks begin abruptly, include intense apprehension, fear, or terror often associated with feelings of impending doom and may last minutes to days. The disorder often begins in late adolescence to mid-adult life (DSM-III, 1980) and, as mentioned previously, probably has a biological basis. Treatment of panic attacks is directed towards one of two conditions: prophylaxis of the acute attacks, or treatment of the acute attack after one is underway. Imipramine, an antidepressant, is often effective for prophylaxis of the acute anxiety attack. The mechanism of the anti- panic action is distinct from the antidepressant effects. The anti- anxiety effect generally occurs within hours of the first dose and at dosages that are often below those effective as an antidepressant.

Alprazolam is reported effective both for prophylaxis of the acute attacks and for treatment of an acute attack (Sheehan, Bao *et al.*, 1984).

Patients subject to panic attacks often develop secondary anticipatory anxiety, or agoraphobia, and after several years, such patients appear to have chronic anxiety.

CHRONIC ANXIETY STATES

Some patients are chronically anxious, a condition classified under American Psychiatric Association's (DSM-III) category as generalized anxiety disorder. This is largely a diagnosis of exclusion, and excludes anxiety due to other diagnosable mental and physical conditions.

Differential Diagnosis of Chronic Anxiety
The distinction between panic attacks, phobias, anticipatory anxiety, depression, stress, tension, and anxiety produced by other disease is important as pharmacological treatment is different.

Depression Anxiety and agitation are frequent concomitants of clinical depression. Anxiety that is the product of depression often subsides as the depression remits, and treatment with a sedating antidepressant - sometimes with the initial addition of a low dose of a benzodiazepine - is a rational pharmacological approach.

Thyrotoxicosis may present as chronic anxiety and must always be considered in the differential diagnosis of causes of chronic anxiety. Treatment is control of hyperthyroidism not anxiolytics.

High dose caffeine or stimulant abuse Caffeine consumption can also be the cause anxiety (Greden, Fontaine *et al.*, 1978), as can abuse of cocaine or amphetamine. Withdrawal syndromes from stimulants can also include anxiety and insomnia.

Stress, the response to external events or life circumstances, can also produce anxiety. The more easily identified stressors – death of a spouse or child, illness, losing a job or economic reversals – are readily acknowledged and recognized as stressful. Not everyone realizes, however, that positive life events are also stressors. Marriage, the birth of a child, the purchase of a home, or a job promotion, because they are desirable, are often not recognized as sources of significant stress.

The body's response to stress is complex and is influenced by the total quantity of stress, coping style, genetic constitution, intelligence, problem-solving ability, past mastery of stressful situations, and the amount of support available. The relationship of stress to disease is complex, and similar stresses can produce a variety of diseases in different people. Benzodiazepines may be an appropriate adjunct in treatment.

A post-traumatic stress syndrome A psychologically healthy person may respond to a severe traumatic event with psychological and physiological symptoms. For months-to-years following the traumatic event, a person may be subject to intrusive images of the stressful situation, nightmares, dysphoria, emotional blunting, and a variety of autonomic hyperarousal states. Benzodiazepines have an adjunctive role while psychological treatment is being pursued.

ANTIDEPRESSANTS USED IN TREATMENT OF ANXIETY

Tricyclic antidepressants are sometimes prescribed for their anti- anxiety properties. As anxiety often accompanies agitated depression, the patient's anxiety may initially improve just due to non-specific sedative effects of antidepressants. Amitriptyline, imipramine and doxepin all have consider-able sedative properties. Additional improvement in anxiety may occur as the mood component of depression improves.

The use of imipramine in the treatment of panic attacks has already been discussed.

BETA ADRENERGIC BLOCKING AS TREATMENT OF ANXIETY

Beta adrenergic blocking medications (e.g., propranolol) can be useful in the treatment of anxiety and panic states (Heiser & Defrancisco, 1976). In a placebo-controlled cross-over study in 25 chronically anxious outpatients, the combination of diazepam and propranolol was found superior to diazepam alone (Hallstrom, Treasaden, Edwards, Ladner, 1981; Pitts, 1984). Beta adrenergic blockade reduces the somatic manifestations of anxiety, particularly tremor and tachycardia.

SOME PRESCRIBING CONSIDERATIONS

Although careful diagnostic assessment of the patient and appropriate selection of medication is important, the role of non-specific factors, such as "doctor warmth", have an important influence on treatment outcome and, sometimes contribute an effect comparable in magnitude to the pharmacological actions of the medication (Rickels, 1973).

Research studies of anti-anxiety medications are not always designed to demonstrate the medication's optimal use. Hollister (1973), for example, noted that the fixed dosing schedules used in many controlled studies concerning the treatment of acute anxiety are inappropriate. A design which would more closely approximate much clinical prescription would be an "as needed" regimen in which the medications were used for a limited period of time (days to weeks). Because of the importance of non-specific treatment factors, the placebo-controlled study remains necessary for assessment of pharmacological effects.

The prescription of psychotropic drugs should always include an assessment of the benefit/risk ratio. Although acute and chronic anxiety reactions are subjectively unpleasant, anxiety is rarely life- threatening, unless the patient has pre-existing illness or attempts to escape the anxiety attack through suicide or drug overdose. For many patients, having access to sedatives and tranquilizers improves the quality of their life and may facilitate their capacity to cope with life stresses and adversities.

The risks of prescribing benzodiazepines for anxiety go beyond that of drug toxicity. Some patients will become psychologically dependent on medications in response to life discomforts. Sometimes the risk extends to people other than the patient for whom the medication was prescribed. For example, many patients share their medications with friends.

Toxicity, side effects, and pharmacological considerations in prescription of benzodiazepines are discussed in Chapter 16. Compared to the tricyclic antidepressants and phenothiazines (and other neuroleptics sometimes prescribed for anxiety), the benzodiazepines have a significantly lower frequency of side effects and allergic reactions. They are not associated with the development of tardive dyskinesia as are the neuroleptics.

A SOME PRACTICAL GUIDELINES FOR PRESCRIBING ANXIOLYTIC DRUGS

In Chapter 5, Hollister presents 7 principles for prescription of benzodiazepines that are generally applicable for treatment of anxiety. Additional emphasis is given here to principles that apply specifically to anxiety.

1. Before prescribing psychotropic medications, the first effort should be to identify life stresses that are causing or aggravating anxiety which may be responsive to counseling, active environmental manipulation, or psychotherapy. Even when the situation appears to be unalterable, such as a reaction to an acute loss, working through the grief reaction at a

psychological level may be assisted with appropriate psychotherapeutic techniques. Medication treatment should be explained to the patient as being only one part of the overall intervention strategy.

2. For chronic anxiety, anxiolytic medications should be prescribed on a fixed dosage schedule instead of *as needed*. This pattern of medication use is analogous to that used for the treatment of chronic pain in which the contingency relationship between the symptom of pain and receiving narcotics is broken.

3. The skilled combination of medical and psychological treatment is frequently more effective than either medical or psychological treatment alone, especially for psychosomatic illnesses.

4. When problems which initially present as self-limited situational reactions do not respond as predicted, the failure to respond should be used as part of the explanation to the patient why referral for non-psychotropic treatment, sometimes in combination with medication, should be undertaken.

5. To decrease the development of tolerance, patients should be encouraged to take periodic holidays from taking psychotropic medications. With longer-acting benzodiazepines, drug-free periods should be for a week or more to allow the benzodiazepine metabolites to clear from the body. Symptoms which are suppressed by the medication may return, however the patient is instructed to tolerate symptoms for this "holiday" period. A break in the patient's ingestion of medication will serve both to decrease tolerance and allow assessment of the need for continued medication. The patient should be aware of the purpose of the "holidays" and be reassured that medication will be restarted if needed.

6. Whenever the patient has been daily taking benzodiazepine medications for several months or more, a gradual tapering of the dosage is indicated before initiating drug holidays. This will minimize physiological rebound and the possibility of precipitating a drug-withdrawal reaction.

7. In spite of counsel, some patients will steadfastly refuse to take medication holidays, will refuse psychiatric referral, and may use medications in a destructive manner. This cannot always be prevented, however physicians should not knowingly prescribe medications to patients who use them as intoxicants or who consistently take them at variance from the prescriptive directions.

Sometimes it is in the best interest of the patient for the physician to refuse further prescription. In such instances, the patient's threat to obtain "street drugs" or get them from another physician should not cajole the physician into continued prescription.

References

Conell LJ, Berlin RM: Withdrawal after substitution of a short-acting for a long-acting benzodiazepine. *JAMA* 1983;250:2838-2840.

Diagnostic and Statistical Manual of Mental Disorders III: American Psychiatric Association, Washington, D.C., 1980.

Greden JF, Fontaine P, Lubetsky M, *et al*: Anxiety and depression associated with caffeinism among psychiatric inpatients. *Am J Psychiatry* 1978;135:963-966.

Hallstrom C, Treasaden I, Edwards JG, Ladner M: Diazepam, propranolol and their combination in the management of chronic anxiety. *Br J Psychiatry* 1981;139:417-421.

Heiser JF and Defrancisco D: The treatment of pathologic panic states with propranolol. *American Journal of Psychiatry* 1976;133:1389-1394.

Hollister LE: *Clinical Use of Psychotherapeutic Drugs*. Springfield, Charles C. Thomas, 1973.

Insel TR, Ninan PT, Aloi J, Jimerson DC, Skolnick P, Paul, SM: A benzodiazepine receptor-mediated model of anxiety: Studies in nonhuman primates and clinical implications. *Arch Gen Psychiatry* 1984;41:741- 750.

Pitts FN: Lactate, beta-antagonist, beta-blockers and anxiety. *J Clin Psychiatry Monograph* 1984;2:25-39.

Reiman EM, Raichle ME, Butler FK, Herscovitch P, Robins E: A focal brain abnormality in panic disorder, a severe form of anxiety. *Nature* 1984;310:683-685.

Rickels K: Predictors of response to benzodiazepines in anxious outpatients, in Garattini S, Mussini E, Randall LO (eds): *The Benzodiazepines: Monographs of the Mario Negri Institute for Pharmacological Research*. New York, Raven Press, 1973, pp 391-404.

Rickels K, Case WG, Downing RW and Winokur A: Long-term diazepam therapy and clinical outcome. *J Am Med Assoc* 1983:250:767-771.

Shader RI, Goodman M, Gever J, *et.al.*: Panic disorders: current perspectives. *J Clin Psychopharmacol.* 1982;2(suppl):2-10.

Sheehan, DV, Coleman JH, Greenblatt, DJ, Jones, KJ, Levine, PH, *et. al.*: Some biochemical correlates of panic attacks with agoraphobia and their response to a new treatment. *J Clin Psychopharm.* 1984;4:66-75.

Weiss KJ, Rosenberg, DJ: Prevalence of anxiety disorder among alcoholics. *J Clin Psychiatry* 1985;46:3-5.

8
Clinical Comparison of Benzodiazepine Hypnotics With Short and Long Elimination Half-Lives

Anthony Kales, MD, Constantin R. Soldatos, MD,
Antonio Vela-Bueno, MD

Over the last few years, articles in both the medical literature and popular press stressing the negative consequences of using hypnotic medication may have made physicians unjustifiably hesitant to prescribe these drugs (Kales & Kales, 1984). Frequently, such articles contend that sleeping pills are prescribed too often. However, these concerns may be exaggerated, as illustrated by the following data.

About one-third of the general population has some type of complaint of disturbed sleep (Bixler et al., 1979a), and only half of these individuals, or approximately 15 percent, seek help from a physician (Bixler, Kales & Soldatos, 1979; Gallup Organization, 1979). These patients probably represent, for the most part, individuals with complaints of severe insomnia (Mellinger & Balter, 1981), who have much higher degrees of psychopathology (Kales & Kales, 1984; Kales et al., 1983a). Physicians prescribe hypnotic drugs for about half of these insomniac patients or 7.5 percent of the population (Bixler et al., 1976). Of this group, 60 percent or about 5 percent of the population are reported to take the drug over a period of a month or longer (Bixler, Kales & Soldatos, 1979), while only about 20 percent, or 1 percent of the general population, take medication each night for at least a month (Bixler, Kales & Soldatos, 1979; Bixler et al., 1979a). This latter estimate is supported by other survey data, showing that approximately 1 percent of the general population uses hypnotic drugs nightly for longer than a two-month period (Mellinger & Balter, 1981; Balter & Bauer, 1975).

Thus, while the frequency of use of hypnotic drugs does not appear to be excessive, physicians may misuse these agents by overrelying on them and consequently prescribing them for nightly use for prolonged periods of time. They may neglect to evaluate the patient thoroughly; whereas to use hypnotic drugs properly in the treatment of insomnia, the physician must first determine if they will complement the overall therapeutic approach. Simply prescribing a hypnotic drug will seldom be of lasting benefit to the patient if the underlying causes of insomnia are not identified and treated. In fact, such an approach actually may create additional serious problems, such as an undue reliance on hypnotic drugs, or even drug dependency. The overall effectiveness of these drugs in treating insomnia usually depends upon how they are used as an adjunct along with other treatments for this condition.

Today, benzodiazepine hypnotics are the drugs of choice. However, when selecting a hypnotic, physicians can not assume that all benzodiazepine hypnotics are essentially alike in their clinical effects. In reality, these drugs have considerable differences in their pharmacokinetic properties, many of which directly affect the drugs' clinical profiles, as is the case for the benzodiazepine anxiolytics (Greenblatt et al., 1982a; Breimer & Jochemsen, 1981). Some of the most important pharmacokinetic properties of the benzodiazepine hypnotics involve their rates of absorption and elimination half-lives.

Rate of absorption is critical in relation to whether a hypnotic is effective for inducing sleep as opposed to maintaining sleep (Greenblatt et al., 1982a; Breimer & Jochemsen, 1981). Elimination half-life determines a drug's potential for accumulation with consequent carry-over effectiveness, daytime anxiolytic effect, and daytime sedation (Kales & Kales, 1984). Further, the potential for a drug to produce early morning insomnia (Kales et al., 1983b) and increased daytime anxiety (Kales et al., 1983b; Morgan & Oswald, 1982) during administration, and rebound insomnia (an intense worsening of sleep above pre-drug baseline levels) and rebound anxiety (significantly increased levels of daytime anxiety) (Kales et al., 1983c; Kales et al., 1979; Kales, Scharf & Kales, 1978) following withdrawal is also determined largely by how rapidly it is eliminated from the body.

Given the high prevalence of insomnia and the need for multidimensional treatment modes, which may include the use of hypnotic drugs, it is clear that physicians would benefit from information regarding the evaluation of insomniac patients and the adjunctive use of hypnotic medication in treatment (Kales et al., 1980a). Our purpose, then, is to enhance the physician's effectiveness in treating insomnia by discussing its multiple etiologic factors, the need for a thorough evaluation, and the differences in effectiveness, side effects, and withdrawal effects between benzodiazepine hypnotics with short and long elimination half-lives.

THE CONDITION OF INSOMNIA

Insomnia is a symptom that may be due to a variety of underlying factors (Kales & Kales, 1984). We have found that psychological factors play a predominant etiologic role in patients with chronic insomnia. In fact, about 70 to 80 percent of patients with insomnia seen in our Sleep Disorders Clinic have one or more abnormally elevated scales on the Minnesota Multiphasic Personality Inventory (MMPI) (Kales et al., 1983a; Kales et al., 1976b). Scales for depression, conversion hysteria, and psychasthenia are the most frequently elevated in these patients, who have strikingly similar personality patterns characterized by internalization of emotions. In retrospective studies, insomniac patients were found to have more emotional difficulties, a lower self-image, and more interpersonal and health problems than control subjects both during childhood and prior to developing sleep difficulty (Healey et al., 1981). Also, they report a peak in life-stress events during the year preceding the onset of their insomnia, suggesting that chronic insomnia develops when life-stress factors are prevalent in individuals who are predisposed by inadequate coping mechanisms (Healey et al., 1981).

Disturbed sleep is often associated with medical conditions accompanied by pain, physical discomfort, anxiety, or depression (Kales & Kales, 1984; Kales, Soldatos & Kales, 1982; Kales, Soldatos & Kales, 1981; Soldatos, Kales & Kales, 1979). Aging also contributes to disturbed sleep: the elderly sleep less and have very little of the "deeper" stages 3 and 4 sleep (Bixler et al., 1984; Williams, Karacan & Hursch, 1974; Feinberg & Carlson, 1968; Agnew, Webb & Williams, 1967). Also, their sleep often reverts to a more polyphasic pattern, with periods of sleepiness during the day and frequent nap taking.

Drugs themselves can cause or contribute to poor sleep. Specifically, stimulant drugs (Smith et al., 1979), steroids, energizing antidepressants (Kales et al., 1977b), or beta-adrenergic blockers (Stephen, 1966) can aggravate or induce insomnia, particularly when taken close to bedtime. Drinking coffee (Karacan et al., 1976) or cola or even smoking (Soldatos et al., 1980) close to bedtime may cause difficulty, usually in initially falling asleep, whereas alcohol consumption can contribute to difficulty staying asleep, mainly in the form of early morning awakenings. Ironically, certain hypnotic drugs may themselves cause sleep difficulty. Benzodiazepine hypnotics with rapid elimination rates may produce early morning insomnia (Kales et al., 1983b) and daytime anxiety (Kales et al., 1983b; Morgan & Oswald, 1982). This syndrome, consisting of a worsening of sleep during the last few hours of drug nights and increased daytime anxiety and tension, appears after 1 to 2 weeks of nightly use when tolerance begins to develop. Further, withdrawal of benzodiazepines with short-to-intermediate elimination half-lives may produce both rebound insomnia and rebound anxiety

(Kales et al., 1983c; Kales et al., 1979; Kales, Scharf & Kales, 1978).

Because of the multiplicity of factors that may underlie the condition of chronic insomnia, a thorough evaluation of these patients should include histories of sleep difficulty (Kales, Soldatos & Kales, 1979), drug use, and psychiatric problems (Kales & Kales, 1984; Kales, Soldatos & Kales, 1982; Kales, Soldatos & Kales, 1981; Soldatos, Kales & Kales, 1979). A thorough sleep history defines the specific sleep problem and any coexisting sleep disorder, assesses its clinical course, evaluates sleep/wakefulness patterns, includes reports from the bed partner, and evaluates the impact of the sleep problem on the patient's life (Kales, Soldatos & Kales, 1979).

A drug history describes the current use of any prescribed and nonprescribed medication, as well as the timing of their administration, particularly in relation to bedtime (Kales & Kales, 1984; Kales, Soldatos & Kales, 1982; Kales, Soldatos & Kales, 1981; Soldatos, Kales & Kales, 1979). If the patient gives a history of using hypnotic drugs that are relatively rapidly eliminated, the physician should assess for the presence of early morning insomnia (Kales et al., 1983b), daytime anxiety (Kales et al., 1983b; Morgan & Oswald, 1982), rebound insomnia, and rebound anxiety (Kales et al., 1983c; Kales et al., 1979; Kales, Scharf & Kales, 1978).

Because psychiatric factors play a major role in the development of insomnia (Kales et al., 1984; Tan et al., 1984; Kales et al., 1983a; Kales et al., 1976b), a thorough assessment of emotional factors often reveals a clear association between the development of certain psychological conflicts or life stresses and the onset of sleep difficulty (Healey et al., 1981). Examination of the patient's mental status may reveal and delineate patterns of depression, anxiety, rumination, obsessive-compulsiveness, hypochondriasis, and, in the elderly, organicity (Kales & Kales, 1984; Kales, Soldatos & Kales, 1982; Kales, Soldatos & Kales, 1981; Soldatos, Kales & Kales, 1979).

PHARMACOKINETIC ISSUES

Onset of Action

The rapidity of a hypnotic drug's sleep-inducing action is a critical issue in treating patients with chronic insomnia because difficulty falling asleep is their most prevalent complaint (Kales et al., 1984; Kales & Kales, 1984). In turn, the most important factor determining the onset of action is the drug's rate of absorption. Of the three hypnotics commercially available in the United States, (flurazepam, temazepam, and triazolam), flurazepam is absorbed most quickly (Greenblatt et al., 1982b). It has an intermediate rate of absorption, followed by triazolam, then temazepam, with an extremely slow rate. Peak concentrations of temazepam are not reached until 2 to 3 hours after administration (Greenblatt et al., 1982b). Thus, one could predict from their pharmacokinetics that flurazepam and triazolam would be effective for inducing sleep, while temazepam would have little efficacy for this type of insomniac complaint unless taken an hour or two before bedtime. Temazepam's slow absorption apparently is due to the particular formulation available in this country, a hard gelatin capsule which has a much slower rate of absorption than the formulation used in Europe (Greenblatt *et al.*, 1982a,b; Divoll *et al.*, 1981; Fuccella *et al.*, 1977).

Elimination Half-Life

Drug accumulation and the consequent potential for producing carryover effectiveness, daytime anxiolytic effects, or daytime sedation are determined primarily by a drug's elimination half-life and total metabolic clearance (Kales & Kales, 1984; Greenblatt *et al.*, 1982b; Breimer & Jochemsen, 1981; Kales *et al.*, 1976a). Obviously, the rate of elimination of a given drug is affected by the presence of active metabolites and their rates of elimination. If the elimination half-life of the parent compound and active metabolites is short, there will be a minimum of drug accumulation, and, thus, less potential for such a drug to produce daytime sedation and performance decrements (Johnson & Chernik, 1982; Church & Johnson, 1979; Oswald *et al.*, 1979). However, these short half-life drugs have a greater potential for producing early morning insomnia (Kales *et al.*, 1983b) and daytime anxiety during administration (Kales *et al.*, 1983b; Morgan & Oswald, 1982) and rebound insomnia and rebound anxiety following abrupt withdrawal (Kales *et al.*, 1983c; Kales *et al.*, 1979; Kales, Scharf & Kales, 1978). On the other hand, drugs with long elimination half-lives accumulate and consequently have less potential for producing early morning insomnia, rebound insomnia, or increases in daytime levels of anxiety (Kales & Kales, 1984; Kales & Kales, 1983). Instead, they are more likely to produce carryover effectiveness, daytime anxiolytic effects, and daytime sedation.

Three different components contribute to the activity of flurazepam (Amrein *et al.*, 1983; Eckert *et al.*, 1983; Greenblatt *et al.*, 1982a; Breimer & Jochemsen, 1981; Greenblatt *et al.*, 1981a; Kaplan *et al.*, 1973). The fast-acting hydroxyethyl flurazepam and flurazepam aldehyde metabolites are responsible for the drug's efficacy for sleep induction and are eliminated rapidly. The desalkylflurazepam metabolite, however, is eliminated very slowly (50–100 hours), accumulating with consecutive nightly administration. Temazepam has an intermediate elimination half-life (a mean of about 15 hours) (Greenblatt *et al.*, 1982a; Divoll *et al.*, 1981), and, therefore, an intermediate degree of accumulation. Finally, triazolam has an ultrashort elimination half-life, with essentially no accumulation with consecutive nights of administration (Eberts, Philopolous & Reineke, 1981; Greenblatt *et al.*, 1981b).

HYPNOTIC DRUG ADMINISTRATION

Efficacy

The effectiveness of flurazepam, which was the first benzodiazepine hypnotic to become commercially available in the United States, is well established. Sleep laboratory studies show that with short-term administration of flurazepam sleep is significantly improved on the first night. Because of the carryover effect of the desalkylflurazepam metabolite, effectiveness is further increased to a slight degree with continued administration so that peak improvement occurs on the second and third consecutive nights of use. Flurazepam continues to be effective both for inducing and maintaining sleep, not only with intermediate-term use (Kales *et al.*, 1982b; Kales *et al.*, 1976a; Kales *et al.*, 1975; Kales *et al.*, 1970), but also with long-term use (one month of consecutive nightly administration) (Kales *et al.*, 1982b; Kales *et al.*, 1976a; Kales *et al.*, 1975). Our initial finding of the maintenance of flurazepam's effectiveness over lengthy periods of administration has been confirmed in a number of studies (Oswald *et al.*, 1979; Dement *et al.*, 1978).

These findings for flurazepam led to the assumption that other benzodiazepine hypnotics too would induce a relatively slow development of tolerance to their efficacy. Our studies, however, have shown that this is not the case; rather, benzodiazepine hypnotics with relatively short elimination half-lives may show a rapid development of tolerance and loss of efficacy. In separate sleep laboratory studies, we evaluated the efficacy of nine benzodiazepine hypnotics: two with long elimination half-lives [flurazepam, 30 mg (Kales *et al.*, 1982b; Kales *et al.*, 1976a; Kales *et al.*, 1975; Kales *et al.*, 1971; Kales *et al.*, 1970) and quazepam, 30 mg (Kales *et al.*, 1982b; Kales *et al.*, 1981; Kales *et al.*, 1980b)], three with intermediate elimination half-lives [flunitrazepam, 2 mg (Scharf *et al.*, 1979; Bixler *et al.*, 1977); nitrazepam, 10 mg (Soldatos, Kales & Bixler, in press); and temazepam, 30 mg (Bixler *et al.*, 1978)], and three with relatively short elimination half-lives [lormetazepam, 1.5 mg (Kales *et al.*, 1982a); midazolam, 20 mg (Kales *et al.*, 1983d); and triazolam, 0.5 mg (Kales *et al.*, 1976c)].

With short-term administration, each of these benzodiazepine hypnotics (with the exception of temazepam) produced a statistically significant improvement of sleep when values for total wake time were compared with their respective placebo-baseline values (Figure 1). While temazepam showed some efficacy for decreasing wake time after sleep onset, the drug had no effect whatsoever on sleep latency (Bixler *et al.*, 1978). This lack of efficacy for sleep induction, exactly what one would predict from the drug's extremely slow rate of absorption (Greenblatt *et al.*, 1982b; Divoll *et al.*, 1981), has been confirmed in other sleep laboratory studies (Mitler *et al.*, 1979; FDA, 1978 & 1980).

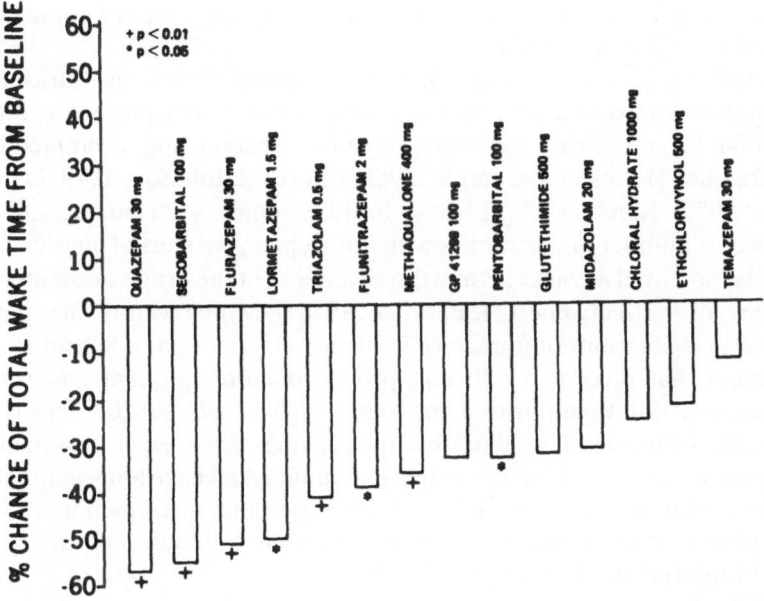

Figure 1 Short-term efficacy of hypnotic drugs. Values for each drug are the mean values for the first three nights of drug administration (Kales, 1982).

Each of the benzodiazepine hypnotics was given on consecutive nights for at least one week. The values in Figure 2 illustrate that the two benzodiazepines with long elimination half-lives show the least degree of loss of efficacy with continued use (Kales & Kales, 1983; Kales, 1982; Kales *et al.*, 1977a). In fact, flurazepam showed no loss of efficacy with continued use and was the only drug to produce a significant decrease in total wake time as compared to baseline. These data demonstrate that benzodiazepine hypnotics with relatively short elimination half-lives may rapidly lose their effectiveness, while those with long elimination half-lives, particularly flurazepam, induce a much slower development of tolerance.

Side Effects

Daytime Sedation

Daytime sedation is not an unexpected side effect with hypnotic drugs because it represents a direct extension of the drugs' therapeutic effects (Kales & Kales, 1984). It is surprising that the three hypnotic drugs that are available commercially (each with a different elimination half-life) do not appear to differ markedly from each other in terms of adverse sedative side effects (FDA package insert for temazepam; FDA package insert for triazolam; Flurazepam, new drug application submission). Thus, daytime sedation may be related more to dose than to a drug's rate of elimination (Johnson & Chernik, 1982).

Nonetheless, because benzodiazepine hypnotics such as flurazepam accumulate with consecutive nightly administration, they present a greater potential for producing excessive daytime sedation and decrements in performance (Johnson & Chernik, 1982; Church & Johnson, 1979; Oswald et al., 1979; Kales et al., 1976a). In 1976, when we summarized and reviewed a number of our studies with flurazepam, we alerted physicians to both the potential advantages and disadvantages of the drug's accumulation and carryover effectiveness (Kales et al., 1976a). More recently, in separate long-term evaluations of flurazepam, 30 mg, and quazepam, 30 and 15 mg, we found that quazepam, 30 mg, produced more frequent and severe daytime sedation than flurazepam, 30 mg (Kales et al., 1982b). This is not surprising when one considers that quazepam's three active components (the parent compound and two active metabolites) all have long elimination half-lives (Chung et al., 1984). We also reported that quazepam in a 15-mg dose produced less frequent and severe daytime sedation than the 30-mg dose of quazepam (Kales et al., 1982b).

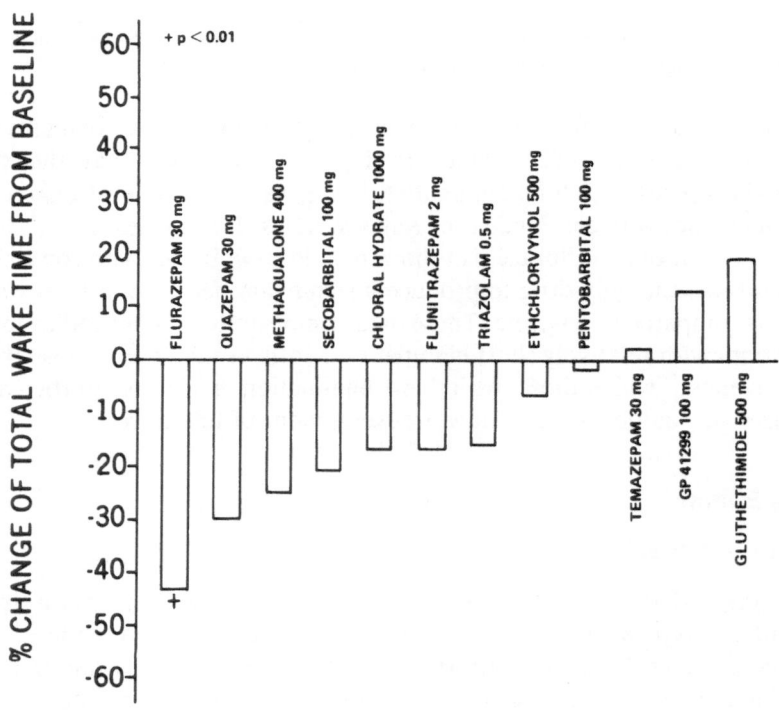

Figure 2 Intermediate-term efficacy of hypnotic drugs. Note the considerable loss in effectiveness for most of the drugs compared to short-term use (Figure 1) (Kales, 1982).

Finally, it should be noted that most of the studies of temazepam's effects on performance were conducted in Europe with the soft gelatin capsule preparation unavailable in the U.S., and usually in lower doses (10-mg or 20-mg) than the 30-mg dose commonly used in this country. Compared with the European formulation, the higher dose and slower absorption rate of the U.S. preparation would be expected to produce more residual drowsiness and daytime sedation and an increased potential for performance decrements (Greenblatt et al., 1982a).

Memory Impairment

There are now a number of reports on cases of varying degrees of memory impairment with benzodiazepine hypnotics extending to episodes of anterograde amnesia (Kales et al., 1983d; Regestein, 1983; Shader & Greenblatt, 1983; Vogel & Vogel, 1983; Spinweber & Johnson, 1982; Poitras, 1980; Roth et al., 1980; Bixler et al., 1979b; Brown et al., 1979; Van der Kroef, 1979; Kales et al., 1976c). Compared with flurazepam and temazepam, triazolam produces, by far, the greatest degree of memory impairment. In one study comparing triazolam, flurazepam, and lorazepam, both triazolam and lorazepam (both low-dose, high-potency benzodiazepines with relatively short elimination half-lives) produced significantly greater memory impairment than flurazepam (Roth et al., 1980). In our own sleep laboratory evaluation of triazolam, two patients had episodes of anterograde amnesia (Kales et al., 1976c). We also noted similar findings in a study of midazolam (Kales et al., 1983d), another benzodiazepine drug with an ultrashort elimination half-life.

Early Morning Insomnia and Daytime Anxiety

More recently, several studies have reported the occurrence of early morning insomnia (Kales et al., 1983b) or daytime anxiety (Kales et al., 1983b; Carskadon et al., 1982; Morgan & Oswald, 1982) during administration of triazolam, 0.5 mg. We have also demonstrated the occurrence of these two phenomena with the use of midazolam (Kales et al., 1983b; Kales et al., 1983d) (Fig. 3). To us, an important aspect of the side effects of early morning insomnia and daytime anxiety is that they are unexpected by the patient because they are the opposite of the drug's therapeutic effects and for that reason, most disturbing and unlikely to be attributed to the drug. It has been noted clinically that two patients for whom triazolam was prescribed for their insomnia experienced daytime anxiety and began using additional doses of the drug during the day to suppress this anxiety (Smith, 1984). Thus, early morning insomnia and rebound anxiety may reinforce drug-taking behavior and ultimately lead to dependence.

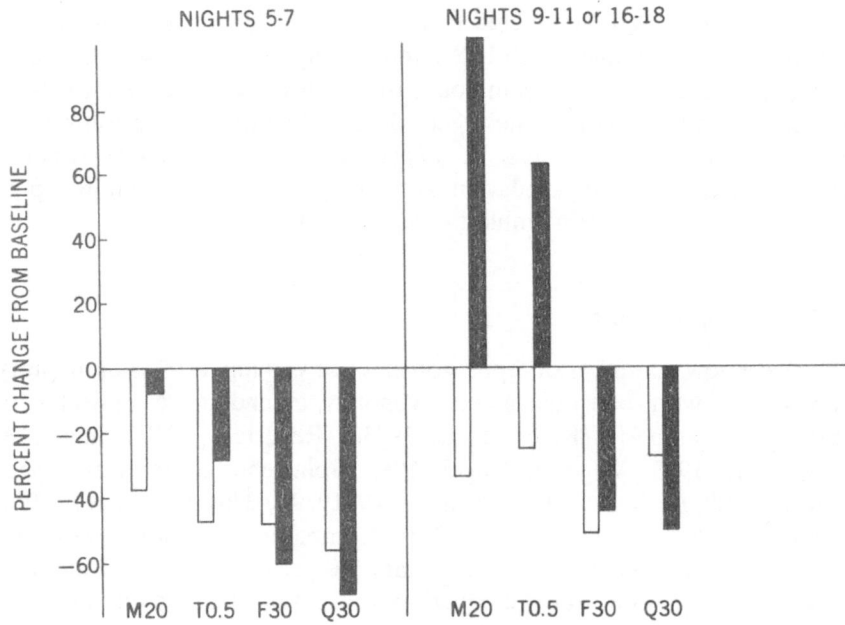

Figure 3: Early morning insomnia with rapidly eliminated benzodiazepine hypnotics. For each drug, the mean wake time for the first six hours of sleep is represented by the clear vertical bar and the mean wake time for the last two hours by the shaded vertical bar. On the first set of drug nights (5–7), the two drugs with short elimination half–lives (midazolam, 20 mg, and triazolam, 0.5 mg) show a considerable loss of effectiveness in the last two hours of the night. On the second set of drug nights (9–11 for midazolam and 16–18 for triazolam), early morning insomnia occurs, as evidenced by a marked increase in wake time above the baseline value. Both long elimination half–life drugs (flurazepam, 30 mg, and quazepam, 30 mg) maintain efficacy throughout the night at both time points (Kales & Kales, 1984).

In contrast to these changes seen with short elimination half-life benzodiazepine hypnotics, drugs that are slowly eliminated, such as flurazepam, do not cause early morning insomnia, and produce decreases rather than increases in daytime anxiety and tension because of their carryover effectiveness. The daytime anxiolytic effects of flurazepam were clearly demonstrated in a study comparing this drug with triazolam (Carskadon *et al.*, 1982). Whereas triazolam produced a 70 percent increase in daytime anxiety, flurazepam significantly improved this variable as well as several other measures of mood. In the same study, the authors reported that neither flurazepam nor triazolam produced increases in daytime sedation as measured by the Stanford Sleepiness Scale (SSS). Yet, they concluded that flurazepam produced more daytime sedation than triazolam because flurazepam subjects had shorter sleep latencies when allowed to sleep during the day (Multiple Sleep Latency Test) (Carskadon *et al.*, 1982). To us, however, the lack of daytime sedation with flurazepam as measured by the SSS and the marked global improvement in daytime mood factors, including a lessening of tension and anxiety, probably indicates that the subjects receiving flurazepam were able to fall asleep quickly because they were more relaxed, not because they were overly sedated. In contrast, triazolam subjects probably had more difficulty trying to sleep during the daytime tests because they were experiencing marked increases in tension and anxiety.

Serious Behavioral Changes

In a controversy regarding triazolam and its side effects (Drost, 1980; Dukes, 1980; Ladimir, 1980; Lasagna, 1980; Offerhaus, 1980; Ayd *et al.*, 1979; MacLeod & Kratochvil, 1979; Van der Kroef, 1979), a Dutch physician reported the occurrence of a number of serious behavioral side effects, including psychotic-like reactions with triazolam administration (Van der Kroef, 1979). These findings led to the suspension of the drug's license in the Netherlands (Dukes, 1980) and to the manufacturer's voluntary withdrawal of the 1-mg tablet from the world market. Halluci-nations with triazolam use have been reported in case reports from Canada (Einarson & Yoder, 1982; Einarson, 1980). We feel that some of these adverse psychological effects can be explained by the phenomena of amnesia, early morning insomnia, daytime anxiety, and rebound insomnia occurring in patients with predisposing psychological vulnerabilities and reactions (Kales & Kales, 1984; Kales & Kales, 1983). In the package insert for triazolam, the FDA indicates that the drug may have a narrow margin of safety between the therapeutic dose level (0.5 mg) and levels associated with serious behavioral changes (1-2 mg), which are only two to four times higher.

HYPNOTIC DRUG WITHDRAWAL

Rebound Insomnia

It has long been recognized that continued use of large doses of non-benzodiazepine sedative hypnotics for prolonged periods of time leads to dependence and withdrawal syndromes (Kales *et al.*, 1974; Kalant, LeBlanc & Gibbons, 1971; Essig, 1964; Swanson & Okada, 1963; Johnson & Van Buren, 1962; Lloyd & Clark, 1959; Frazer *et al.*, 1958; Frazer *et al.*, 1954; Fraser *et al.*, 1953; Isbell, 1950; Isbell *et al.*, 1950). There have been numerous reports of withdrawal reactions with benzodiazepine anxiolytics and hypnotics, as well (Berlin & Conell, 1983; Lader, 1983; Rickels *et al.*, 1983; Tyrer, Owen & Dawling, 1983; Hollister, 1981; Tyrer, Rutherford & Huggett, 1981; Khan, Joyce & Jones, 1980; Winokur *et al.*, 1980; Jacob & Sellers, 1979; Pevnick, Jasinski & Haertzen, 1978; Hollister, 1977; Preskorn & Denner, 1977; Hanna, 1972). In many cases, the withdrawal reactions

131

reported for benzodiazepines have also followed their prolonged use in high doses. More recently, however, withdrawal symptoms have been noted after use of relatively low doses of benzodiazepines, but for extended periods (Berlin & Conell, 1983; Lader, 1983; Rickels *et al.*, 1983; Winokur *et al.*, 1980; Pevnick, Jasinski & Haertzen, 1978). We have extended these observations through the striking finding that a definite withdrawal syndrome, rebound insomnia and anxiety, may occur not only with discontinuation of a low daily dose of a drug but even after relatively short periods of administration (Kales *et al.*, 1983b; Kales *et al.*, 1983c; Kales, Scharf & Kales, 1979).

Soon after flurazepam was introduced in the U.S., we reported that following withdrawal of the drug, there is a carryover effectiveness for the first night or two (Kales *et al.*, 1971). Sleep usually continues to be improved slightly to moderately on these early withdrawal nights compared to baseline measures (Kales *et al.*, 1982b; Kales *et al.*, 1976a; Kales *et al.*, 1975). Studies of other investigators confirmed these findings, showing that abrupt withdrawal of flurazepam did not produce any significant worsening of sleep (Oswald *et al.*, 1979; Dement *et al.*, 1978).

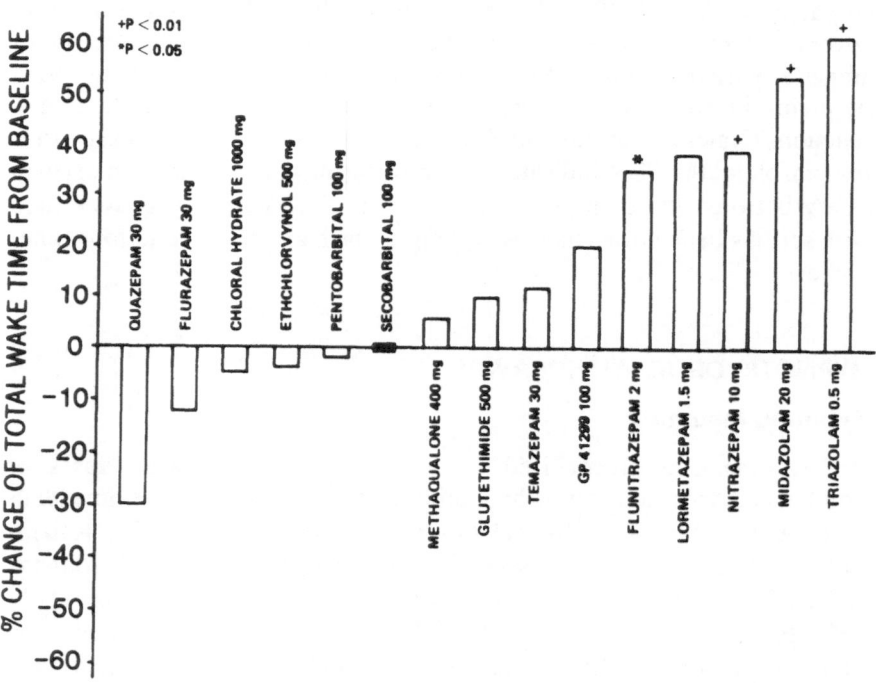

Figure 4: Rebound insomnia with benzodiazepine hypnotics. Following withdrawal of triazolam, midazolam, nitrazepam, lormetazepam, and flunitrazepam, there is a marked worsening of sleep above baseline levels, while with quazepam and flurazepam, sleep continues to be somewhat improved. For seven of the drugs, withdrawal values approximate those of baseline (Kales *et al.*, 1983c).

Subsequently, our separate studies of eight benzodiazepine hypnotics showed that withdrawal of drugs with rapid or intermediate elimination rates resulted in rebound insomnia at night as well as rebound anxiety during the day (Kales *et al.*, 1983c; Kales & Kales, 1983; Kales, 1982). Rebound insomnia occurred with five of the benzodiazepine hypnotics studied even when mean values for the first three withdrawal nights were considered (Fig. 4). All of these drugs produced either 40 percent or statistically significant increases in total wake time compared to baseline (Kales *et al.*, 1983c). The drugs and doses in order of the greatest degree of rebound insomnia were triazolam, 0.5 mg; midazolam, 20 mg; nitrazepam, 10 mg; lormetazepam, 1.5 mg; and flunitrazepam, 2 mg, with increases in total wake time above baseline ranging from 60 percent for triazolam to 35 percent for flunitrazepam. In contrast, the values for total wake time for the flurazepam and quazepam groups were below baseline levels, i.e., sleep was actually slightly to moderately improved on the first three withdrawal nights.

Figure 5 illustrates for each drug group the mean values for total wake time on the single night that showed the greatest percentage increase over baseline among the first three withdrawal nights (Kales *et al.*, 1983c). Again, striking increases in wakefulness were shown for the same five benzodiazepine drugs with short or intermediate elimination half-lives, with triazolam producing by far the greatest increase in total wake time over baseline (130%).

In an effort to rule out a delayed occurence of a rebound phenomenon with flurazepam and quazepam, we extended the withdrawal period to 15 consecutive nights, all of which were evaluated in the sleep laboratory (Kales *et al.*, 1982b). Increases in total wake time were slight for both drugs, with the greatest degree of worsening for flurazepam (22%) occurring on nights 4 and 14 of the withdrawal period, and for quazepam (4.5%) occurring on the fifteenth withdrawal night.

Role of Dose and Individual Rates of Metabolism

In examining the relationship between dose and the occurrence of rebound insomnia we studied the withdrawal of three doses of the rapidly eliminated benzodiazepine hypnotic, midazolam (10, 20, and 30 mg), four doses of lormetazepam (0.5, 1.0, 1.5, and 2.0 mg), a short-to-intermediate half-life benzodiazepine, and 7.5-, 15-, and 30-mg doses of quazepam, a benzodiazepine hypnotic with a long elimination half-life. For midazolam the mean values for the percent change from baseline in total wake time for the three increasing doses were 0.6% (N.S.), 52.6% (p<0.01), and 88.4% (p<0.01). Likewise, withdrawal of the four doses of lormetazepam produced successively greater increases in rebound insomnia with values for percent change in total wake time of 9.9% (N.S.), 27.2% (N.S.), 38.2%

(N.S.), and 73.1% (p<0.01). In contrast, the values for percent change in total wake time following withdrawal of the three doses of quazepam showed no rebound insomnia. In fact, the opposite trend was demonstrated, with greater degrees of carryover effectiveness related to increasing dose. Across all of our studies of benzodiazepine hypnotics in various doses, the highest degree of withdrawal sleep disturbance for each drug occurred with the following doses (listed in order of decreasing severity of rebound insomnia): midazolam, 30 mg; lormetazepam, 2 mg; triazolam, 0.5 mg; nitrazepam, 10 mg; and flunitrazepam, 2 mg, with the increase in total wake time above baseline ranging from 88 percent for midazolam to 35 percent for flunitrazepam (mean values for first three withdrawal nights).

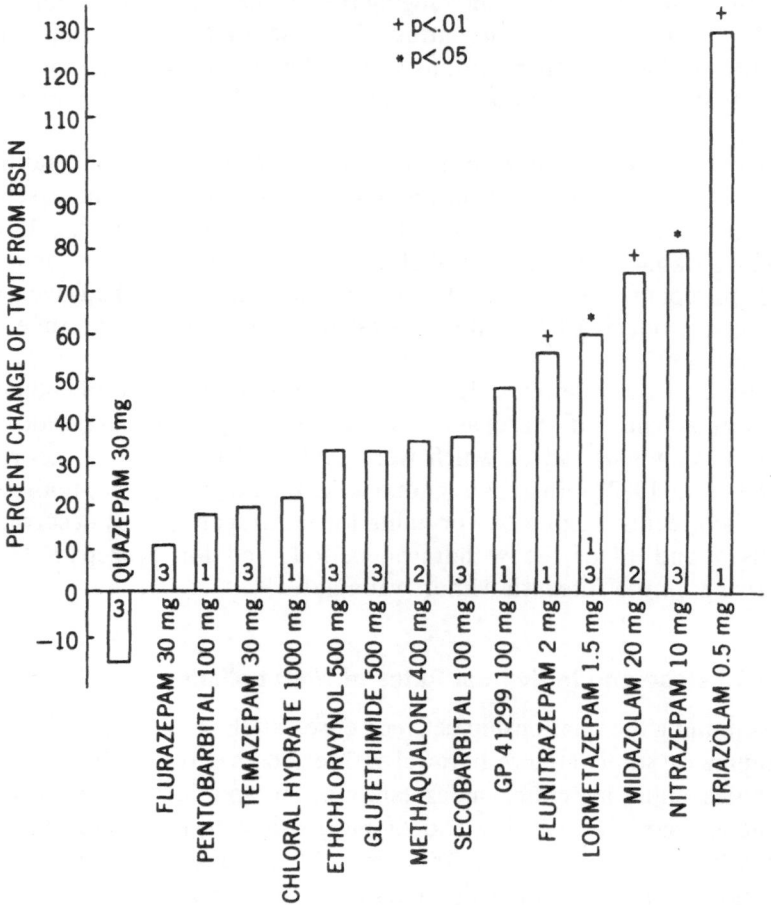

Figure 5 Rebound insomnia with benzodiazepine hypnotics. Looking at the single withdrawal night within each drug group that showed the greatest mean wake time, five of the drugs (triazolam, lormetazepam, nitrazepam, midazolam, and flunitrazepam) showed a marked and significant increase in total wake time. The withdrawal night on which the greatest increase in total wake time occurred for each drug is indicated by a number at the base of each vertical bar (Kales *et al.*, 1983c).

The possibility has been raised that, due to individual differences in rates of metabolism, marked sleep disturbances following withdrawal of the slowly eliminated drugs could go undetected if group mean values are analyzed, because they could occur at varying times from subject to subject. To resolve this issue, we evaluated the presence of rebound insomnia on individual subject nights following withdrawal of five benzodiazepine hypnotics in comparison to a placebo group (Bixler et al., in press). Remarkably, the same relationships were observed between rebound insomnia and both elimination half-life and dose whether the data are analyzed by individual subject nights or as group condition means. Specifically, significant sleep difficulty was identified on 61.9% of the individual subject nights following withdrawal of the rapidly eliminated drug, triazolam, 0.5 mg, compared to only 13.3% for the placebo control group (p<0.01). Likewise, group mean values for withdrawal of triazolam showed nearly a 60% increase in total wake time over baseline (p<0.01) (Table 1). For the three doses of midazolam the same dose-related increases in rebound insomnia were apparent in both group mean values and in the percentage of individual subject nights with significant sleep disturbance (range, 11.1%, N.S., to 66.7%, p<0.01). Similarly, withdrawal of the four doses of lormetazepam, produced successively greater increases in rebound insomnia in both group mean values and in individual subject values for the percentage of nights with significant sleep disturbance (range, 27.8%, N.S., to 55.6%, p<0.01).

In contrast, for the extended 15-night withdrawal period of the long half-life hypnotics, flurazepam and quazepam, both in 30-mg doses, no rebound insomnia was demonstrated in either group mean values or in individual subject night rates. The rates for the flurazepam and quazepam subjects not only approximated to the value of the placebo group for the first three nights of withdrawal (as listed in the table), but also remained similar to the placebo value throughout the 15-night withdrawal period.

Agreement with Other Studies

There is strong agreement that sleep withdrawal difficulties are frequently present, and to a strong degree, with the rapidly eliminated drugs (Adam, Oswald & Shapiro, in press; Mamelak, Csima & Price, in press; Mamelak, Csima & Price, 1984; Bliwise et al., 1984; Vela-Bueno et al., 1983; Monti et al., 1982; Scharf et al., 1982; Oswald et al., 1979; Roth, Kramer & Lutz, 1976; Vogel et al., 1976; Vogel et al., 1975) and infrequently present and, if so, to a milder degree with the slowly eliminated drugs (Mamelak, Csima & Price, 1984; Bliwise et al., 1984; Oswald et al., 1979; Dement et al., 1978). In fact, no investigator has demonstrated rebound insomnia following the withdrawal of flurazepam of quazepam. In the three studies reporting any sleep disturbance following withdrawal of slowly eliminated drugs, only mild degrees of sleep disturbance have been noted. For example, one study reported only an 8-minute increase in wakefulness over baseline levels (Greenblatt *et al.*, 1981). A second study reported a mild degree of sleep disturbance based only on the changes seen in one subjective mood scale (Mendelson *et al*, 1982), while the objective data showed only a 4.5-minute increase in sleep latency (although this was termed "rebound"), and an actual 12-minute improvement in total wake time. Additionally, in our study (Kales *et al.*, 1982b) in which we monitored patients for 15 consecutive nights following withdrawal of flurazepam and quazepam, the greatest increase in total wake time for flurazepam occurred on the fourth withdrawal night (22%) and for quazepam on the fifteenth withdrawal night (4.5%). Finally, one study (Mitler *et al.*, 1984) reported on withdrawal data based on individual subject nights. The conclusions of this study are not valid, however, because data from only one drug group were analyzed by subject nights, while data for the other drug group and placebo group were analyzed using group mean values. In our recent study (Bixler *et al.*, in press), we did apply the same criteria for assessing individual subject nights across each drug evaluated as well as for a separate placebo group. We found extremely high rates of rebound insomnia for rapidly eliminated drugs (triazolam, midazolam, and lormetazepam) and low rates for slowly eliminated drugs (flurazepam and quazepam) which were similar to that of the placebo control group (Table 1) throughout the extended 2-week with-drawal period.

Table 1 Sleep disturbance on first three nights of withdrawal

	Rebound insomnia rate for individual subject nights[a]		Minutes of TWT for overall condition[b]	
	Percent	*Base line*	*Withdrawal*	*% Change*
Short half-life				
Triazolam, 0.5 mg	61.9†	94.2	150.5†	59.8†
Long half-life				
Flurazepam, 30 mg	11.1	100.6	87.4	−13.1
Quazepam, 30 mg	5.6	70.7	49.3	−30.3
Placebo	13.3	67.9	70.6	4.0

[a] All rates are compared to the placebo group rate using the Dunn Multiple Comparison *t*-test
[b] All comparisons are made between the mean minutes of total wake time on baseline and withdrawal within each individual study
†*p*<0.01
(Adapted from Bixler *et al.*, in press)

In summary, our findings indicate that following withdrawal of a benzodiazepine with a short half-life, rebound insomnia usually occurs on the first withdrawal night and is of an intense degree; with an intermediate half-life benzodiazepine, it frequently occurs and is of a moderate degree; and with a benzodiazepine with a long half-life, it may occur, but infrequently, on a delayed basis, and be of a lesser degree (Kales & Kales, 1983; Kales et al., 1983c; Kales, 1982).

One could speculate that the rebound insomnia occurring following the withdrawal of benzodiazepine drugs with short and intermediate half-lives is a phenomenon that is not specific to this drug class but rather related only to the rate of elimination of these CNS-depressant drugs from the body. If this were the case, one would expect to observe rebound insomnia following the withdrawal of non-benzodiazepine drugs that are relatively rapidly eliminated. However, our studies of non-benzodiazepine hypnotics did not demonstrate rebound insomnia following withdrawal of clinical doses that had been administered nightly for two week periods (Kales & Kales, 1984; Kales et al., 1983c). In fact, the greatest increase in total wake time over baseline for the first three nights of withdrawal was only ten percent (for glutethimide). Even when considering the withdrawal night for each drug group with the single highest value for total wake time, none of the non-benzodiazepine drugs' withdrawal produced rebound insomnia, although values for four of the drugs were about 35 percent above baseline (Kales & Kales, 1984; Kales et al., 1983c).

HYPNOTIC DRUGS IN THE ADJUNCTIVE TREATMENT OF INSOMNIA

The adjunctive use of hypnotic medication, particularly beyond a short term period, is indicated primarily for patients with chronic insomnia (Kales & Kales, 1984; Kales, Soldatos & Kales, 1982; Kales, Soldatos & Kales, 1981; Kales et al., 1980a; Soldatos, Kales & Kales, 1979). In cases of transient insomnia, hypnotic medication may or may not be used. The primary focus in transient insomnia is to remove or relieve the stress-generating situation which precipitated the onset of sleeplessness. If the stressful situation cannot be eliminated, the physician is best able to help the patient by identifying and strengthening adaptive coping mechanisms. When sleep difficulty is due to conflicts in scheduling and disturbance of biological rhythms, as with jet lag, drug use should be avoided, and instead, adjustments should be made in scheduling activities to accommodate the person's circadian needs.

In patients with chronic insomnia, the internalization of emotions (Kales & Kales, 1984; Kales, Soldatos & Kales, 1981; Kales et al., 1976b) leads to emotional arousal (Kales et al., 1976b; Coursey, Buchsbaum & Frankel,

1975) that, in turn, results in physiological activation (Freedman & Sattler, 1982; Haynes, Adams & Franzen, 1981; Haynes, Follingstad & McGowan, 1974; Monroe, 1967) and insomnia. Soon, a fear of sleeplessness and its consequences develops, leading to a vicious circle of physiological activation, sleeplessness, more fear of sleeplessness, further emotional arousal and still further sleeplessness (Kales & Kales, 1984; Kales, Soldatos & Kales, 1981; Kales *et al.*, 1976b). Only a small percentage of patients with chronic insomnia have major or endogenous depression (Tan *et al.*, 1984), for which a tricyclic antidepressant with sedative side effects would be the drug of choice (Kales & Kales, 1984). Thus, for the majority of patients with chronic insomnia, hypnotic medication may be indicated as an adjunct to break the vicious circle which perpetuates their sleep difficulty and to facilitate the physician's overall therapeutic approach.

When a hypnotic is indicated as an adjunctive treatment, the benzodiazepines are the drugs of choice (Kales & Kales, 1984; Kales *et al.*, 1980a). The non-benzodiazepine hypnotics, barbiturate and non-barbiturate, have a narrow margin of safety; although patients develop considerable tolerance to these drugs' therapeutic effects with chronic use, it appears that only minimal tolerance develops to their lethal effects. The barbiturate drugs, in particular, are strong respiratory depressants (Cooper, 1977). These facts are especially important because these drugs are frequently used in suicide attempts (Cooper, 1977). Further, certain non-barbiturate non-benzodiazepines may present special hazards in successfully treating an overdose; one example is glutethimide, which has high lipid solubility and anticholinergic activity.

Within the benzodiazepine class of currently available hypnotic drugs, the overall experimental findings and clinical experience would favor flurazepam as the hypnotic medication to be used adjunctively in most cases of insomnia. This drug has been on the market for over ten years, and its efficacy, side effects, and withdrawal effects are well established (Kales & Kales, 1984; Kales *et al.*, 1976a).

In terms of its effectiveness, it is at least as effective as triazolam with short-term use (Kales *et al.*, 1982b; Kales *et al.*, 1976a; Kales *et al.*, 1976c; Kales *et al.*, 1970) and superior to temazepam (Bixler *et al.*, 1978), which has a marked delay in reaching peak plasma concentration due to its slow rate of dissolution and absorption (Greenblatt *et al.*, 1982a) This problem is clearly identified in the drug's package insert, which states that sleep laboratory studies have not been able to establish the drug's efficacy for inducing sleep, even when given 30 minutes before bedtime. This limitation greatly restricts temazepam's usefulness in clinical practice because it must be given one to two hours before bedtime to produce efficacy for sleep induction. This practice itself may increase the drug's potential for producing side effects such as incoordination and accidental falls, especially in the elderly.

138

With continued consecutive nightly use, flurazepam is clearly more effective than either triazolam or temazepam (Kales *et al.*, 1982b; Bixler *et al.*, 1978; Kales *et al.*, 1976a; Kales *et al.*, 1976c; Kales *et al.*, 1970). Temazepam's lack of efficacy for sleep induction continues to be a problem with prolonged use (Bixler *et al.*, 1978), while triazolam loses much of its effectiveness within a two- to three-week period of administration (Adam, Oswald & Shapiro, in press; Kales *et al.*, 1976c). Several studies have reported that triazolam maintained its efficacy with continued use over a period of several weeks (Pegram, Hyde & Linton, 1980; Roth, Kramer & Lutz, 1976). However, data from these studies show that total sleep time increased by a range of only a few minutes to 15 minutes over baseline values, increases which are not clinically relevant.

In terms of side effects, flurazepam does not produce paradoxical reactions such as early morning insomnia or increases in daytime anxiety or tension levels, as is the case with triazolam and other ultrashort elimination half-life drugs such as midazolam (Kales & Kales, 1983; Kales *et al.*, 1983c; Kales, 1982). Also, it produces significantly less memory impairment than triazolam (Roth *et al.*, 1980). Finally, flurazepam (Kales & Kales, 1984) has not been found to produce behavioral side effects and psychiatric symptoms such as amnesia, confusional states, feelings of depersonalization, or hallucinations as have been reported with triazolam at doses only slightly higher than those recommended (Regestein, 1983; Shader & Greenblatt, 1983; Freedman & Sattler, 1982; Poitras, 1980; Van der Kroef, 1979; Cooper, 1977; Kales *et al.*, 1976c). It is yet to be determined whether triazolam's side effects (other than its rebound phenomena which are related more to its rapid elimination) are a consequence of its high potency nature or its triazolo-ring structure.

For flurazepam, the major disadvantage is drug accumulation and daytime sedation (Kales & Kales, 1984; Greenblatt *et al.*, 1982a; Johnson & Chernik, 1982; Church & Johnson, 1979; Oswald *et al.*, 1979; Kales *et al.*, 1976a). Any hypnotic drug that is efficacious can produce residual drowsiness, daytime sedation, and performance decrements. Thus, patients receiving hypnotic medication should be cautioned regarding these potential side effects, particularly if they drive or perform other tasks for which vigilance is critical (Kales & Kales, 1984; Kales *et al.*, 1980a). Daytime sedation with flurazepam can be greatly minimized by prescribing the 15-mg dose for most patients, not just the elderly (Kales & Kales, 1984; Kales *et al.*, 1980a; Kales *et al.*, 1976a). Both our studies and clinical experience have shown that while there is little daytime sedation with the 15-mg dose, there is a carryover anxiolytic effect that is beneficial to many patients with chronic insomnia who typically manifest varying degrees of anxiety, apprehension, rumination, and somatization (Kales & Kales, 1984). This anxiolytic effect also eliminates the need for an anxiolytic drug during the daytime in most of these patients.

A significant therapeutic dilemma can result when the patient's daytime activities require heightened vigilance. If the physician considers prescribing a rapidly eliminated drug such as triazolam, which does not accumulate, serious daytime difficulty may result because of triazolam's propensity for producing episodes of anterograde amnesia (Regestein, 1983; Shader & Greenblatt, 1983; Poitras, 1980; Van der Kroef, 1979; Kales *et al.*, 1976c). Thus, when optimal daytime performance is required the next day, hypnotic medication should be avoided or, if used, only in the lowest available dose.

During the withdrawal phase of treatment, flurazepam has another considerable advantage over temazepam and triazolam (Kales & Kales, 1984; Kales & Kales, 1983; Kales *et al.*, 1983c; Kales, 1982; Kales *et al.*, 1979; Kales, Scharf & Kales, 1978). Abrupt withdrawal of triazolam frequently produces intense sleep disturbance in the form of rebound insomnia. Temazepam, with its intermediate half-life, produces rebound insomnia somewhat less frequently and of moderate intensity. However, with long half-life drugs such as flurazepam, withdrawal sleep disturbance seldom occurs, and, when present, is of a milder degree. Clearly, it is advantageous for the patient to be able to experience a smooth withdrawal process. In this way, the physician can best enhance in the patient a feeling of mastery that he or she can cope successfully without the indefinite use of sleeping medication.

References

Adam K, Oswald I, Shapiro C: Effects of loprazolam and of triazolam on sleep and overnight urinary cortisol. *Psychopharmacology*, in press.

Agnew HW, Jr, Webb WW, Williams RL: Sleep patterns in late middle age males: an EEG study. *Electroencephalogr Clin Neurophysiol* 1967;23:168-171.

Amrein R, Bovey F, Cano JP, *et al*: Pharmacokinetics and pharcodynamics of flurazepam in man, Part II. *Drugs Exp Clin Res* 1983;9:95-99.

Ayd FJ, Jr, Barclay WR, Curran WJ, *et al*: Behavioral reactions to triazolam (letter to editor). *Lancet* 1979;2:1018.

Balter MB, Bauer ML: Patterns of prescribing and use of hypnotic drugs in the United States, in Clift AD (ed): *Sleep Disturbance and Hypnotic Drug Dependence*. New York, Excerpta Medica, 1975, pp 261-293.

Berlin RM, Connel LJ: Withdrawal symptoms after long-term treatment with therapeutic doses of flurazepam: a case report. *Am J Psychiatry* 1983;140:488-490.

Bixler EO, Kales A, Jacoby JA, *et al*: Nocturnal sleep and wakefulness: effects of age and sex in normal sleepers. *Int J Neurosci* 1984;23:33-42.

Bixler EO, Kales A, Soldatos CR: Sleep disorders encountered in medical practice: a national survey of physicians. *Behav Med* 1979;6:1-6.

Bixler EO, Kales A, Soldatos CR, et al: Flunitrazepam, an investigational hypnotic drug: sleep laboratory evaluations. J Clin Pharmacol 1977;17:569-578.

Bixler EO, Kales A, Soldatos CR, et al: Effectiveness of temazepam with short-, intermediate-, and long-term use: sleep laboratory evaluation. J Clin Pharmacol 1978;18:110-118.

Bixler EO, Kales JD, Kales A, et al: Rebound insomnia and elimination half-life: assessment of individual subject response. J Clin Pharmacol; in press.

Bixler EO, Kales JD, Kales A, et al: Hypnotic drug prescription patterns: two physician surveys. Sleep Res 1976;5:62.

Bixler EO, Kales JD, Soldatos CR, et al: Prevalence of sleep disorders in the Los Angeles metropolitan area. Am J Psychiatry 1979a;136:1257-1262.

Bixler EO, Scharf MB, Soldatos CR, et al: Effects of hypnotic drugs on memory. Life Sci 1979b;25:1379-1388.

Bliwise D, Seidel W, Greenblatt DJ, et al: Nighttime and daytime efficacy of flurazepam and oxazepam in chronic insomnia. Am J Psychiatry 1984;141:191-195.

Breimer DD, Jochemsen R: Pharmacokinetics of hypnotic drugs, in Wheatley D (ed): Psychopharmacology of Sleep. New York, Raven Press, 1981, pp 135-152.

Brown CR, Sarnquist FH, Canup CA, et al: Clinical, electroencephalographic, and pharmacokinetic studies of a water-soluble benzodiazepine, midazolam maleate. Anesthesiology 1979;50:467-470.

Carskadon MA, Seidel WF, Greenblatt DJ, et al: Daytime carry-over of triazolam and flurazepam in elderly insomniacs. Sleep 1982;5:361-371.

Chung M, Hilbert JM, Gural RP, et al: Multiple-dose quazepam kinetics. Clin Pharmacol Ther 1984;35:520-524.

Church MW, Johnson LC: Mood and performance of poor sleepers during repeated use with flurazepam. Psychopharmacology 1979;61:309-316.

Cooper JR (ed): Sedative-hypnotic Drugs: Risks and Benefits. National Institute on Drug Abuse Report, U.S. D.H.E.W. No. [ADM] 79-592. Washington, D.C., U.S. Government Printing Office, 1977.

Coursey RD, Buchsbaum M, Frankel BL: Personality measures and evoked responses in chronic insomniacs. J Abnorm Psychol 1975;84:239-249.

Dement WC, Carskadon MA, Mitler MM, et al: Prolonged use of flurazepam: a sleep laboratory study. Behav Med 1978;5:25-31.

Divoll M, Greenblatt DJ, Harmatz JS, et al: Effect of age and gender on disposition of temazepam. J Pharm Sci 1981;70:1104-1107.

Drost RA: The Halcion story (letter to editor). Lancet 1980;1:1027-1028.

Dukes, MNG: The van der Kroef syndrome, in Dukes MNG (ed): Side Effects of Drugs Annual IV. Amsterdam, Excerpta Medica, 1980.

Eberts FS, Philopolous Y, Reineke LM: Triazolam disposition. Clin Pharmacol Ther 1981;29:81-93.

Eckert M, Ziegler WH, Cano JP, et al: Pharmacokinetics and pharmacodynamics of flurazepam in man, part I. *Drugs Exp Clin Res* 1983;9:77-84.

Einarson TR: Hallucinations from triazolam. *Drug Intell Clin Pharmacol* 1980;14:714.

Einarson TR, Yoder ES: Triazolam psychosis – a syndrome? *Drug Intell Clin Pharmacol* 1982;16:330.

Essig CF: Addiction to nonbarbiturate sedative and tranquilizing drugs. *Clin Pharmacol Ther* 1964;5:334-343.

Feinberg I, Carlson VR: Sleep variables as a function of age in man. *Arch Gen Psychiatry* 1968;18:239-250.

Flurazepam, new drug application submission.

Food and Drug Administration (FDA)a. Package insert for triazolam (Halcion).

Food and Drug Administration (FDA)b. Package insert for temazepam (Restoril).

Food and Drug Administration (FDA): Psychopharmacologic Drugs Advisory Meeting Minutes on Evaluation of Temazepam. Washington, D.C., 1978 and 1980.

Fraser HF, Isbell H, Eisenman AJ, et al: Chronic barbiturate intoxication. *Arch Int Med* 1954;94:34-41.

Fraser HF, Shaver MR, Maxwell ES, et al: Death due to withdrawal of barbiturates. *Ann Int Med* 1953;38:1319-1325.

Fraser HF, Wikler A, Essig CF, et al: Degree of physical dependence induced by secobarbital or pentobarbital. *J Am Med Assoc* 1958;166:126-129.

Freedman RR, Sattler HL: Physiological and psychological factors in sleep-onset insomnia. *J Abnorm Psychol* 1982;91:380-389.

Fuccella LM, Bolcioni G, Tamassia V, et al: Human pharmacokinetcs and bioavailability of temazepam administered in soft gelatin capsules. *Eur J Clin Pharmacol* 1977;12:383-386.

The Gallup Organization: *The Gallup Study of Sleeping Habits*. Princeton, N.J., Gallup, 1979.

Greenblatt DJ, Divoll M, Abernethy DR, et al: Benzodiazepine hypnotics: kinetic and therapeutic options. *Sleep* 1982a;5:S18-S27.

Greenblatt DJ, Divoll M, Harmatz JS, et al: Kinetics and clinical effects of flurazepam in young and elderly non-insomniacs. *Clin Pharmacol Ther* 1981a;30:475-486.

Greenblatt DJ, Divoll M, Moshitto LJ, et al: Electron-capture gas chromatographic analysis of the triazolobenzodiazepine alprazolam and triazolam. *J Chromatogr* 1981b;225:202-207.

Greenblatt DJ, Shader RI, Abernethy DR, et al: Benzodiazepines and the challenge of pharmacokinetic taxonomy, in Usdin E, Skolnick P, Tallman JF, Jr, et al (eds): *Pharmacology of Benzodiazepines*. London, The Macmillan Press, Ltd., Scientific and Medical Division, 1982b, pp 257-269.

Hanna SM: A case of oxazepam (Serenid D) dependence. *Br J Psychiatry* 1972;120:443-445.

Haynes SN, Follingstad DR, McGowan WT: Insomnia: sleep patterns and anxiety level. *J Psychosom Res* 1974;18:69-74.

Haynes SN, Adams A, Franzen M: The effects of presleep stress on sleep-onset insomnia. *J Abnorm Psychol* 1981;90:601-606.

Healey ES, Kales A, Monroe LJ, *et al*: Onset of insomnia: role of life-stress events. *Psychom Med* 1981;43:439-451.

Hollister LE: Pharmacology and pharmacokinetics of the minor tranquilizers. *Psychiatr Ann* 1981;11(supp):26-31.

Hollister LE: Withdrawal from benzodiazepine therapy. *J Am Med Assoc* 1977;237:1432.

Isbell H: Addiction to barbiturates and the barbiturate abstinence syndrome. *Ann Int Med* 1950;33:108-121.

Isbell H, Altschul S, Kornetsky CH, *et al*: Chronic barbiturate intoxication: an experimental study. *Am Med Assoc Arch Neurol Psychiatry* 1950;64:1-28.

Jacob MS, Sellers EM: Use of drugs with dependence liability. *Can Med Assoc J* 1979;121:717-724.

Johnson FA, Van Buren HC: Abstinence syndrome following glutethimide intoxication. *J Am Med Assoc* 1962;180:1024-1027.

Johnson LC, Chernik DA: Sedative-hypnotics and human performance. *Psychopharmacology* 1982;76:101-113.

Kalant H, LeBlanc A, Gibbons R: Tolerance to, and dependence on, some non-opiate psychotropic drugs. *Pharmacol Rev* 1971;23:135-191.

Kales A: Benzodiazepines in the treatment of insomnia, in Usdin E, Skolnick P, Tallman J, *et al* (eds): *Pharmacology of Benzodiazepines*. London, The Macmillan Press, Ltd., Scientific and Medical Division, 1982, pp. 199-217.

Kales A, Allen C, Scharf MB, *et al*: Hypnotic drugs and their effectiveness. *Arch Gen Psychiatry* 1970;23:226-232.

Kales A, Bixler EO, Kales JD, *et al*: Comparative effectiveness of nine hypnotic drugs: sleep laboratory studies. *J Clin Pharmacol* 1977a;17:207-213.

Kales A, Bixler EO, Scharf MB, *et al*: Sleep laboratory studies of flurazepam: a model for evaluating hypnotic drugs. *Clin Pharmacol Ther* 1976a;19:576-583.

Kales A, Bixler EO, Soldatos CR, *et al*: Dose-response studies of lormetazepam: efficacy, side effects, and rebound insomnia. *J Clin Pharmacol* 1982a;22:520-530.

Kales A, Bixler EO, Soldatos CR, *et al*: Quazepam and flurazepam: long-term use and extended withdrawal. *Clin Pharmacol Ther* 1982b;32:781-788.

Kales A, Bixler EO, Tan T-L, *et al*: Chronic hypnotic-drug use: ineffectiveness, drug-withdrawal insomnia, and dependence. *J Am Med Assoc* 1974;227:513-517.

Kales A, Caldwell AB, Preston TA, *et al*: Personality patterns in insomnia. *Arch Gen Psychiatry* 1976b;33:1128-1134.

Kales A, Caldwell AB, Soldatos CR, *et al*: Biopsychobehavioral correlates of insomnia, II: pattern specificity and consistency with the Minnesota Multiphasic Personality Inventory. *Psychosom Med* 1983a;45:341-356.

Kales A, Kales JD: Sleep laboratory studies of hypnotic drugs: efficacy and withdrawal effects. *J Clin Psychopharmacol* 1983;3:140-150.

Kales A, Kales JD: *Evaluation and Treatment of Insomnia*. New York, Oxford University Press, 1984.

Kales A, Kales JD, Bixler EO, *et al*: Effectiveness of hypnotic drugs with prolonged use: flurazepam and pentobarbital. *Clin Pharmacol Ther* 1975;18:356-363.

Kales A, Kales JD, Bixler EO, *et al*: Hypnotic efficacy of triazolam: sleep laboratory evaluation of intermediate-term effectiveness. *J Clin Pharmacol* 1976c;16:399-406.

Kales A, Kales JD, Jacobson A, *et al*: Effects of imipramine on enuretic frequency and sleep stages. *Pediatrics* 1977b;60:431-436.

Kales A, Kales JD, Scharf MB, *et al*: The prescription of hypnotic drugs, in Buchwald C, Cohen S, Katz D, *et al* (eds): *Frequently Prescribed and Abused Drugs: Their Indications, Efficacy, and Rational Prescribing* (N.T.S. Medical Monograph Series, vol. 1, no. 1). New York, Career Teacher Center, 1980a, pp 57-75.

Kales A, Scharf MB, Bixler EO, *et al*: Dose-response studies of quazepam. *Clin Pharmacol Ther* 1981;30:194-200.

Kales A, Scharf MB, Kales JD: Rebound insomnia: a new clinical syndrome. *Science* 1978;201:1039-1041.

Kales A, Scharf MB, Kales JD, *et al*: Rebound insomnia: a potential hazard following withdrawal of certain benzodiazepines. *J Am Med Assoc* 1979;241:1692-1695.

Kales A, Scharf MB, Soldatos CR, *et al*: Quazepam: a new benzodiazepine hypnotic: intermediate-term sleep laboratory evaluation. *J Clin Pharmacol* 1980 b;20:184-192.

Kales A, Soldatos CR, Bixler EO, *et al*: Early morning insomnia with rapidly eliminated benzodiazepines. *Science* 1983b;220:95-97.

Kales A, Soldatos CR, Bixler EO, *et al*: Rebound insomnia and rebound anxiety: a review. *Pharmacology* 1983c;26:121-137.

Kales A, Soldatos CR, Bixler EO, *et al*: Midazolam: dose-response studies of effectiveness and rebound insomnia. *Pharmacology* 1983d;26:138-149.

Kales A, Soldatos CR, Kales JD: Sleep disorders: evaluation and management in the office setting, in Arieti S, Brodie HKH (eds): *American Handbook of Psychiatry*, vol. 7, ed. 2. New York, Basic Books, 1981, pp 423-454.

Kales A, Soldatos CR, Kales JD: Taking a sleep history. *Am Fam Physician* 1979;22:101-108.

Kales J, Kales A, Bixler EO, *et al*: Effects of placebo and flurazepam on sleep patterns in insomniac subjects. *Clin Pharmacol Ther* 1971;12:691-697.

Kales JD, Kales A, Bixler EO, *et al*: Biopsychobehavioral correlates of insomnia, V: clinical characteristics and behavioral correlates. *Am J Psychiatry*, 1984;141:1371-1376.

Kales JD, Soldatos CR, Kales A: Diagnosis and treatment of sleep disorders, in Greist JH, Jefferson W, Spitzer RL (eds): *Treatment of Mental Disorders*. New York, Oxford University Press, 1982, pp 473-500.

Kaplan SA, de Silva JAF, Jack ML, et al: Blood level profile in man following chronic oral administration of flurazepam hydrochloride. *J Pharm Sci* 1973;62:1932-1935.

Karacan I, Thornby JI, Anch AM, et al: Dose-related sleep disturbances induced by coffee and caffeine. *Clin Pharmacol Ther* 1976;20:682-689.

Khan A, Joyce P, Jones AV: Benzodiazepine withdrawal syndromes. *NZ Med J* 1980 ;92:94-96.

Lader M: Dependence on benzodiazepines. *J Clin Psychiatry* 1983;44:121-127.

Ladimir I: Trials and tribulations of triazolam (commentary). *J Clin Pharm* 1980;20:159-161.

Lasagna L: The Halcion story: trial by media. *Lancet* 1980;1:815-816.

Lloyd EA, Clark LD: Convulsions and delirium incident to glutethimide (Doriden) withdrawal. *Dis Ner Syst* 1959;20:524-526.

MacLeod N, Kratochvil CH: Behavioural reactions to triazolam. *Lancet* 1979;2:638-639.

Mamelak M, Csima A, Price V: A comparative 25-night sleep laboratory study on the effects of quazepam and triazolam on the sleep of chronic insomniacs. *J Clin Pharmacol* 1984;24:65-75.

Mamelak M, Csima A, Price V: The effects of brotizolam on the sleep of chronic insomniacs. *Br J Clin Pharmacol*, in press.

Mellinger GD, Balter MB: Prevalence and patterns of use of psychotherapeutic drugs: results from a 1979 national survey of American adults, in Pognoni G, Bellantuoano C, Lader M (eds): *Epidemiological Impact of Psychotropic Drug*. Amsterdam, Elsevier/North-Holland Biomedical Press, 1981.

Mendelson WB, Weingartner H, Greenblatt DJ, et al: A clinical study of flurazepam. *Sleep* 1982;5:350-360.

Mitler MM, Carskadon MA, Phillips RL, et al: Hypnotic efficacy of temazepam: a long-term sleep laboratory evaluation. *Br J Clin Pharmacol* 1979;8:63S-68S.

Mitler MM, Seidel WF, van den Hoed J, et al: Comparative hypnotic effects of flurazepam, triazolam, and placebo: a long-term simultaneous nighttime and daytime study. *J Clin Psychopharmacol* 1984;4:2-13.

Monroe LJ: Psychological and physiological differences between good and poor sleepers. *J Abnorm Psychol* 1967;72:255-264.

Monti JM, Debellis J, Gratadoux E, et al: Sleep laboratory study of the effects of midazolam in insomniac patients. *Eur J Clin Pharmacol* 1982;21:479-484.

Morgan K, Oswald I: Anxiety caused by a short-life hypnotic. *Br Med J* 1982;284:942.

Offerhaus L: Trials and tribulations of triazolam. *J Clin Pharmacol* 1980;20:700-701.

Oswald I, Adam K, Borrow S, et al: The effects of two hypnotics on sleep, subjective feelings and skilled performance, in Passouant P, Oswald I (eds): *Pharmacology of the States of Alertness*. New York, Pergamon Press, 1979, pp 51-63.

Pegram V, Hyde P, Linton P: Chronic use of triazolam: the effects on the sleep patterns of insomniacs. *J Int Med Res* 1980;8:224-231.

Pevnick J, Jasinski D, Haertzen A: Abrupt withdrawal from therapeutically administered diazepam. *Arch Gen Psychiatry* 1978;35:995-998.

Poitras R: A propos d'episodes d'amnesies anterogrades associes a l'utilisation du triazolam. *Union Med Can* 1980;109:427-429.

Preskorn SH, Denner LJ: Benzodiazepines and withdrawal psychosis. *J Am Med Assoc* 1977;237:36-38.

Regestein QR: Commentary 2. *Pharmacotherapy* 1983;3:146.

Rickels K, Case WG, Downing RW, *et al*: Long-term diazepam therapy and clinical outcome. *J Am Med Assoc* 1983;250:767-771.

Roth T, Hartse KM, Saab PG, *et al*: The effects of flurazepam, lorazepam, triazolam on sleep and memory. *Psychopharmacology* 1980;70:231-237.

Roth T, Kramer M, Lutz T: Intermediate use of triazolam: a sleep laboratory study. *J Int Med Res* 1976;4:59-62.

Scharf MB, Bixler EO, Kales A, *et al*: Long-term sleep laboratory evaluation of flunitrazepam. *Pharmacology* 1979;19:173-181.

Scharf MB, Kales A, Bixler EO, *et al*: Lorazepam: efficacy, side effects, and rebound phenomena. *Clin Pharmacol Ther* 1982;31:175-179.

Shader RI, Greenblatt DJ: Triazolam and anterograde amnesia: all is not well in the Z-zone (editorial). *J Clin Psychopharmacol* 1983;3:272.

Smith DE, Wesson DR, Buxton ME, *et al*: Amphetamine use, misuse, and abuse, in *Proceedings of the National Amphetamine Conference*. Boston, G.K. Hall and Co., 1979.

Soldatos CR, Kales A, Bixler EO: Effectiveness of flunitrazepam and nitrazepam. *Pharmacology*, in press.

Soldatos CR, Kales A, Kales JD: Management of insomnia. *Annu Rev Med* 1979;30:301-312.

Soldatos CR, Kales JD, Scharf MB, *et al*: Cigarette smoking associated with sleep difficulty. *Science* 1980;207:551-553.

Spinweber CL, Johnson LC: Effects of triazolam (0.5 mg) on sleep, performance, memory, and arousal threshold. *Psychopharmacology* 1982;76:5-12.

Stephen S: Unwanted effects of propranolol. *Am J Cardiol* 1966;18:463-468.

Swanson LA, Okada T: Death after withdrawal of meprobamate. *J Am Med Assoc* 1963;184:780-781.

Tan TL, Kales JD, Kales A, *et al*: Biopsychobehavioral correlates of insomnia, IV: diagnosis based on DSM-III. *Am J Psychiatry* 1984;141:357-362.

Tyrer P, Owen R, Dawling S: Gradual withdrawal of diazepam after long-term therapy. *Lancet* 1983;1:1402-1406.

Tyrer P, Rutherford D, Huggett T: Benzodiazepine withdrawal symptoms and propranolol. *Lancet* 1981;1:520-522.

Van der Kroef C: Reactions to triazolam (letter to editor). *Lancet* 1979;2:526.

146

Vela-Bueno A, Oliveros JC, Dobladez-Blanco B, *et al*: Brotizolam: a sleep laboratory evaluation. *Eur J Clin Pharmacol* 1983;25:53-56.

Vogel GW, Vogel F: Effect of midazolam on sleep of insomniacs. *Br J Clin Pharmacol* 1983;16(Supp 1):103S-108S.

Vogel GW, Barker K, Gibbons P, *et al*: A comparison of the effects of flurazepam 30 mg and triazolam 0.5 mg on the sleep of insomniacs. *Psychopharmacology* 1976;47:81-86.

Vogel GW, Thurmond A, Gibbons P, *et al*: The effect of triazolam on the sleep of insomniacs. *Psychopharmacology* 1975;41:65-69.

Williams RL, Karacan I, Hursch C: *EEG of Human Sleep: Clinical Applications*. New York, John Wiley & Sons, 1974.

Winokur A, Rickels K, Greenblatt DJ, *et al*: Withdrawal reaction from long-term, low-dosage administration of diazepam. *Arch Gen Psychiatry* 1980;37:101-105.

9
Seizure Disorders

Walter Ling, MD
Donald R. Wesson, MD

INTRODUCTION

Benzodiazepines are used for treatment of seizures in three ways: (1) parenterally in the treatment of status epilepticus, (2) in chronic maintenance for seizure prophylaxis and (3) during alcohol withdrawal, for prevention of the withdrawal syndrome, which includes grand mal seizures. The anticonvulsant properties vary between the different benzodiazepine analogs. Some benzodiazepines are marketed with the primary indication of treating seizure disorders.

The preclinical studies of benzodiazepine's anticonvulsant effects are reviewed in Chapter 11. Benzodiazepines are potent anticonvulsants in experimentally induced seizures and the anticonvulsant effects of benzodiazepines are due primarily to the prevention of spread of eliptiform electrical activity. Benzodiazepines have little effect on abnormal electrical activity from the seizure focus.

This chapter briefly reviews the history of clinical use of selected benzodiazepines in the treatment of seizure disorders and presents guidelines for their use in treatment of seizures and in management of seizure disorders.

BENZODIAZEPINES IN STATUS EPILEPTICUS

Diazepam, clorazepam and lorazepam have all been successfully used in the treatment of status epilepticus.

Diazepam

Diazepam was reported to be effective for the treatment of status epilepticus in the mid-1960's (Gastaut *et al.*, 1965; Lombroso, 1966;

Prensky *et al.*, 1967). Diazepam is still considered to be the drug of choice by many clinicians for the initial control of seizures during status epilepticus. Although intravenous phenytoin itself is effective in controlling seizures (Cranford *et al.*, 1979), diazepam is generally preferred because of its more rapid onset of anticonvulsant effects. Given intravenously, diazepam has a very rapid onset of clinical activity. In 80% of the patients treated, cessation of seizures occurred within 5 minutes of injection, and in a third of them, seizures stopped within 3 minutes (Delgado-Escueta *et al.*, 1982).

Diazepam is effective against most types of status epilepticus, but is especially effective against absence seizures (also known as simple petit mal, pure petit mal and pyknoepilepsy) and absence status (Browne & Penry, 1973). It is less effective in stopping other forms of status: psychomotor, tonic and clonic, and infantile myoclonic.

One recommended regimen in treatment of status epilepticus in adults is to infuse diazepam at a rate not to exceed 2 mg/minute for an initial dose of 10 mg and in subsequent 10 mg increments at 15 to 20 minute intervals until seizures stop or up to a total of 40 mg. Because of rapid tissue distribution, the anticonvulsant effect of diazepam is short-lived and its use must be promptly followed by administration of phenytoin to maintain seizure control. Careful monitoring of cardiorespiratory function is essential with infusion of diazepam because of its central nervous system and cardiorespiratory depressant effects. Apnea and cardiac arrest may occur in the elderly and in those who are acutely medically ill. Patients treated simultaneously with barbiturates are especially prone to develop severe hypotension. Slowing the rate of infusion may prevent this from occurring. If barbiturates must be used after diazepam infusion, Mattson (1972) recommends that an hour be allowed between the administration of the benzodiazepine and the barbiturate.

Delgado-Escueta *et al.* (1982) recommend a stepwise approach to drug treatment of tonic–clonic status epilepticus. If seizures fail to stop after an initial infusion of 20 mg of diazepam and 18 mg/kg of phenytoin, one possible next step of management is to administer 100 mg of diazepam diluted in 500 ml of 5% dextrose in water given intravenously at the rate of 40 mg/hr (said to ensure a diazepam serum level of 0.2–0.8 u/ml). With diazepam levels within this range and a phenytoin level of 15–20 µg/ml maintained by i.v. drip, seizures will be stopped in 88 percent of patients (Delgado-Escueta *et al.*, 1982).

Clonazepam

Gastaut *et al.* (1971) showed that clonazepam was an even more potent anticonvulsant than diazepam. An intravenous dose of 0.25–4.0 mg of clonazepam is equivalent to 5–25 mg of diazepam in controlling seizures. Some investigators consider intravenous clonazepam to be the most effective agent available in the treatment of status epilepticus (Gregoriades & Frangos, 1977).

Two techniques of administration have been recommended for clonazepam: a slow intravenous infusion of one-half mg to 1 mg in children (1 mg in adults) in 2 minutes or one-fourth mg bolus at 30 second intervals in both adults and children. Additionally, clonazepam can be administered in young children by rubbing 3–5 drops of a 0.25% solution into the buccal mucosa. It can also be given as a suppository (Overweg & Binnie, 1983).

Lorazepam

Lorazepam has potent anticonvulsant activities and in some studies, has shown advantages over diazepam. Waltregny and Dargent (1975) reported on its effectiveness for treatment of status epilepticus. Its onset of action is rapid, but because of its slower rate of tissue distribution, its anticonvulsant activity is prolonged compared to diazepam (Walker et al., 1979; Griffith, 1980).

In a randomized double-blind trial comparing 10 mg intravenous diazepam to 4 mg lorazepam, lorazepam was found to be equally efficacious to diazepam in controlling seizures in status epilepticus from various causes. Eighty-nine percent of seizure episodes were stopped after 1 or 2 doses of lorazepam while 76% stopped after treatment with diazepam. Respiratory depression, a major complication of intravenous benzodiazepines, occurred in four patients in both the diazepam and lorazepam group; those showing adverse effects to lorazepam were noted to be older and had more concomitant medical illnesses than those who reacted adversely to diazepam (Leppik et al., 1983).

In normal patients and in patients with chronic obstructive pulmonary disease, the depressant effect of lorazepam on the cardiorespiratory system has been reported to be minimal (Cormack, Milledge & Hanning, 1977; Elliott et al., 1971; Denaut, 1975). However, in a more recent review of literature and on their own clinical experience with lorazepam in status epilepticus, Levy and Krall (1984) noted some instances of respiratory depression with lorazepam. They suggested that more seriously ill patients may be more sensitive to the adverse effects of lorazepam.

Both generalized and partial status epilepticus appear to respond favorably to lorazepam. It may be possible to reduce the frequency of cardiorespiratory complications by using smaller doses (e.g., 2 mg at 5 minute intervals to a total of 8 mg).

With its rapid onset and longer duration of action, lorazepam may prove in time to be the preferred benzodiazepine for treatment of status epilepticus. In Levy and Krall's (1984) experience, no patients resistant to lorazepam responded to subsequent administration of diazepam. This suggested to them that lorazepam may be the preferred initial medication to use.

BENZODIAZEPINES IN OTHER SEIZURE DISORDERS

Unlike its intravenous use in status epilepticus, oral benzodiazepines have only a limited role in the long-term management of seizure disorders. The promising early results (Browne & Penry, 1973) have not been substantiated by subsequent clinical experiences. Today, benzodiazepines are not considered a drug of first choice in the long-term management of epilepsies.

Clonazepam

Clonazepam is a particularly potent anticonvulsant. In early clinical trials, it was effective in various types of seizures in adults and children, but especially in seizures associated with myoclonus and in photosensitive seizures (O'Donohoe & Paes, 1977; Nanda et al., 1977). The major side effects were drowsiness, ataxia and drooling, especially during the first few days of treatment. Drooling and hypersecretion appear to be dose related and are particularly prone to occur in retarded patients. Clonazepam has variable effects on the behavior of patients.

There is a wide range of serum concentration after oral administration of clonazepam and, unlike phenytoin, there is little correlation between serum benzodiazepine serum level and the clinical anti-epileptic effect (Nanda et al., 1977).

Because of initial excessive drowsiness, clonazepam must be started gradually. The recommended initial dose for adults is 1.5 mg per day in divided doses with gradual increments of 0.5–1 mg at 3 day intervals to a maximum of 20 mg per day. In young children, 0.01–0.03 mg per kilogram per day is the recommended initial dose. Maintenance doses range from 0.1 mg to 0.2 mg per kilogram per day.

Tolerance and adaptation develop quickly with continued administration of clonazepam leading to loss of anticonvulsant activities. This occurs in up to 30% of patients within 1–6 months of initiation of therapy. Breakthrough seizures are frequent requiring frequent dosage adjustments or complete withdrawal of the medication. In some patients, clonazepam has a paradoxical effect resulting in worsening of grand mal seizures. Tonic seizures and absence status have been reported after withdrawal of clonazepam. When discontinuing clonazepam, it is tapered at the rate of 0.25 mg per day.

Clonazepam may interact with other anticonvulsants. On rare occasions, the concurrent administration of clonazepam and valproic acid has led to emergence of absence status necessitating withdrawal from the medications (Jeavons, 1977). Iavanainen and Himberg (1982), on the other hand, have successfully combined clonazepam and valproic acid in patients with progressive myoclonus epilepsy.

At present, clonazepam appears to rank behind ethosuximide and valproic acid in treatment of absence seizures and myoclonic seizures.

However, it remains a useful alternative for cases resistant to these other medications.

Clorazepate

Clorazepate appears to be a useful, not as the only, primary anticonvulsant but as an adjunctive medication, in some patients with a variety of seizure disorders in whom seizures are not fully controlled by conventional anti-epileptic regimens. It is well accepted and well tolerated by patients in doses up to 3 mg per kilogram per day given in divided doses (Troupin *et al.*, 1980; Berchou, Rodin & Russell, 1981). In a double-blind study, it appeared to compare favorably to phenobarbital as a secondary anticonvulsant (Wilensky *et al.*, 1981).

Clorazepate is available in the United States as an anti-anxiety agent, but is not labeled in the package insert for use in treatment of seizures. As an adjunctive anticonvulsant, it may be especially useful in epileptic patients in whom anxiety is a significant factor in the precipitation of seizure attacks.

Nitrazepam

Nitrazepam appears to be an effective agent for myoclonic seizures in children, especially in those with hypsarrhythmia and infantile myoclonic spasms (Markham, 1964; Gibbs & Anderson, 1965). The results of early clinical experience were judged to be exceedingly favorable in myoclonic seizures with and without classical hypsarrhythmia. A 50% or more reduction in seizure frequency was reported in over half the patients (Browne & Penry, 1973). It appeared to be comparable to ACTH in its ability to suppress seizures (Grossi-Bianchi & Pistone, 1968) and it carries none of the risks of corticosteroids. It does, however, have some disadvantages of its own, chiefly drowsiness and hypersalivation. Toleration develops to its anticonvulsant effects, as is true with all benzodiazepines, and seems to occur more often in patients with myoclonic seizures (Browne & Penry, 1973).

Interest in the anticonvulsant effects of nitrazepam appears to have diminished with the wide availability of clonazepam and the introduction of valproic acid.

Nitrazepam is available in most countries, chiefly as a hypnotic, but is not marketed in the United States.

Clobazam

Clobazam has been shown to be a potent anticonvulsant effective against a variety of seizures including myoclonic and complex partial seizures (Gastaut & Low, 1979; Critchley *et al.*, 1981). It has been used successfully to prevent the cyclical exacerbation of seizures associated with menstrual cycles in doses of 20–30 mg per day (Feely, Calvert & Gibson, 1982).

153

Clobazam is generally well accepted and well tolerated by patients. There is less sedation and less effect on psychomotor performance compared to other benzodiazepines but, like all other benzodiazepines, tolerance to its anticonvulsant effect develops with continued oral administration. Other side effects are few, although mid-cycle galactorrhea was noted in a patient in the Feely, Calvery & Gibson study and a case of neologistic jargon dysphasia has been reported recently (Wilson *et al.*, 1983).

BENZODIAZEPINES IN ECLAMPTIC SEIZURES

Chlordiazepoxide and diazepam used intravenously have been shown to be effective for eclamptic seizures by many investigators (Lean *et al.*, 1968; Hohenbleicher, 1969; Elliott, 1970; Kasturilal & Shetti, 1975). In the series of 90 patients reported by Lean and his coworkers, only 2 had recurrent eclamptic seizures after receiving benzodiazepines. These results compared favorably to the use of other sedative medications. Good sedation was achieved without loss of consciousness. The hypotensive effect of benzodiazepines appears to be an added advantage in this situation.

BENZODIAZEPINES IN ALCOHOL WITHDRAWAL SEIZURES

Benzodiazepines are effective in controlling seizure activities and in preventing their emergence in acute alcoholic withdrawal (Nicol *et al.*, 1969; Golbert *et al.*, 1967; Kaim *et al.*, 1969). Most acute alcohol treatment regimens now include a benzodiazepine for sedation and for prevention of the more severe withdrawal symptoms (Sellers & Kalant, 1976; Sellers *et al.*, 1982). Chlordiazepoxide and diazepam are equally efficacious in equivalent doses. Other benzodiazepines can also be used provided that the effective half-life of the benzodiazepine is taken into account.

Both diazepam and chlordiazepoxide are well absorbed when given orally, whereas absorption after intramuscular administration is much more erratic. It is generally preferrable to give either diazepam or chlordiazepoxide intravenously if parenteral administration is necessary. One current recommendation is to give a single 20 mg dose orally or intravenously at hourly intervals until the desired level of tranquilization is achieved, monitoring the cardiorespiratory effects with each injection. Alternatively, smaller doses (2.5–5.0 mg diazepam or 12.5–25 mg chlordiazepoxide) can be given at frequent intervals of every 5–10 minutes with simple precautions.

Although alcohol withdrawal is the most common cause of seizures during the immediate withdrawal period, the clinician must continue to be vigilant for other possible causes: severe head trauma with or without subdural hematoma, metabolic derangements and central nervous system infections.

CONCLUSIONS

Intravenous benzodiazepines are highly effective for treatment of status epilepticus. Diazepam and lorazepam appears to be equally efficacious, however lorazepam may be preferred due to its longer duration of action.

Benzodiazepines are effective medications for treatment of eclamptic and alcohol withdrawal seizures.

Additionally, benzodiazepines are the first choice in initial treatment of status epilepticus, however their role among the anticonvulsants for seizure prophylaxis is adjunctive. When the subject was reviewed a decade ago (Browne & Penry, 1973), it was recognized that development of tolerance to the anticonvulsant effects of orally administered benzodiazepines limited their long-term use as anticonvulsants.

Nevertheless, benzodiazepines have a definite place in the armamentarium of medications for the treatment of different types of seizures. Diazepam remains an initial drug of choice for status epilepticus of various etiologies. Several other benzodiazepines are useful adjuncts in many treatment regimens in seizure disorders of children and adults.

Oral benzodiazepines may have a role in treatment of some seizure patients in whom seizure attacks are frequently preceded by a considerable period of anxiety. In our own experience, drug abuse and drug dependence have not been problems in these patients.

References

Berchou RC, Rodin EA, Russell ME: Clorazepate therapy for refractory seizures. *Neurology* 1981;31:1483-1485.

Brown TR, Penry JK: Benzodiazepines in the treatment of epilepsy. *Epilepsia* 1973;14:277-310.

Cormack RS, Milledge JS, Hanning CD: Respiratory effects and amnesia after premedication with morphine or lorazepam. *Br J Anaesth* 1977;49:351-361.

Cranford RE, Leppik IE, Patrick B, *et al*: Intravenous phenytoin in acute treatment of seizures. *Neurology* 1979;29:1474-1479.

Critchley EM, Vakil SD, Hayward HW, *et al*: Double-blind clinical trial of clobazam in refractory epilepsy and the effect of clobazam on blood levels of phenobarbitone, phenytoin and carbamazepine. *Royal Soc Med Intl Sympos Series* 1981;43:159-164.

Denaut M, Yernault JC, De Coster A: Double-blind comparison of the respiratory effects of parenteral lorazepam and diazepam in patients with chronic obstructive lung disease. *Curr Med Res Opin* 1975;2:611-615.

Delgado-Escueta AV, Treiman DM, Walsh GO: The treatable epilepsies. *N Engl J Med* 1983;308:1508-1514, 1576-1584.

Delgado-Escueta AV, Westertain C, Treiman DM, *et al*: Current concepts in neurology: management of status epilepticus. *N Engl J Med* 1982;306:1337-1340.

Elliott HW, Nomoj N, Navarro G, *et al*: Central nervous system and cardiovascular effects of lorazepam in man. *Clin Pharmacol Ther* 1971;12:468-481.

Elliott PM: The management of eclampsia with intravenous diazepam and protoveratrine. *Aust NZ J Obstet Gynaecol* 1970;10:99-100.

Feely M, Calvert R, Gibson J: Clobazam in catamenial epilepsy. *Lancet* 1982;2:71-73.

Gastaut H, Courjon J, Poire R, *et al*: Treatment of status epilepticus with a new benzodiazepine more active than diazepam. *Epilepsia* 1971;12:197-214.

Gastaut H, Low MD: Antiepileptic properties of clobazam, a 1-5 benzodiazepine, in man. *Epilepsia* 1979;20:437-446.

Gastaut H, Naquet R, Poire R, *et al*: Treatment of status epilepticus with diazepam (Valium). *Epilepsia* 1965;6:167-182.

Gibbs FA, Anderson EM: **Treatment of hypsarrhythmia and infantile spasms with a Librium** analogue. *Neurology* 1965;15:1173-1176.

Golbert TM, Sanz CJ, Rose HD, *et al*: Comparative evaluation in treatment of alcohol withdrawal syndromes. *J Am Med Assoc* 1967;201:99-102.

Greenblatt DJ, Shader RI, Abernethy DR: Current status of benzodiazepines. *N Engl J Med* 1983;309:354-358,410-416.

Gregoriades AD, Frango EG: Clinical observations on clonazepam in intractible epilepsy, in Penry JK (ed): *Epilepsy: The Eighth International Symposium*. New York, Raven Press, 1977, pp 169-175.

Griffith PA, Karp HR: Lorazepam in therapy for status epilepticus. *Ann Neurol* 1980;7:493.

Grossi-Bianchi ML, Pistone FM: Comparison of treatment with ACTH and nitrazepam in some forms of infantile convulsive syndromes. *RiV Clin Pediatr* 1968;81:233-234.

Hohenbleicher R: Twenty-three convulsions after Caeserian section without fatal outcome with administration of diazepam. *Med Klin* 1969;64:434-435.

Iiavanainen M, Himberg J-J: Valproate and clonazepam in treatment of severe progressive myoclonus epilepsy. *Arch Neurol* 1982;39:236-238.

Jeavons PM: Choice of drug therapy in epilepsy. *Practitioner* 1977;219:542-556.

Kaim SC, Klett CJ, Rothfeld B: Treatment of the acute alcohol withdrawal state: a comparison of four drugs. *Am J Psychiatry* 1969;125:1640-1646.

Kasturilal FICS, Shetti RN: Role of diazepam in the management of eclampsia. *Curr Ther Res* 1975;18:627-635.

Lean TH, Ratnau SS, Sivasamboo R: Use of benzodiazepines in the management of eclampsia. *J Obstet Gynaecol Br Emp* 1968;75:856-862.

Leppik IE, Derivan AT, Homan RW, *et al*: Double-blind study of lorazepam and diazepam in status epilepticus. *J Am Med Assoc* 1983;249:1452-1454.

Levy RJ, Krall RL: Treatment of status epilepticus with lorazepam. *Arch Neurol* 1984;41:605-611.

Lombrosa CT: Treatment of status epilepticus with diazepam. *Neurology* 1966;16:629-634.

Markham CH: The treatment of myoclonic seizures of infancy and childhood with LA-1. *Pediatrics* 1964;34:511-518.

Mattson RH: The benzodiazepines, in Woodbury DM, Penry JK, Schmidt RP (eds): *Antiepileptic Drugs*. New York, Raven Press, 1972, p 510.

Nanda RN, Johnson RH, Keogh HJ, *et al*: Treatment of chronic epilepsy for 1 to 2 years with clonazepam, in Penry JK (ed): *Epilepsy: The Eighth International Symposium*. New York, Raven Press, 1977, pp 163-168.

Nicol CF, Tutton JC, Smith BH: Parenteral diazepam in status epilepticus. *Neurology* 1969;19:332-343.

O'Donohoe NV, Paes BA: A trial of clonazepam in the treatment of severe epilepsy in infancy and childhood, in Penry JK (ed): *Epilepsy: Eighth International Symposium*. New York, Raven Press, 1977, pp 159-162.

Overweg J, Binnie CD: Benzodiazepines in neurological disorders, in Costa E (ed): *The Benzodiazepines: From Molecular Biology to Clinical Practice*. New York, Raven Press, 1983, pp 339-347.

Prensky AL, Roff MC, Moore MJ, *et al*: Intravenous diazepam in the treatment of prolonged seizure activity. *N Engl J Med* 1967;276:779-784.

Sellers EM, Kalant H: Alcohol intoxication and withdrawal. *N Engl J Med* 1976;294:757-762.

Sellers EM, Naranjo CA, Harrison M, *et al*: Simplifying treatment of alcohol withdrawal: diazepam loading. *Clin Pharmacol Ther* 1982;31:268 abstract.

Troupin AS, Wilensky AJ, Friel P, *et al*: Clorazepate as an anticonvulsant, in Johannessen SJ, *et al* (eds): *Antiepileptic Therapy: Advances in Drug Monitoring*. New York, Raven Press, 1980, pp 291-298.

Walker JE, Homan RW, Vasko MR, *et al*: Lorazepam in status epilepticus. *Ann Neurol* 1979;6:207-213.

Waltregny A, Dargent J: Preliminary study of parenteral lorazepam in status epilepticus. *Acta Neurol Belg* 1975;75:219-229.

Wilensky AJ, Ojemann LM, Tenkin NR, *et al*: Clorazepate and phenytoin as antiepileptic drugs: a double-blind study. *Neurology* 1981;31:1271-1276.

Wilson A, Petty R, Perry A, *et al*: Paroxysmal language disturbance in an epileptic treated with clobazam. *Neurology* 1983;33:652-654.

10
Alcohol and Other Drug Withdrawals

Donald R. Wesson, MD
David E. Smith, MD

Drug withdrawal is the process of weaning a patient from a drug to which their body has undergone cellular adaptation, i.e., physical dependence. The goal of drug withdrawal is to accomplish the weaning process with safety while reducing symptoms to a tolerable level. Although withdrawal is often a necessary step in the treatment of addictive disease drug withdrawal alone, no matter how skillfully executed, is not adequate treatment for 'addictive disease'.

Neither patients nor their physicians should expect symptom-free withdrawal. The reversal of the cellular adaptation to the drug of dependency generates symptoms, and *no* symptoms suggest that the diagnosis of physical dependency may have been in error. Patients who expect symptom-free withdrawal become frightened when symptoms develop and may conclude that their withdrawal is not proceeding well. Although physicians are reluctant to discuss withdrawal symptoms, fearing that symptoms will be induced by suggestion or expectation the advantages of anticipatory guidance and justifying some level of symptoms as an expected and necessary part of withdrawal outweighs the possibility of symptom generation by suggestion.

Since the goal is to reverse the cellular adaptation in a controlled manner, the principle is to use withdrawal medications which are long-acting and thus, with stepwise reduction in administered doses, provide a smooth decrease in blood and tissue levels. Diazepam and chlordiazepoxide have become the standard treatment of alcohol withdrawal, and benzodiazepines are commonly adjunctively employed in other types of drug withdrawal.

BENZODIAZEPINE DETOXIFICATION

Benzodiazepine withdrawal, covered in detail in Chapter 17, is more complex than withdrawal of other sedative–hypnotics. Excepting slow taper of therapeutically prescribed benzodiazepines to prevent symptom rebound in individuals who are still in control of their use (e.g., physically dependent without addictive disease), benzodiazepines are not first choice of withdrawal medications for benzodiazepine withdrawal.

ALCOHOL WITHDRAWAL

Withdrawal from sedative–hypnotics, including alcohol, can result in seizures, psychosis, hyperpyrexia and death. Two pharmacological principals guide pharmacological management of sedative–hypnotic withdrawal: (1) do not abruptly stop sedative–hypnotics, and (2) substitute long acting sedative–hypnotics for rapidly metabolized or excreted sedative–hypnotics during withdrawal. All sedative–hypnotics are cross-tolerant allowing the clinician to choose a long-acting withdrawal sedative as the withdrawal medication.

Benzodiazepines have become the standard pharmacological treatment for alcohol withdrawal, and use of other medications in alcohol withdrawal without defensible medical justification raises potential medical–legal liability. The use of chlordiazepoxide in treatment of acute alcohol withdrawal was one of earliest clinical applications of chlordiazepoxide. (Kaim, 1973). Clinicians develop preferences for different benzodiazepines based on familiarity, pharmacologic characteristics or beliefs about addiction or therapeutic properties. Brown (1983) for example, prefers oxazepam because it is metabolized to an inactive form, thus preventing accumulation. If a *mixed* sedative–hypnotic (including benzodiazepine) dependency exists, we prefer using phenobarbital as the withdrawal medication, substituting phenobarbital for both alcohol and the other sedative–hypnotics.

For alcohol withdrawal, we use chlordiazepoxide as the withdrawal medication. During the first 24 hours, chlordiazepoxide 25 mg by mouth is administered every 4 hours until the patient is sedated, sleeping or has sustained horizontal nystagmus. If the patient is grossly tremulous, hyperreflexic, diaphoretic and vomiting, we give an immediate dose of 100 mg of chlordiazepoxide intramuscularly followed by chlordiazepoxide 50 mg intramuscularly every hour until signs and symptoms of acute alcohol withdrawal have abated. If the patient has significant gastritis, we concomitantly administer cimetidine (Tagamet[R]) 300 mg i.m. with the chlordiazepoxide, keeping in mind that cimetidine inhibits demethylation of chlordiazepoxide (Klotz, Anttila & Reimann, 1979; Desmond, Patwardham & Schenker, 1980). We avoid using phenothiazine antinauseants as they lower seizure threshold. Intravenous fluids are used only if there is clinically significant dehydration due to vomiting and diarrhea.

Following the first 24 hours of treatment, the total amount of chlordiazepoxide given during the first 24 hours is decreased 25 mg each day. If the patient is sleeping soundly at the time a dosage is due, the dose is omitted. If sleep onset insomnia, continues in a patient who shows no other signs of alcohol withdrawal, insomnia is treated with L-tryptophan 2–4 gm given 30 minutes before bedtime.

STIMULANT WITHDRAWAL

In the first 24-72 hours following cessation of chronic use of cocaine, amphetamine and nicotine, patients experience dysphoria, "nervousness", restlessness, sleep onset insomnia, increased dream intensity, and dysphoria – a symptom cluster which overlap diagnostic criteria for agitated depression. During the first few days of stimulant withdrawal, patients crave tranquilization, and benzodiazepines or tricyclic antidepressants are commonly prescribed. Chronic methamphetamine administration to Rhesus monkey depletes 30 to 50 percent of whole brain norepinephrine (Seiden, Fischman & Schuster, 1975), a fact used to rationalize clinical trials with desipramine, a potent blocker of norepinephrine reuptake by presynaptic neurons as treatment for cocaine and amphetamine withdrawal. In our experience L-tryptophan, the amino acid precursor of serotonin, in doses of 2 gm three times daily and 4 gm at bedtime, works as well as benzodiazepines in counteracting anxiety, restlessness, and sleep disturbances, avoids the behavioral decompensation sometimes observed with sedatives, and does not introduce the risk of initiating sedative dependence. The most common side effect to tryptophan is mild gastrointestinal upset, usually alleviated by giving the tryptophan dose with a small carbohydrate snack. Failure of tryptophan to modulate symptoms is usually the result of inadequate tryptophan dose or taking the tryptophan with a protein-containing meal. When taken with other amino acids, tryptophan is not efficiently transported across blood–brain barrier as the amino acids share the same transport mechanism across the blood–brain barrier.

OPIATE WITHDRAWAL

Methadone is the usual withdrawal medication used for opiate withdrawal. Regulations governing use of methadone are restrictive and its use in the U.S. for opiate withdrawal is restrictd to specially-licensed programs. Symptomatic treatment of opiate withdrawal symptoms using a variety of non-narcotic sedatives, anticholinergics (e.g. Lomotil[R]) or propoxyphene (Darvon[R]) is pharmacologically rational. However, clonidine (Catapres[R]) has largely supplanted other medications for symptomatic treatment of narcotic withdrawal.

SUMMARY

The only established role of benzodiazepines in treatment of drug withdrawal is for alcohol detoxification. A medical rationale for ancillary use of benzodiazepines in management of other types of drug withdrawal can be made, but in general, benzodiazepines are not the treatment of first choice.

References

Brown CG: The alcohol-withdrawal syndrome. *West J Med* 1983;138:579-581.

Desmond PV, Patwardham RV, Schenker S, *et al*: Cimetidine impairs elimination of chlordiazepoxide (Librium) in man. *Ann Int Med* 1980;93:266-268.

Kaim SC: Benzodiazepines in the treatment of alcohol withdrawal states, in Garattini S, Mussini E, Randall LO (eds.) *The Benzodiazepines*. New York: Raven Press, 1973.

Klotz U, Antilla VJ, Reimann I: Cimetidine/diazepam interaction. *Lancet* 1979;2:699.

Seiden LS, Fischman MW, Schuster CR: Long-term methamphetamine induced changes in brain catecholamines in tolerant Rhesus monkeys. *Drug Alcohol Depend* 1975;1:215-219.

Wagner GC, Seiden LS, Schuster CR: Methamphetamine-induced changes in brain catecholamines in rats and guinea pigs. *Drug Alcohol Depend* 1979;4:435-438.

11
Additional Clinical Uses of Benzodiazepines

Donald R. Wesson, MD

Previous chapters have discussed standard uses of benzodiazepines. Some other uses of benzodiazepines which are new, under investigation, or applicable to unusual clinical situations are reviewed in this chapter.

SCHIZOPHRENIA

The role of benzodiazepines in the treatment of schizophrenia is being re-examined. The impetus for taking a fresh look resulted from new knowledge about the relationship between GABA neuronal activity and dopaminergic activity. Enhanced dopaminergic activity is thought responsible, at least in part, for some symptoms that occur in schizophrenics. With the knowledge that GABA neuronal activity modulates dopaminergic activity and that benzodiazepines facilitate GABA neurotransmission, it is reasonable to postulate that benzodiazepines could be beneficial in the treatment of schizophrenia by dampening dopaminergic activity.

Early controlled studies of benzodiazepines in treatment of schizophrenia were not encouraging, and the clinical consensus evolved that benzodiazepines were ineffective in treating the psychotic manifestations of schizophrenia. Nestoros (1980), who reviewed published controlled studies utilizing benzodiazepines alone or in combination with neuroleptics in treatment of schizophrenia, concluded that doses of benzodiazepines in studies showing no beneficial effects were probably too small. Currently trials are underway in many sites using high doses of high-milligram potency benzodiazepines and benzodiazepine derivatives (e.g. Astrup & Vatten, 1984).

MANIA

Lithium is the standard treatment for manic-depressive illness, however the

163

onset of lithium's antimanic effects often requires several days to take effect. Therefore, during the acute manic phase of their illness, patients are often treated with both lithium and a neuroleptic, and neuroleptic-induced parkinsonism often occurs. Therefore, alternatives to neuroleptics would be desirable.

In a study of 12 patients with acute mania, clonazepam was compared to lithium using a 10-day double-blind crossover design. Six patients received clonazepam for 10 days followed by lithium, and the other 6 patients received lithium followed by clonazepam. Clonazepam, in doses of 4–16 mg, was found significantly more efficacious than lithium in reducing symptoms of motor overactivity and logorrhea (Chouinard, Young & Annable, 1983). These investigators cite clonazepam's rapid onset of action, sedation, and reduced need for neuroleptics as advantages in the treatment of acute mania.

DEPRESSION

Although benzodiazepines as a class have not proven generally effective as antidepressants (Schatzberg & Cole, 1978), alprazolam has been reported in controlled studies to compare favorably with imipramine (Feighner, Meredith et al.; Kales et al., 1982)

NIGHT TERROR/NIGHTMARE SYNDROME

Nightmares consist of at least two types of dream disturbances: the night terror/nightmare syndrome and dream anxiety attack. Night terror nightmares are not associated with REM sleep and occur during stage 4 sleep, usually early in the sleep period. They are associated with motor activity, and recall is usually limited to fragments. Benzodiazepines, because they reduce stage 4 sleep, have been suggested as effective therapy for night terror nightmares (Kramer, 1979).

In the post-traumatic stress syndrome, sleep–dream disturbances are sometimes associated with recurrent intrusive imagery during stage 4 sleep. Benzodiazepines have been suggested as one adjunct to therapy (Friedman, 1981).

NOCTURNAL MYOCLONUS

Frequent repetitive leg jerks due to nocturnal myoclonus can be severe and a cause of insomnia. Case reports support the use of clonazepam in doses of either 0.5 mg at bedtime or 0.5 mg three times daily in nocturnal myoclonus and a variant, "restless legs syndrome" (Boghew, 1980; Matthews, 1979).

TIC DOULOUREUX

Tic douloureux is a disorder in which a person has paroxysms of severe pain in one or more branches of the trigeminal nerve. The usual treatment is carbamazepine, an anticonvulsant.

Clonazepam, whose anticonvulsant uses are described in Chapter 9, has also been used to treat tic douloureux. In an open label clinical trial of clonazepam in 25 patients with tic douloureux, the paroxysms of pain disappeared in 40% of patients, and 23% were improved. Of 16 patients whose pain had not responded to carbamazepine, eight responded favorably to clonazepam. Side effects of clonazepam, e.g. somnolence and ataxia, were severe, leading the investigators to conclude that clonazepam should be considered a second choice to carbamazepine (Court and Kase, 1976).

Anesthesia

Benzodiazepines are useful adjuncts to anesthesia. They are often used for preoperative medications to allay anxiety and induce sedation. For very short procedures, such as electric cardioversion, injectable benzodiazepines alone can provide sufficient anesthesia and, in addition, produce amnesia for the procedure (Kanto and Klotz, 1982).

CONCLUSION

In addition to the applications discussed here and in other chapters, many additional uses are suggested by scattered case reports. Some will eventally find their way into standard use, and others, which look promising in uncontrolled trials, will be rejected by careful controlled study.

References

Astrup C. Vatten L: Effects of the benzodiazepine derivative estazolam in schizophrenia. *Biol Psychiatry* 1984;19:85-88.

Boghew D: Successful treatment of restless legs with clonazepam (letter). *Ann Neurol* 1980;8:341.

Chouinard G, Young SN, Annable L: Antimanic effects of clonazepam. *Biol Psychiatry* 1983;18:451-466.

Court JE, Kase CS: Treatment of tic douloureux with a new anticonvulsant (clonazepam). *J Neurol Neurosurg Psychiatry* 1976;39:297-299.

Friedman MJ: Post-Vietnam syndrome. *Psychosomatics* 1981;22:931-941.

Kanto J, Klotz U: Intravenous benzodiazepines as anaesthetic agents: pharmacokinetics and clinical consequences. *Acta Anaesth Scand* 1982;26:554-569.

Kramer M: Dream disturbances. *Psychiatr Ann* 1979;9:50-68.

Matthews WB: Treatment of restless legs syndrome with clonazepam (letter). *Br Med J* 1979;1:751.

Nestoros JN: Benzodiazepines in schizophrenia: a need for reassessment. *Int Pharmacopsychiatry* 1980;15:171-179.

Rickels K, Cohen D, Csanalosi I, Harris H, Koepke H, Weblowsky J: Alprazolam and imipramine in depressed outpatients: A controlled study. *Current Therapeutic Research* 1982;32:157-164.

Schatzberg AF, Cole JO: Benzodiazepines in depressive disorders. *Arch Gen Psychiatry* 1978;35:1359-1365.

12
Vital Uses of Diazepam in Third World Countries

John Ward, BA

The World Health Organization (WHO) has placed diazepam in the 'list of essential drugs', recommending that all countries include it among the approximately 250 indispensable medicaments to have available to patients (Anonymous, 1983). In many developing countries, diazepam is used for life-saving indications. In addition to its use in the treatment of anxiety and psychiatric disorders, diazepam has a vital role in the treatment of tetanus, status epilepticus, febrile seizures, eclampsia, cerebral malaria, alcohol withdrawal and chloroquine intoxication. Use of benzodiazepines in the treatment of status epilepticus is discussed in Chapter 9. Uses of diazepam that are unique to the Third World countries are discussed in the subsequent text.

PSYCHIATRIC DISORDERS

Carstairs (1973) surveyed the psychiatric problems of developing countries, summarized the literature, and predicted that the incidence of psychiatric disorders in the Third World would soon be equal to that in the developed world.

Subsequent epidemiological studies have shown that the prevalence of serious mental diseases in developing countries is the same as in developed countries (Busnello, 1980; Anonymous, 1975). As Carstairs predicted, their relationship to important life events is similar to US and European experience (Vadher, 1981). Harding et al. (1980), applying stringent criteria in a carefully standardized two-stage screening procedure, found that about 14% of patients seeking primary health care in 4 representative Third World countries have significant psychiatric morbidity. The figure is confirmed by another WHO study (Busnello, 1980). The great majority of the complaints were of neurotic origin.

The important potential role of psychotropic drugs in this situation has

167

been emphasized by Olatawura (1979), and Odejide (1980). Johnson (1976) and Busnello (1980) have reported on WHO studies confirming their importance. Whereas the role of antipsychotic, antidepressant and anti-epileptic treatment for the people of developing countries has long been recognized, it is now becoming apparent that the anxiolytic drugs are just as important for treating the so-called "minor emotional disturbances".

Haworth (1982) reviewed the rationale and justification for according any priority to treatment of minor psychiatric illness when resources are limited: when there may not even be enough antimalarials for all patients with malaria and children are dying of malnutrition and infectious diseases. He presents data that minor ailments are assuming relatively greater importance and that their alleviation may enable patients to better cope with more serious problems. To enhance therapeutic effectiveness and minimize toxicity, medical assistants or nurse practitioners can be trained to prescribe benzodiazepines rather than having them available as over-the-counter medications.

Haworth (1982) emphasizes that the manifestations of neurotic illness differ considerably from one culture to another but that the prevalence of neuroses is similar.

A multicentre study, conducted under the auspices of the Division of Mental Health of WHO at their centers in Bombay (India), Ibadan (Nigeria), London (England) and Tokyo (Japan), is assessing the role of diazepam in treating such emotional disturbances in different populations (WHO, 1980b).

Apart from the treatment of neurotic anxiety and its manifestations, diazepam has been extensively used in Third World countries as an adjunct to lithium and haloperidol in the early therapy of mania (Heinrich, 1977). Chakrabarti (1983) stresses the problem of treating acute mania in a general hospital ward, where these patients are difficult to manage. They can be quickly sedated by an intravenous injection of a neuroleptic, such as haloperidol, followed by diazepam 20 mg intravenously. On awakening, patients are usually quite amenable to an oral treatment regimen. This style of management is much more in keeping with the community-based tradition in these countries than the alternative of a locked mental ward.

TETANUS

Injectable diazepam is of great value in the control of muscle spasms associated with tetanus. The usual adult dose is 5–10 mg intramuscularly or intravenously initially, repeated as necessary every 3 or 4 hours. In infants over 30 days of age, 1–2 mg of diazepam are given intramuscularly or by slow intravenous injection, repeated every 3 to 4 hours as necessary. Children 5 years or older may need the same dose as adults to control tetanus spasms.

In some cases, dosages up to 40 mg/kg/day have been given to control spasms without untoward effects (Femi-Pearse, 1966). When using diazepam intravenously, respiratory assistance should always be available.

Treatment of tetanus remains difficult and the mortality rate high. However, comparison of mortality rates in the Congo, before and after substitution of injectable diazepam for pentobarbital in tetanus showed a highly significant reduction in mortality (Norredam & Hainau, 1970). With pentobarbital as the sedative and muscle relaxant, mortality was 67% and tracheotomies. Other studies from Haiti to South Vietnam have reported a diazepam, mortality was reduced to 39% and only 15% of patients required tracheostomies. Other studies from Haiti to South Vietnam have reported a reduced mortality rate when Valium substituted for multiple drug regimens (Garnier *et al.*, 1975, Linh, 1975). In Sierra Leone, the use of diazepam has helped ensure the survival of half the children afflicted, although other factors including better nursing care and immunization programs have certainly contributed to the falling death rate (Muller, 1982).

The survival rate varies with the severity of the tetanus. Using diazepam as the sole muscle-relaxant agent, one study of patients aged 3 to 79 years in Haiti showed survival rates of 63% in severe tetanus, 95% in moderate tetanus, and 100% in mild tetanus (Garnier, 1975). Survival rates in childhood tetanus have been particularly impressive when injectable diazepam was used alone or combined with other medications: a 90% survival rate was reported in 42 children aged 1 month to 3 years, and addition of diazepam to a sedative–anticonvulsant regimen increased survival rates from 68% to 81% in children aged 1 month to 12 years (Phatak & Shah, 1970).

Although controlled or double-blind studies in the treatment of tetanus are difficult to perform, the evidence supports the clinical opinion that injectable diazepam is a useful adjunctive therapy in tetanus.

MALARIA

Although diazepam has no action against the malaria parasite, it is an important adjunct for managing patients in the acute phase of malaria when they may be delirious and disruptive to a medical ward.

Cerebral Malaria

Up to one in every 10 patients contracting malaria develops the cerebral form (Gentilini & Charmot, 1980) which, if it proceeds to coma, is rapidly fatal (Langer & Stemberger, 1979). Children are especially susceptible to the cerebral form (Gentilini & Charmot, 1980).

Emergency treatment includes sedation, often with a phenothiazine

(Barbotin, Thomas & Andre, 1970; Dao, 1970), but if convulsions are occurring, phenothiazines are contraindicated because they lower the seizure threshold, and a barbiturate (Gentilini & Charmot, 1980; Okouoyo, 1981; Swai *et al.*, 1983), paraldehyde (Gilles, 1980; Hall, 1976; Swai *et al.*, 1983) or diazepam by intravenous injection is recommended (Gentilini & Charmot, 1980). Good results have been reported with this technique from African countries – Senegal, Gabon, Morocco, Tanzania and Madagascar – and from Thailand (Hall, 1976; White & Warrell, 1983). With the ease and frequency of intercontinental air travel, the interest in this type of emergency and its treatment is expected to increase also in non-endemic areas (Gentilini & Charmot, 1980; Gilles, 1980; Loseke *et al.*, 1980; Vachon, Carbon & Gibert, 1974; White *et al.*, 1983).

In adults, doses of 100 mg diazepam may be given by slow intravenous injection (Diop Mar *et al.*, 1977); other authors propose 0.2 mg of diazepam for each kilogram of bodyweight repeated every 4 hours (Barbotin, Thomas & Andre, 1970; Swai *et al.*, 1983). If the initial injection does not succeed in controlling the seizures, it may be repeated after 5-15 minutes (Swai *et al.*, 1983). Somewhat lower doses – 30 mg by continuous I.V. infusion – have been given to control other central nervous system symptoms such as rigidity and hyperthermia (Thonnier *et al.*, 1979).

Children's doses range from 0.5 to 1.0 mg per kilogram of bodyweight, given by perfusion, up to 6 times a day (Okouoyo, 1981).

CHLOROQUINE TOXICITY

One of the most effective and widely used medications for prevention and treatment of acute malarial attacks is chloroquine. Unfortunately chloroquine in overdose is extremely toxic and is a frequent cause of death in many African countries.

Records from Abidjan (Bondurand *et al.*, 1980) show a steady increase in cases of intoxication since 1970 (Figure 1). Since the introduction of diazepam treatment for chloroquine toxicity, the death rate has been cut from 35% to 5% or less.

Study of this treatment in Abidjan as well as Nigeria (Okonkwo *et al.*, 1981) suggests that the injection of diazepam displaces the toxin from nerve cells, improving the chances of the successful use of heart massage in case of cardiac arrest. Bondurand (1980) observes: "So long as we had time to inject diazepam, and the blood flow was sufficient to ensure its adequate distribution, cardiac massage was always successful and recovery uneventful.

"The dose of diazepam needed to neutralize the toxicity of chloroquine is proportionate to the amount of chloroquine ingested. In the muscle preparation studied experimentally, the optimum proportion is 1 mg diazepam to every 9 mg chloroquine. But the proportion is not the same in man. Clinical experience appears to show that the optimum clinical dose is 1 mg diazepam to 30 mg chloroquine". Using this treatment, there have never been any signs of re-intoxication.

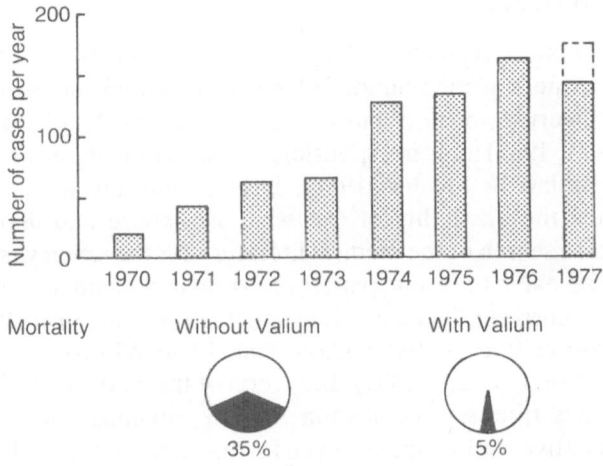

Figure 1 Incidence of chloroquine intoxication in Abidjan and reduction of mortality by diazepam.

ECLAMPSIA

Eclampsia is rare as a cause of death in Western countries today, but it remains one of the major causes of maternal and perinatal mortality in the Third World. A study from Zambia (Thakker & Wacha, 1981) shows that diazepam, because of its sedative and anticonvulsant properties, has a significant role in the management of eclampsia. The use of diazepam combined with a less conservative approach to caesarian section than previously used in the unit led to a marked improvement in outcome. Perinatal mortality at 20% was lower than previous series reported from African and other developing countries, and comparable with European figures. Maternal mortality was also low: of the 3 mothers who died (out of 46), two were moribund on admission, having refused earlier hospitalization. Diazepam was considered very effective in reducing the recurrence of convulsions. Also, diazepam is easy to inject, relatively inexpensive and does not entail special nursing care, all features which recommend it for use in the circumstances prevailing in Third World countries.

ANESTHESIA

Diazepam is also widely used in *operative and diagnostic procedures*

(Aderoju *et al.*, 1979; Yanov & Kujan, 1981), where its benefits to the patient, its safety, the simple management and saving of anesthetics are of particular advantage in developing countries.

ABUSE AND DEPENDENCE

The controversy surrounding diazepam and other benzodiazepines in Europe and America, compounded of few documented and many anecdotal reports of "overuse, misuse and abuse" on the one hand (Marks, 1978; Owen & Tyrer, 1983) and "irresponsible and sensational journalism" on the other (Greenblatt & Shader, 1981), has not entirely missed the Third World. While the possibility of excessive use, abuse and dependence of course exists, a search of the medical literature for the seven years up to the end of 1983 revealed only nine papers referring to dependence and abuse in developing countries (Acuda & Muhangi, 1979; Kusumanto, 1979; Smith, 1982; Thakker & Wacha, 1981; Thongchai, 1979; Widjono, 1975; Anonymous, 1981; Anonymous, 1980a). In several of these, the term "abuse" was applied to describe self-medication – with vitamins, the "pill", antimalarials, sedatives or hypnotics – even for appropriate medical indications. Yet in many of these countries, the absence of a prescription system and the resort to over-the-counter pharmacy purchase – or even the street market – for many forms of medication is the norm rather than the antisocial exception implied by the term "abuse" in the western sense.

The isolated reports of true abuse or dependence on benzodiazepines in developing countries (Acuda & Muhangi, 1979; Kusumanto, 1979; Teo, Chee & Tan, 1979; Thongchai, 1979; Widjono, 1975) emphasize that they have occurred in connection with the use of heroin, marihuana or alcohol, often for the "quasitherapeutic" purpose of controlling the undesirable effects of the primary drugs (Smith, 1982). Alcohol, marihuana and the opiates still constitute the major abuse problems of the Third World (Comlavi, 1981; Anonymous, 1980a), and the benzodiazepines rarely cause this type of difficulty (Anonymous, 1981).

CONCLUSION

There is certainly need for more information on the appropriate use of benzodiazepines and other psychotropic agents, addressed specifically to the requirements of developing countries (Busnello, 1980). The substantial and continuing educational effort which must be made if problems are to be avoided in the future can best be met by close cooperation between health professionals, manufacturers, consumers, and national and international health agencies. Such cooperation will help to ensure that the particular benefits of diazepam to the Third World continue to outweigh possible drawbacks due to overenthusiastic or inappropriate use.

References

Acuda SW, Muhangi J: Diazepam addiction in Kenya. *E Afr Med J* 1979;56:76-79.

Aderoju EA, Lewis EA, Ayoola EA, *et al*: Fiberoptic endoscopy in upper gastrointestinal bleeding: Experience in Ibadan, Nigeria. *E Afr Med J* 1979;55:420-424.

Barbotin M, Thomas J, Andre LL: Données actuelles sur l'accès pernicieux palustre. *Med Trop* 1970;30:530-541.

Bondurand A, M'Dri K, Coffi S, *et al*: L'intoxication au chloroquine au Centre Hospitalier Universitaire Abidjan. *Afr Med* 1980;19:239-242.

Busnello ED: Psychosocial aspects of mental health care in developing countries – the role of the benzodiazepines, in Priest, Vianno Filho, Amrein, *et al*: *The Benzodiazepines Today and Tomorrow*. Lancaster, MTP Press, 1980.

Carstairs GM: Psychiatric problems of developing countries. *Br J Psychiatry* 1973;123:271-277.

Chakrabarti GN: Rapid relief of psychotic states by intravenous administration of haloperidol followed by i.v. diazepam, in Abstracts 7th World Congress of Psychiatry, July 11-16, 1983, Vienna/Austria, p.573, Abstr No 706, Society of Austrian Neurologists and Psychiatrists. Vienna Austria, July, 1983.

Comlavi PI: Legislation, prescription and importation. *Proc Afr Seminar on Problems of Drug Dependence*, Lagos, 1980, pp.120-121 (International Council on Alcohol and Addictions, Lausanne 1981).

Dao C: Paludisme signes, diagnostics, traitment. *Gaz Med Fr* 1970;77:6503-6510.

Diop Mar I, Banastier H, Sow A, *et al*: Paludisme neurologique de l'adulte autochtone en zone d'hypoendémie. *Bulletin de la Société Médicale d'Afrique Noir de Langue Français* 1977;22:6-29.

Femi-Pearse D: Experience with diazepam in tetanus. *Br Med J* 1966;2:862-865.

Garnier MJ, Davidson KJ, Marshall FN, *et al*: Tetanus in Haiti. *Lancet* 1975;1:383-386.

Garnier MJ: Tetanus in patients three years of age and up: a personal series of 230 consecutive patients. *Am J Surg* 1975;129:459-463.

Gentilini M, Charmot G: Therapie der cerebralen Formen der Malaria, in Dietrich M *et al*. (eds): *Malaria: Diagnose - Klinik - Therapie* (Congress, May 10-11, 1979, Hahnenklee-Harz, Germany). Basel, Switzerland, Roche, 1980, pp 201-215.

Gilles HM: The management and treatment of malaria (a personal view). *Annales de la Société Belge de Médecine Tropicale* 1980;60:129-136.

Greenblatt DJ, Shader RJ: Clinical use of the benzodiazepines. *Rat Drug Therapy* 1981;15:2-6.

Harding JW, De Arango MV, Baltazar J, *et al*: Mental disorders in primary health care: a study of their frequency and diagnosis in four developing countries. *Psychol Med* 1980;10:231-241.

Hall AP: The treatment of malaria. *Br Med J* 1976;1:323-328.

Haworth A: The usefulness of benzodiazepines in the management of various disorders in developing countries: sociological and health planning issues. *Report of the Working Group on the Use and Abuse of Psychotropic Substances in Developing Countries with Special Reference to Benzodiazepines.* ICAA-Cipat Publication, October 10-15, 1982, pp 22-30.

Heinrich K: Die psychiatrische Frühklinik bei Psychotischen Störungen. *Therapiewoche* 1977;27:6453-6454,6456-6459.

Johnson BCA: Mental disorders other than schizophrenia and depression, in *Advances in the drug therapy of mental illness.* Geneva, WHO, 1976, pp 83-91.

Kusumanto S: Drug abuse in Indonesia. *J Psychiatr Assoc Thailand* 1979;24:24-34.

Langer G, Stemberger H: Malaria-Koma beim Säugling. *Wien Med Wochenschr* 1979;129:301-303.

Linh NN: Tetanus in South Vietnam – Review of 164 cases. *Southeast Asian J Trop Med Publ Hlth* 1975;5:430-434.

Loseke N, Nenayer P, Retif J, et al: L'encephalopathie malarique à propos d'une observation. *Revue Méd de Bruxelles* 1980;1:263-266.

Marks J: *The Benzodiazepines: Use, Overuse, Misuse, Abuse?* Lancaster, MTP Press, 1978.

Muller, M: *The Health of Nations. A North – South Investigation.* London, Faber & Faber, 1982, pp. 17-19.

Norredam K, Hainau B: Treatment of tetanus in tropical Africa: a comparison between a barbiturate and diazepam in the treatment of neonatal tetanus. *Ann Soc Belge Med Trop* 1970;50:239-246.

Odejide AD: Patterns of psychotropic drug use in Nigerian outpatient clinic. *Int Pharmaco-psychiatr* 1980;15:14-23.

Okonkwo P, Eta I, Oguakwa J, et al: Chloroquine – Immunoassays and radioisotopic studies, in *Proceedings of the 7th International Congress of Pharmacology.* Paris, France, 1978, Part 2, p 937.

Okouoyo E: Neuropaludisme du nourisson et de l'enfant: à propos de 4 observations à l'hôpital pédiatrique d'Owendo (Libreville, Gabon). *Méd Afr Noire* 1981;28:177-184.

Olatawura MO: Perspectives in the treatment of mental disorders in developing countries: Africa. *Prog Neuro-Psychopharmacol* 1979;3:119-123.

Owen RT, Tyrer P: Benzodiazepine dependence: a review of the evidence. *Drugs* 1983;25:385-398.

Phatak AT, Shah SH: Diazepam as adjuvant therapy in childhood tetanus: 477 patients with tetanus in Baroda. *Clin Pediatr* 1970;9:573-576.

Smith DE: Are the benzodiazepines being overprescribed? Panel discussion, in *Proc Symp on Benzodiazepines from Molecular Biology to Clinical Practice* 3rd Wld Congr of Biological Psychiatry, Stockholm 1981. New York, Raven Press, 1982.

Swai ABM, Palangyo K, Kihamia CM, et al: Clinical management of acute falciparum malaria in Tanzania. *Tropical Doctor* 1983;13:159-163.

Teo SH, Chee KT, Tan CT: Psychiatric complications of Rohypnol abuse. *Singapore Med J* 1979;20:270-273.

Thakker U, Wacha DSO: Eclampsia in Lusaka. *Med J Zambia* 1981;15:59-64.

Thongchai Uneklabh (Rangsit): Drug abuse of non-narcotic types: an incidence in Thailand. *3rd National Workshop on Drug Dependent Treatment,* Pattaya, 1979.

Thonnier C, Bruneu A, Valmary J, *et al*: Accès pernicieux palustre et insuffisance rénale chez une femme enceinte de 5 mois: utilisation des prostaglandines pour la délivrance. *Méd Trop* 1979;29:323-327.

Vachon F, Carbon C, Gibert C: Diagnostic et traitment du paludisme cérébral en zone non endémique. *Bull Wld Health Organiz* 1974;50:169-175.

Vadher A, Ndetei DM: Life events and depression in a Kenyan setting. *Br J Psychiatr* 1981;139:134-137.

White NJ, Warrell DA, Chanthanvanich P, *et al*: Severe hypoglycemia and hyperinsulinemia in falciparum malaria. *N Engl J Med* 1983;309:61-66.

Widjono E: Drug dependence in Indonesia. *Indones Psychiatr Q* 1975;8:57-62.

Yanov E, Kujan S: Evaluation of some methods of intravenous anaesthesia in gynaecological outpatients. *Ethiop Med J* 1981;19:109.

Anonymous: Mental health in developing countries. *Br Med J* 1975;2:187-188.

Anonymous: Report of the 3rd WHO Travelling Seminar in the USSR on the Safe Use of Psychotropic and Narcotic Substances, Moscow and Tashkent 1981, Report MNH/81-34. Geneva, WHO, 1981.

Anonymous: Colloque international sur les problèmes de la drogue dans les pays africains d'expression française. Dakar 1980a. Actes de travaux, CIPAT. Lausanne.

Anonymous: Psychopharmacology – an area of research to improve mental health care. *WHO Chron* 1980b;34:465-469.

Anonymous: *The Selection of Essential Drugs.* Third Report of WHO Expert Committee. Technical Report Series 685. Geneva, WHO, 1983.

III. Non-medical Use, Misuse and Abuse

13
Abuse and Dependency: An International Perspective

David E. Smith, MD
John Marks, MD

The abuse liability and dependency characteristics of the benzodiazepines have produced substantial controversy. One reason for divergent opinions has been the comparison of benzodiazepine abuse with recreational drug abuse: cocaine, heroin or sedative-hypnotics such as methaqualone or secobarbital which are euphoriants used for recreational purposes. The comparison is misleading. Benzodiazepines are not powerful euphoriants, and most benzodiazepine abuse (even in committed recreational drug abusers) is secondary drug abuse: self-medication of adverse effects of other drugs (e.g. to reduce the nervousness induced by cocaine, or self-medication of heroin withdrawal symptoms). Because of benzodiazepines' effectiveness in ameliorating symptoms induced by other drugs or withdrawal, benzodiazepines have drug value in the illicit drug marketplace. Other medications used in treatment of drug withdrawal, such as clonidine which is used for the treatment of opiate withdrawal, have drug black market value even though such drugs themselves are not drugs of abuse. Although benzodiazepine abuse by recreational drug abusers occurs, the problem is not of primary public health importance anywhere in the world.

Of more compelling public health significance is physical or psychological dependency on benzodiazepines arising from misprescription of benzodiazepines. Problems are of two types: 1) prescription for inappropriate reasons and to patients for whom benzodiazepines are contraindicated, and 2) excessive prescription – either in duration or amount.

Considerable controversy also arises about the prescription of benzodiazepines to individuals who are alcoholic or recovering from alcoholism. If benzodiazepines complicate or worsen the disease of alcoholism, this is of major public health importance as alcoholism affects millions of people worldwide.

Additionally, there is concern about benzodiazepine dependency emanating from therapeutic prescription in therapeutic dosages even for approved medical indications. This concern takes the forms of widespread criticism about the reliance of medicine on pharmacological solutions, with the conclusion that physicians overtranquilize their patients; and case reports of benzodiazepine withdrawal symptoms developing in patients who have been taking benzodiazepines chronically.

The purpose of this chapter is to put benzodiazepine use and dependence in a rational perspective. Since there are many forces, the most powerful of which is the media, that counter development of a scientific viewpoint, we will begin by examining the contribution which the media makes.

THE MEDIA

Any drug use pattern is a complicated interaction of physical, psychological, pharmacolgical and socio-cultural variables. Complicated issues are impossible to condense to the form and simplicity required by popular media. The usual result is that the media focuses on one manageable aspect of benzodiazepines such as dependence or overprescription. The media's need for intensity and personal interest focus has resulted in the media overplaying a few dramatic cases of benzodiazepine dependence or emphasizing the theme of an over-tranquilized society, with excessive physician prescription of benzodiazepines as the cause of benzodiazepine dependence in their patients. Especially in the last ten years, the notion of overprescription has become ascendant, although physicians' prescriptions for the benzodiazepines are actually declining (Rickels, 1983; Marks, 1983) and, for some therapeutic uses such as chronic anxiety, there is evidence that the benzodiazepines may be underutilized (Marks, 1983). The primary media attention about benzodiazepine dependence has focused on diazepam, with a tacit, if not overt, theme that the other benzodiazepines are less likely to be dependence-prone. As a result, physicians have switched their patients to other benzodiazepines, believing that the other benzodiazepines would not produce physical dependence. The benzodiazepines, however, vary only in degree and are not qualitatively different. All benzodiazepines attach to specific receptor sites. Quantitative differences are due to metabolic half-life, receptor site affinity and lipophilia.

INTERNATIONAL DEFINITIONS OF ABUSE AND DEPENDENCE

A major source of confusion regarding benzodiazepine abuse and dependence has been the lack of agreed upon definitions of abuse and dependence. Understanding can proceed only with a strict adherence to definitions. We have adopted the definitions proposed by the World Health Organization (1969):

Drug Dependence: A state, psychic and sometimes also physical, which results from the interaction between a living organism and a drug, which is characterized by behavioral and other responses that always include compulsion to take the drug on a continuous or periodic basis in order to experience its psychic effects and sometimes to avoid the discomfort of its absence. Tolerance may be present.

Used in this way, the term *dependence* covers both dependence arising in a therapeutic treatment attempt as well as that which may evolve from recreation drug use.

Misuse and Abuse: The use of a drug for non-medical purposes or for unapproved medical indications deemed inappropriate by the majority.

Drug abuse refers to drug use which interferes with the individual's health, economic or social functioning. An individual can misuse a drug for non-medical purposes, but unless the drug misuse induces dysfunction, it is not abuse.

Overuse: Excessive medical or lay use of a drug, in terms of length of therapy or severity of the disorder treated, but always within the framework of use for diseases in which there is medically accepted evidence of therapeutic effect.

Tolerance: The need to use increasing doses of a drug in order to produce the same effect. This may depend on altered sensitivity in the cell receptor, or increased rates of metabolism of the drug, or changes in cell transmitter substance.

The definitions of terms presented here are not universally accepted. Navaratnam (1982), at the United Nations Research and Training Center in Drug Dependence, combines under "abuse" what is defined here as "misuse" and "abuse".

The substance abuse disorder classification used by the American Psychiatric Association's *Diagnostic and Statistical Manual* (DSM III) distinguishes between *non-pathological substance abuse* and *pathological drug abuse*. A pathological pattern (APA, 1980) includes:

a. A pattern of pathological drug abuse manifested by intoxication throughout the day.

b. Inability to cut down or stop use.

c. Repeated attempts to control use with periods of temporary abstinence or restriction of use to certain times of the day.

d. Continuation of substance abuse despite a serious physical disorder aggravated by the use of the substance.

e. The need for regular use of the substance for adequate functioning.

f. An episode of complications as a result of intoxication (such as alcoholic blackout or opiate overdose).

The World Health Organization has also devised a classification scheme based on patterns:

1. *Experimental use* is defined as short-term, non-patterned trials of a drug. The users are primarily motivated by curiosity and a desire to experience the anticipated effects. Experimental use generally begins among close friends.

2. *Social–recreational* use occurs in social settings among friends or acquaintances wanting to share an experience perceived as acceptable and pleasurable. These "users" primary motivation is social, and use is voluntary.

3. *Circumstantial–situational* use is defined as task-specific, self-limited use which is variably patterned, differing in frequency, intensity and duration. Use is motivated by the perceived need to achieve a known and anticipated drug effect deemed desirable to cope with a specific condition or situation.

4. *Intensified use* is characterized by long-term patterned use of at least one episode a day. Such use is motivated by a perceived need or desire to achieve relief from a persistent problem or stressful situation.

5. *Compulsive use* is characterized by high frequency and high intensity levels of relatively long duration, producing some degree of psychological dependence. The dependence is such that the individual user cannot at will discontinue such use without experiencing physical discomfort or psychological disruption (Smith, 1984).

DEPENDENCE IN THERAPEUTIC USE

Benzodiazepine dependence is significantly different depending on whether it develops during therapeutic treatment or from recreational use. Apparently only a small subgroup of patients who take benzodiazepines chronically for therapeutic indication develop dependency on benzodiazepines (Marks, 1978; Marks, 1983a; Smith & Wesson, 1983; Marks, 1983b). Dependence does not manifest itself while therapy is continued, but becomes apparent, because withdrawal signs and symptoms occur when benzodiazepine treatment is stopped.

The presence of a withdrawal reaction does not necessarily imply dependence. Return of anxiety or insomnia (Morgan & Oswald, 1982; Marks, 1983b) may be the unmasking of symptoms which were being suppressed by the benzodiazepine therapy, the return of the original chronic anxiety (Rickels, Case & Diamond, 1980; Rickels *et al.*, 1983), a pseudo-dependence reaction (Winokur & Rickels, 1981; Marks, 1983b), or the "crutch" phenomenon (Marks, 1983a).

The incidence of dependence depends on the length of continuous use and generally requires three to four months of continuous use to develop. There is concern, however, that rebound insomnia may develop in a matter of weeks to some of the newer, shorter-acting, high potency benzo- diazepines, such as triazolam. Dependence is fostered by daily dosage and probably the concomitant use of alcohol (See Chapter 17).

Pharmacological tolerance with dosage escalation is rare in this type of dependence.

Thus the incidence of benzodiazepine dependence will depend upon prescribing standards, which vary from one country to another. In the United States, long-term benzodiazepine therapy is exceptional (Mellinger & Balter, 1981; Marks, 1983b). In Third World countries, therapy is generally of short duration, although the reason may be more economic than standard of practice. In the United Kingdom and other European countries, long-term benzodiazepine is common (Mellinger & Balter, 1981; Marks, 1983b), and the amount of control by practitioners is less (Marks, 1983b). Some authors believe the incidence of benzodiazepine dependency occurring from therapeutic treatment is greater (Tyrer, Rutherford & Huggett, 1981)

Although studies have documented that misuse and overuse of benzodiazepines occurs (Marks, 1978; Marks, 1983a), the prevalance is not as great as suggested by certain sociologists (Twaddle & Sweet, 1970).

In many countries, including the United States and most of Europe, prescriptions for the benzodiazepines are declining because of growing physician and consumer concern over drug dependence. The initial use is generally justified, and therapeutic use is mainly restricted to those with severe emotional problems (Uhlenhuth, Balter & Lipman, 1978; Mellinger *el al.*, 1978; Marks, 1983a). There is more concern about the extent of the *long-term* use of benzodiazepines in many European countries, although it is recognized that many patients suffer from chronic anxiety states and could not otherwise function in the community (Ayd, 1981; Rickels *et al.*, 1983).

PRIMARY BENZODIAZEPINE ABUSE

On a world-wide basis it is clear that primary benzodiazepine abuse is rare. For example, in the World Health Organization 5th Review of Psychotropic

Substances (1981) there is an unsubstantiated statement that there have been reports of primary benzodiazepine abuse in the Philippines, Australia and Malaysia. One of us (J.M.) has visited the Philippines and in discussions with the police and regulatory authorities was told that benzodiazepine abuse itself is rare and is almost always secondary to use of other drugs of abuse. The isolated reports referred to by the WHO appear to be therapeutic misuse rather than abuse. In that same report (WHO, 1981), Thailand had reported 150 cases of reputed primary benzodiazepine abuse; in contrast, however, during the same time period, there were an estimated 400,000 cases of narcotic abuse in Thailand.

In the WHO 6th review (1982), it is specifically accepted that "very few use benzodiazepines as their primary drug of abuse" (page 10). There is one study (Sellars et al., 1982) in which it would appear on first reading that there are a substantial number of cases of primary benzodiazepine abuse. Close examination reveals, however, that though it is not possible to determine the numbers exactly, most represent either suicide attempts (i.e., single overdose users) or multiple drug abusers.

The international situation related to primary benzodiazepine abuse has also been studied by Navaratnam (1982). He stresses that abuse restricted to a benzodiazepine is rare in most countries and quotes as an example the admission figures for Thanyarak Hospital in Thailand where less than 1% of the addiction admissions were for benzodiazepines. He also quotes the Swiss study by Ladewig (see below) in support of this contention.

In the USA, Ayd (1980) has reported that most long-term single benzodiazepine users do so for therapeutic purposes. Drug treatment programs such as the Haight Ashbury Free Medical Clinic do encounter benzodiazepine dependent patients emanating from both therapeutic initiation and self-medication in the illicit drug culture. In the illicit drug culture, however, the benzodiazepines are not used as a primary drug for euphoria, but are clearly a secondary drug used mainly as a form of self-medication in individuals ranging from methadone maintenance clients to cocaine abusers for self-treating stimulant side effects. The amount of primary abuse of the benzodiazepines in the drug culture is minimal although there has been a growing problem of drugs of deception in which a primary drug of abuse such as methaqualone (Quaalude[R]) is counterfeited using diazepam. In these situations, the individual seeks a Quaalude[R] but, in fact, finds that the street Quaalude[R] containing diazepam produces much less disinhibition and euphoria than does a pharmaceutical Quaalude[R] that contains methaqualone – a shorter-acting, more powerful agent that is highly desired in the drug culture.

Whatever the route to dependence however, the physician must be aware that such dependence can occur and that abrupt cessation of administration is contraindicated and poses substantial risk to the patient. The Haight Ashbury Free Medical Clinic has developed phenobarbital substitution and graded reduction schedules that minimize withdrawal sequelae. Other clinicians gradually reduce the dependence producing benzodiazepine itself, usually in an inpatient setting over a 21–28 day period in order to minimize withdrawal sequelae. Again we stress that the dependence and withdrawal severity is seen mainly in the dependence prone patient, which constitutes approximately 10% of the general population exposed to the benzodiazepines in the therapeutic setting.

Within the United Kingdom too the number of cases of primary benzodiazepine abuse is very small indeed (Marks, 1978; Marks, 1983b) and is accepted by the regulatory authorities as no problem. One particular comment (Prescott, 1983) appears to be relevant in this respect "They are not 'fun' drugs..... In Edinburgh drug takers and pushers often break into chemists' shops. They are very discriminating and clear out all the narcotics, barbiturates, methaqualone and amphetamines but leave the benzodiazepines behind".

In Europe there are four reports that require attention (Allgulander, 1978; Kemper, Poser & Poser, 1980; Van Oefele, Wolf & Ruther, 1983; Ladewig, Banziger & Lowenheck, 1981). The first three of these cover a total of some 600 patients. Unfortunately the information given makes it difficult to assess the exact proportion that represent dependence in therapeutic use, the proportion of multiple drug abuse and those that are single drug primary abusers of benzodiazepines. Examination of the papers however shows that the vast proportion represent multiple drug abusers, confirming that in Europe as in other areas, primary benzodiazepine abuse is rare. The fourth paper, a study in Switzerland by Ladewig considers the incidence on the basis of a questionnaire interview of all Swiss physicians. His criterion of abuse is a strict one similar to that which we have used, though probably also embracing some cases that we would class as misuse. Over 70% of the physicians replied and all those who reported observations of abuse were interviewed by telephone following a structured questionnaire. Having excluded unproven cases and those without adequate evidence, Ladewig found an abuse incidence in Switzerland of 434 patients as shown in Table 1. The 41% of primary benzodiazepine abuse is higher than appears to be the case in most countries. On the other hand 180 such cases in a population of 6.1 million or as Ladewig has calculated, two dependence cases per 100,000 prescriptions for benzodiazepines is low. Risk of individual benzodiazepines followed availability and as Ladewig noted "It was not possible to identify any increase in the inappropriate use of a particular compound. Among those found to be misused were both drugs with short half-life and those with long half-life, so that, from the epidemiological point of view, it is not possible to establish a connection between half-life and abuse risk". This is the conclusion that we have reached from other evidence (Marks, 1983b).

Table 1 Incidence of abuse benzodiazepine in Switzerland. Based on Ladewig. Banziger & Lowenheck, 1981

Primary isolated benzodiazepine abuse	180 patients	41%
Changeover isolated abuse from other drugs	14 patients	
Alcohol plus benzodiazepines	105 patients	59%
Multiple drug abuse	135 patients	
	434 patients	

In addition to the overall international rarity of the reports it is important to note that such cases are not associated with social, public health or medical sequelae and there is no evidence that benzodiazepine users act as agents for the spread of abuse of these drugs (Navaratnam, 1982; Marks, 1983a; Smith & Wesson, 1983).

SECONDARY BENZODIAZEPINE ABUSE

This is the current abuse pattern and benzodiazepine abuse is a feature of the mixed drug abuse found in many countries at the present time. This applies for the alcoholic, for the "middle class, middle aged" user and for the adolescent drug abuser. The exact pattern of the drugs that are used and particularly the primary drug of abuse depends upon a variety of factors which includes the social class of the group (university students compared with drop-outs in the drug culture), local and national fads and fashions and the availability of drugs in the community at any stage, depending on the effectiveness of policing. In many countries and cultures the narcotics are the primary drugs of abuse, though overall it is probable that alcohol represents a much more extensive problem. In other areas the primary drugs of abuse may be marihuana, solvents or hallucinogenic fungi.

In most cases some form of sedative compound is included within the pattern of the drug mixture and at the present time the benzodiazepines are accepted as the most commonly used sedatives in practice. Navaratnam (1982) points out that part of this secondary abuse should be regarded as iatrogenic since it stems from the subsequent abuse of a benzodiazepine that has been prescribed during a doctor's attempt to withdraw another drug (including alcohol). Most however arise in the socio-recreational use area.

Among the secondary benzodiazepine abusers we must also include drug experimenters as opposed to the habitual drug abusers. The proportion of these is currently unknown (Navaratnam, 1982).

The Extent of Abuse of Benzodiazepines Among Known Narcotic Abusers

The first report that attempted to determine the extent of the problem was that of Woody *et al.* (1975). They found that up to 40% of the narcotic abusers with whom they were concerned were "diazepam users", though their report stresses that the proportion of these that were diazepam "misusers", i.e., were using diazepam, however misguidedly. in a therapeutic sense was far from clear. Since that original report there have been numerous studies that have attempted to determine the proportion that are benzodiazepine users within the abuse scene.

One method for assessing this level is by routine urine testing. Primm (1981) reported a low incidence in random urine samples of a population of heroin addicts in Harlem, as did Senay *et al.* (1977) (3%) among a group on methadone maintenance withdrawal in Chicago. Among a group of alcoholics minor tranquilizers were being used by 12.7% prior to treatment (Sokolow *et al.*, 1981). A study of 6000 Los Angeles County probationers (Budd, 1981) revealed 350 benzodiazepine positive urines (about 6%). Of these 350, 58% were associated with other drugs, mainly narcotics. It is not clear however how many of the 147 urines (i.e. about 2.5% of the total population) who showed only a benzodiazepine on urinalysis were receiving them therapeutically. On the other hand, urine testing of patients in one methadone treatment program gives up to 65% positive results for the simultaneous ingestion of benzodiazepines (WHO, 1981). It is interesting to note that this figure, by far the highest of any reported (as much as a 10-fold factor above most surveys) is based on a study in only 29 patients in two centres and that they may well not be typical. Yet it is this high figure which is quoted by WHO (1982). It has also been pointed out that urine test methods are far from reliable because such patients may produce fake urine samples (Dally, 1983).

An alternative method for determining the level of secondary abuse is to take a careful history from patients though this may not always be reliable. In one such study in various USA centres on a group of 427 admissions to drug abuse treatment programs there were 692 mentions of other drug use during the past year (i.e. several used multiple drugs) and of these 195 mentions were benzodiazepines though this does not indicate the proportion of the admissions who had used benzodiazepines (Brown & Chaitkin, 1981). It would however appear that the abuse of benzodiazepines was irregular, for during the month prior to admission there were only 74 mentions of benzodiazepines.

One of the most extensive recent reviews of multiple drug abuse is that of Kornblith (1981). This covers over 30 papers between 1964 and 1978. It is noteworthy that the use of non-barbiturate sedatives (predominantly benzodiazepines) is in nearly all instances less than that of hallucinogens, barbiturates, alcohol and stimulants among primary narcotic addicts. Specifically, contrary to the WHO report (1982), sedative hypnotic abuse was low in methadone maintenance patients (Senay *et al.*, 1977; Newman, 1977; Perkins & Block, 1970; Kornblith & Shollar, 1978).

The Reasons For Use of Benzodiazepines Among Narcotic Abusers

There would appear to be three reasons for the use of the benzodiazepines in the mixed drug abuse situation. In the individual case one or more of these may be operative at any period.

1. As a substitute drug when the narcotic drug of primary dependence is not available.

Attention to this use is specifically referred to in the WHO (1981, 1982) reports and is also stressed in the study by Navaratnam (1982). It is abundantly clear from many clinical studies that the use of benzodiazepines can reduce the unpleasant withdrawal effects from narcotic substances and the use in this context probably represents an attempt to overcome the withdrawal that would be experienced. Those who have abused narcotics extensively always stress that they do not regard the benzodiazepine as a satisfactory equivalent substitute for the narcotic but that it makes the reduced narcotic dose more tolerable. Clinical interviews at the Haight Ashbury Free Medical Clinic of methadone maintenance patients self-administering benzodiazepines and undergoing withdrawal indicated that these patients use the benzodiazepines not for disinhibition and euphoria but for suppression of psychic distress. The group of methadone maintenance clients who have a high degree of underlying psychological distress and self-medicate with the benzodiazepines may be at risk for secondary benzodiazepine dependence. This group is also at high risk for the abuse of alcohol and seem to vary the dosage of their various drugs in order to manage psychic distress. All the evidence suggests that if the narcotic is available at a reasonable price it will be utilised.

Some measure of the substitution preference can be determined from the differential street price, particularly as benzodiazepines are so widely available in the community that they have virtually no scarcity factor in their price. In the San Francisco drug culture, for example, Valium[R] (diazepam) is available, but is used primarily as a secondary drug, selling at a relatively low price (approximately 50 cents per tablet). By contrast, in the same illicit drug culture, a short-acting sedative hypnotic, such as methaqualone or secobarbital, are primary drugs of abuse, and a pharmaceutical Quaalude[R] may sell for as high as $5.00 per tablet.

One other factor that indicates the low preference rating for the benzodiazepines is that while diazepam has been imported illicitly into the USA, it is not sold in the black market as such but is made to imitate methaqualone tablets which sell "at a higher price than that commanded by benzodiazepines" (WHO, 1982).

While we believe that this does give some representation of the preference rating of the substances we would not wish to generalize from one country to another or even more from one city to a different country. As we shall see later there are vast cultural/national differences in the extent of secondary use.

2. As a euphoriant particularly when combined with methadone (WHO, 1981).

Such a euphoriant effect is a feature of the combination rather than of the individual benzodiazepine when taken alone, although there have been reports that certain of the benzodiazepines may themselves be perceived as being euphoriant by those accustomed to drug recreational use. Moreover it is a feature that is only seen to any extent when the dose of the benzodiazepine is escalated well above the normal therapeutic level. This has become a feature of recent abuse in Thailand (Poshyachinda, 1982). It has been suggested (Stitzer et al., 1981) that this potentiating effect may be the result of altered distribution or metabolism of the methadone or of modulation of the central nervous system endorphin systems, but the mechanism involved is not yet known.

3. To reduce the side effects during narcotic abuse.

In particular a benzodiazepine may be used to overcome the anxiety state provoked by a "bad" trip with heroin or amphetamines. Whether such use, and its extent is unknown, should really be regarded as abuse rather than misuse, is a matter for dispute.

The Benzodiazepines That Are Abused

A study in 1978 (Marks, 1978), updated in 1983 (Marks, 1983b), indicates that most if not all the benzodiazepines that are readily available are abused. The actual drugs differ from one country to another and from one time to another. It would appear that this does not depend to any great extent on any clear preference but on such factors as the availability of the substance within the community, and to a certain extent upon the communication within the members of the street drug scene. The factor which may determine some aspect of preference is the rate of absorption from the alimentary canal. Substances that are slowly absorbed are not, on the whole, perceived as exerting a distinguishable effect, while those that are rapidly absorbed and distributed to the central nervous system appear to be preferred.

Among the ones that are reported to be used fairly commonly in many countries are diazepam and nitrazepam. Chlordiazepoxide was one of the substances abused during the 1970s but this particular substance is now only rarely found, possibly because it is not so widely available. Reports from Germany (Kemper, Poser & Poser, 1980) indicate a wider abuse of bromazepam, though this substance which is equally widely available in some other countries does not seem to have the same abuse level there. Flunitrazepam was abused briefly in Italy but a change in legislation in that country rapidly shifted the preference away from this particular substance.

Navaratnam (1982), on the basis of data reported to the United Nations for 1981/1982 found that 22 out of 57 countries indicated the existence of some benzodiazepine abuse, but of these only 16 suggested that there was a problem causing public health concern. The abuse involved 22 different benzodiazepines (if illicit traffic is taken as an indication of abuse).

He stresses that the information relating to the level of abuse is inadequate but that "The data tend to indicate that benzodiazepine abuse is minor compared to the general drug abuse problem or even opiate abuse... several countries stressed that benzodiazepine abuse was a secondary problem component to the problems associated with narcotic drugs". He also notes the variation which exists from one country to another quoting the cases of diazepam in Thailand, flunitrazepam in Singapore, lorazepam in Mauritius and oxazepam in Australia. On the basis of this international experience and of the recent Ladewig study in Switzerland, Navaratnam suggests that the prevalence of abuse bears a close relationship to the market penetration in a country of the various benzodiazepines.

Experience in the Haight Ashbury Free Medical Clinic Drug Detoxification Program has supported Navaratnam's findings. The Clinic has seen an increased incidence of dependence on the newer benzodiazepines and an increase in patients dependent on the newer benzodiazepines after being shifted from some of the older compounds such as diazepam. Although this represents a minority of the total patients receiving diazepam therapy, studies by the Haight Ashbury Free Medical Clinic have indicated that these patients are shifted or initiated on newer benzodiazepine therapy because both they and their physicians erroneously felt that the new benzodiazepines were non-addicting. We stress that the choice of benzodiazepine should be made on therapeutic grounds as all benzodiazepines that are currently available have qualitatively similar physical dependence producing potential. Whether this will apply to the substances that are currently under study which have an agonist–antagonist activity is a matter for conjecture. In addition, all benzodiazepine dependence will respond to the same phenobarbital detoxification schedule.

The question of trying to assess any differences in abuse potential between the different members of the series by animal experimental methods or human studies is considered later.

FORECASTING DRUG ABUSE POTENTIAL AMONG THE BENZODIAZEPINES BY ANIMAL EXPERIMENTAL STUDIES

The general techniques for the assessment of dependence and abuse liability of sedative–hypnotics are reviewed in a World Health Organization Report (1974) and the results of such studies applied to the benzodiazepines have been reviewed in two recent WHO meetings (1981; 1982), by Woods (1983) and by Navaratnam (1982).

In experimental studies in animals using self-administration techniques, it should be noted that by the oral and intragastric routes none of the benzodiazepines demonstrates clear evidence of reinforcement. By the intravenous route some of the benzodiazepines show a higher self-administration rate than the vehicle but the results are not striking or consistent (Navaratnam, 1982; Woods, 1983). When compared with other substances they show greater reinforcement than neuroleptics and antidepressants but less than barbiturates, alcohol, cocaine and narcotics (Griffiths *et al.*, 1981). These studies which show an apparent low risk for the benzodiazepines as a group probably relate to psychological dependence liability and there is no direct evidence that they have relevance to *abuse* risk.

Examination of the conflicting findings, using different methods, demonstrates that there are currently no good techniques by which the *abuse* liability can be assessed, even if there were really valid human data on differential abuse liability to assess the validity of the animal studies in clinical practice. Currently it appears that each of the benzodiazepines that act purely as agonists on the benzodiazepine cell receptors shows a dependence liability and the risk at equivalent dosage appears to be equal. None of these animal techniques appears to give a reliable indication of the abuse risk. A reliable animal model is clearly one of the desirable aims of future research.

FORECASTING DRUG ABUSE POTENTIAL AMONG THE BENZODIAZEPINES BY HUMAN STUDIES

This aspect is also considered in the WHO technical handbook (1975) and the results reviewed in the WHO recent meetings (1981; 1982) and by Woods (1983).

Though such techniques have been well established for the narcotics, there is little reliable information available so far on which the drug abuse potential can be assessed for sedative–hypnotic substances. Moreover such information that is available is difficult to validate when the clinical abuse liability is not clearly defined.

All such studies must now be undertaken on volunteers. It is important to determine the effect on those who are already familiar with the effects of various substances that have been abused rather than on those who have only used a relatively small number of the substances for purely therapeutic purposes or on normals. Certainly the results that have been determined using the different groups of subjects varies widely (Navaratnam, 1982; Woods, 1983).

The methods currently tested fall into two main groups. Firstly, the ability of substances to substitute for other substances of dependence in those who are already dependent. Secondly, a preference rating for the substance in the field of socio-recreational use. The first of these probably gives a reasonable indication of the dependence liability, mainly testing for physical dependence. There is no evidence that the abuse risk is tied directly or closely to the liability to physical dependence only. Indeed the evidence suggests that other factors are also involved. Hence this particular method must be interpreted with considerable caution.

The alternative method appears to offer greater chance of success in determining the abuse risk. The main difficulty lies in the selection of the test group. The perceived effects and the expectations vary between the groups of abusers depending upon their main substance of abuse and the use to which they are putting their secondary substances. Most of the preference rating therefore give a good indication of the preference rating among primary drugs of abuse. The indications are not as clear for drugs of secondary use.

So far as preference studies for benzodiazepines are concerned, one of the earliest was that by Woody, O'Brien & Greenstein (1975). In this study, all three groups (young whites, young blacks and older blacks) placed diazepam very low on their preference rating. Another study (Cole et al., 1982) to determine preference using the Addiction Research Center Inventory as the measure, suggests that though there is an abuse potential for the benzodiazepines it is substantially less than that for methaqualone.

Inpatient volunteers with documented histories of sedative abuse have been extensively studied by the Griffiths group (Griffiths et al., 1980; Griffiths, Bigelow & Liebson, 1979; Griffiths & Bigelow, 1981; Griffiths et al., 1981) with a view to determining drug preferences. Chlorpromazine shows no preference over placebo. For diazepam and pentobarbital these volunteers, familiar with sedative abuse, preferred the higher doses. While the reinforcing efficacy of diazepam was greater than that of chlorpromazine it was significantly less than that of pentobarbital. On the other hand, in outpatients with minimal psychotropic drug experience (Johanson & Uhlenhuth, 1982), there was a definite preference for placebo compared with both 5 and 10 mg diazepam.

Despite the variations between the techniques, the results appear in general to indicate that the benzodiazepines at normal therapeutic dose levels are poor reinforcers when compared to many other sedative-hypnotics in normals (Johanson & Uhlenhuth, 1982) or anxious subjects (de Wit et al., 1982). At higher dose levels in abusers, or in those with insomnia, there is a clear preference for benzodiazepines over placebo but a lower rating than for example the short-acting barbiturates or methaqualone.

When we come to the question of preference rating by this technique between the benzodiazepines themselves, the results are far less clear. At present, it is probably wise to suggest that there are no clear cut and validated studies which give a true indication of any definite preference rating between the various members of the benzodiazepine group (Navaratnam, 1982).

The evidence of the level of abuse, the preference rating, the level of seizures and the pattern of street abuse all indicate that, taken on an international basis, there is no correlation between the level of abuse and the degree of sedation among the benzodiazepines, the rate of elimination or the lipid solubility. There is indeed no consistent finding suggesting that the abuse liability of any individual benzodiazepine is greater than another. This is also the conclusion reached by Navaratnam (1982).

BEHAVIORAL EFFECTS OF BENZODIAZEPINE ABUSE

The WHO report comments that the abuse of the benzodiazepines leads to a "striking deterioration in personal care and in social interactions" though it gives no references in support of this statement. It is not clear from the context of the statement whether this personal neglect refers to the very few cases of primary abuse of the benzodiazepines or whether to benzodiazepine abuse which comes secondary to abuse of other substances. If the latter, then the conclusion is open to considerable doubt in interpretation for there is "considerable deterioration" associated with the drugs of primary dependence in the majority of such cases. To ascribe differences to the benzodiazepine component is probably not justified on the basis of the currently available evidence.

Examination of the literature reveals little evidence to support the view expressed by the WHO and in the absence of references from WHO there would appear to be considerable doubt whether this statement can be substantiated. For example, Ladewig, Banziger & Lowenheck (1981) in Switzerland in a group that he designated isolated benzodiazepine abuse, i.e., those with primary abuse of only a benzodiazepine, found that there were both positive and negative consequences of the abuse. Positive consequences were the ability to work and social stabilization. Negative consequences were irritability, increased fatigability and loss of interest. In the other group designated as representing secondary benzodiazepine abuse (i.e., multiple drug abuse), Ladewig noted that there were significantly more negative consequences. Particular mention is made of the markedly increased risk of traffic accidents and at work.

It has been suggested (Lader, Ron & Petursson, 1984) that the long term use of benzodiazepines can lead to cortical atrophy of the type that is associated with alcohol abuse. The study by Lader is an uncontrolled one and in a study published by Poser *et al.* (1983) it is reported that this finding could not be substantiated. With all central nervous system depressant compounds this is clearly a fact that requires attention but so far there has not been any clear evidence that it occurs. Moreover, it has been suggested that there may be a deterioration in cognitive skills with the long term use (or abuse) of the benzodiazepines. Here again evidence is far from clear at present.

It is abundantly clear that like all central nervous system active drugs that can lead to disinhibition, the benzodiazepines can lead to adverse behavioural reactions in a very small proportion of people. Perhaps the most extensively catalogued reaction is the paradoxical rage reaction. Whether this is an idiosyncratic reaction is a matter of dispute. What is clear is that these reactions are no more prevalent or florid in those who use the benzodiazepines within the framework of socio-recreational use than in the therapeutic field, particularly when the different personality of the two groups is taken into account.

Within the socio-recreational drug using group, it is clear that some measure of cross-fertilization of benzodiazepine use must be a feature, otherwise it is difficult to understand the high percentage of users that are reported in some clinics. There is no evidence on the other hand that such people encourage abuse outside that particular circle similar to the way narcotics are pushed outside the circle of immediate users.

Another interesting feature of benzodiazepine abuse is the lack of evidence that it leads to the abuse of other drugs. As we have repeatedly stressed this is not a drug of primary abuse but is used almost entirely in a secondary fashion among existing drug abusers.

ABUSE DIFFERS SIGNIFICANTLY FROM THERAPEUTIC DEPENDENCE

As we have noted earlier, there have been suggestions that dependence under therapeutic use and socio-recreational abuse are merely facets of one single drug dependence phenomenon. This we strongly dispute for the following reasons:

1. Though it is true that those who develop dependence during therapeutic use are often those who have been found to be dependent on other sedative substances (either alcohol or hypnotics), therapeutic dependence only extremely rarely leads on to socio-recreational abuse in the case of the benzodiazepines, whereas it is an all too common feature with the narcotics.

2. Dose escalation is very rare during therapeutic dependence but is common during the abuse situation.

3. Since almost all the cases of benzodiazepine abuse come within the type of secondary rather than primary abuse the group of people involved differs significantly from that of the therapeutic long users.

A SOCIO-MEDICAL APPRAISAL OF BENZODIAZEPINE ABUSE

From all the data we reviewed, we draw the following conclusions about the nature of benzodiazepine abuse:

1. It is typically secondary in nature to various other substances of primary abuse.

2. It occurs as the sedative component of mixed drug abuse with the following features:

   a. It may be used to reduce the unwanted effects of the primary drug of abuse.

   b. It may be used as a substitute for narcotics when narcotics are unavailable or to reduce narcotic withdrawal symptoms.

Drug abuse is a multifactorial and complex interaction which involves the personality of the individual, the environmental situation in which the individual is placed and the pharmacological effects of the drugs themselves. The pharmacological effects of the drugs are but one factor and perhaps only a relatively small one. People who abuse drugs for socio-recreational purposes do not readily give up the habit in its entirety but substitute alternative drugs with a clear preference rating for their substitution.

All physicians who prescribe benzodiazepines, however, must be familiar with their dependence producing potential, particularly in high-risk, dependence prone individuals. The therapeutic benefits must be weighed objectively against the potential for abuse and dependence before initiating benzodiazepine therapy.

SUMMARY AND CONCLUSIONS

The current international situation on dependence and abuse of benzodiazepines is reviewed on the basis of the authors' own experience and a critical appraisal of the literature. The following conclusions are drawn:

1. Dependence can occur during therapeutic use with a time/dose relationship; the longer the time of administration, the lower the dose to produce dependence. Dependence is rare with short courses of treatment. The level may rise to a substantial figure after more than one year of continuous administration.

2. The risk of dependence is increased in those with known predisposition to dependence and in the relatives of those with an alcohol problem.

3. Abuse of benzodiazepines is a small problem in a few countries. It is nearly always secondary to abuse of other drugs and the level and pattern of abuse is variable from one country to another.

4. There are significant differences between the dependence in therapeutic use and abuse for socio-recreational purposes. There is evidence that one very rarely leads on to the other.

5. The extent of benzodiazepine dependence and abuse has been overstated by the media.

References

Allgulander C: Dependence on sedative and hypnotic drugs: A comparative clinical and social study. *Acta Psychiat Scand* 1978;270(Suppl).

American Psychiatric Association: *Diagnostic and Statistical Manual of Mental Disorders*, ed.2. Washington, DC, APA, 1980.

Ayd FJ: Benzodiazepines: social issues: misuse and abuse. *Psychosomatics* 1980;21(suppl):21-25.

Ayd FJ: Diazepam – the question of long-term therapy and withdrawal reactions. *Drug Ther* 1981;Special Supplement.

Ayd FJ: Benzodiazepine dependence and withdrawal. *J Psychoactive Drugs* 1983;15:67-70.

Brown BS, Chaitkin L: Use of stimulant/depressant drugs by drug abuse clients in selected metropolitan areas. *Int J Addict* 1981;16:1473-1490.

Budd RD: The use of diazepam and of cocaine in combination with other drugs by Los Angeles county probationers. *Am J Drug Alcohol Abuse* 1981;8:249-255.

Cohen S: Valium: its use and abuse. *Drug Abuse Alcohol Newsl* 1976;5.

Cole JO, Orzack MH, Benes FM, *et al*: Subjective effects of benzodiazepines and methaqualone in recreational sedative users. *Psychopharmacol Bull* 1982;18:87-96.

De Wit H, Johanson CE, Uhlenhuth EH, *et al*: The effects of two non-pharmacological variables on drug preference in humans. Read before the CPPD Meeting, Toronto, June, 1982.

Griffiths RR, Bigelow GE: Human self-administration of sedative and stimulant drugs. *Psychopharmacol Bull* 1981;17:138-140.

Griffiths RR, Bigelow GE, Liebson I: Human drug self-administration: double-blind comparison of pentobarbital, diazepam, chlorpromazine and placebo. *J Pharmacol Exp Ther* 1979;210:301-310.

Griffiths RR, Bigelow GE, Liebson I, *et al*: Drug preference in humans: double-blind choice comparison of pentobarbital, diazepam and placebo. *J Pharmacol Exp Ther* 1980;215:649-661.

Griffiths RR, Lucas S, Bradford LD, *et al*: Self-injection of barbiturates and benzodiazepines in baboons. *Psychopharmacol* 1981;75:101-109.

Hayner G, Inaba D: A pharmacological approach to outpatient benzodiazepine detoxification. *J Psychoactive Drugs* 1983;15:99-104.

Hollister LE: Principles of therapeutic applications of benzodiazepines. *J Psychoactive Drugs* 1983;15:41-44.

Johanson CE, Uhlenhuth EH: Drug preferences in humans. *Fed Proc* 1982;41:228-233.

Kemper N, Poser W, Poser S: Benzodiazepin-Abhangigkeit. *Dtsch Med Wochenschr* 1980;105:1707-1712.

Kornblith AB: Multiple drug abuse involving nonopiate, nonalcoholic substances: I. Prevalence. *Int J Addict* 1981;16:197-232.

Kornblith AB, Shollar E: The effect of chronic medical conditions in methadone maintenance patients on the course of their rehabilitation, in Smith D (ed): *A Multicultural View of Drug Abuse: Proceedings of the National Drug Abuse Conference.* Cambridge, Mass. Schenkman, 1978.

Lader M, Ron M, Petursson H: Computed axial brain tomography in long-term benzodiazepine users. *Psychol Med* 1984;14:203-206.

Ladewig D, Banziger W, Lowenheck M: Tranquilizer abuse – results of a nationwide Swiss survey. *TGO tijdschrift voor beneesmiddelenonderzoek* 1981;6:1132-1137.

Marks J: *The Benzodiazepines: Use, Overuse, Misuse, Abuse?* Lancaster, MTP Press, 1978.

Marks J: The benzodiazepines: an international perspective. *J Psychoactive Drugs* 1983a;15:137-149.

Marks J: Benzodiazepines – for good or evil. *Neuropsychobiology* 1983b;10:115-126.

Mellinger GD: Use of licit drugs and other coping alternatives: some personal observations on the hazards of living, in Lettiere DJ (ed): *Drugs and Suicide – When Other Coping Strategies Fail.* Beverly Hills, CA, Sage Publications, 1978.

Mellinger GD, Balter MB: Prevalence and patterns of use of psychotherapeutic drugs: results from a 1979 national survey of American adults. Read before the International Seminar on the Epidemiological Impact of Psychotropic Drugs, Milan, June 24-26, 1981.

Mellinger GD, Balter MB, Manheimer DI, *et al*: Psychic distress, life crisis and the use of psychotherapeutic medications. *Arch Gen Psychiatry* 1978;35:1045-1052.

Morgan K, Oswald I: Anxiety caused by a short-life hypnotic. *Br Med J* 1982;284:942.

Navaratnam V: Impact of scheduling drugs under the 1971 Convention on Psychotropic Substances – the benzodiazepines reappraised. United Nations Research and Training Centre in Drug Dependence, National Drug Research Centre, Univ Science Malaysia, Minden, Penang, Malaysia 1982.

Newman RG: *Methadone Treatment in Narcotic Addiction: Program Management, Findings and Prospects For the Future.* New York, Academic Press, 1977.

Newsome J, Seymour R: Benzodiazepines and the treatment of alcohol abuse. *J Psychoactive Drugs* 1983;15:97-98.

Perkins Abuse Advisory Committee, Rockville, MD, May 15, 1981.

Rickels K: Benzodiazepines in the treatment of anxiety: North American experience, in Costa E (ed): *The Benzodiazepines: From Molecular Biology to Clinical Practice*. New York, Raven Press, 1983, pp 295-310.

Rickels K, Case WG, Diamond L: Relapse after short-term drug therapy in neurotic outpatients. *Int Pharmacopsychiatry* 1980;15:186-192.

Rickels K, Case G, Downing R, *et al*: Long-term diazepam therapy and clinical outcome. *J Am Med Assoc* 1983;250:767-771.

Sellers EM, Marsham JA, Kaplan HL, *et al*: Acute and chronic drug abuse emergencies in Metropolitan Toronto. *Int J Addict* 1981;16:283-303.

Senay EC, Harvey WH, Oss JN, *et al*: Adjunctive drug use by methadone patients. *Am J Drug Alcohol Abuse* 1977;4:533-541.

Smith DE: Introduction: the benzodiazepines. *J Psychoactive Drugs* 1983;15:1-8.

Smith DE, Wesson DR: Benzodiazepine dependency syndromes. *J Psychoactive Drugs* 1983;15:85-96.

Smith DE: Substance abuse disorders: drugs and alcohol. In: *Review of General Psychiatry*, Lange Medical Publishers, Los Altos, 1984, pp 278-297.

Sokolow L, Welte J, Hynes G, *et al*: Multiple substance use by alcoholics. *Br J Addict* 1981;76:147-158.

Stitzer ML, Griffiths RR, McLellan AT, *et al*: Diazepam use among methadone maintenance patients: patterns and dosages. *Drug Alcohol Depend* 1981;8:189-199.

Twaddle AC, Sweet RH: Characteristics & experiences of patients with preventable hospital admission. *Soc Sci Med* 1970;4:141-145.

Tyrer P, Owen R, Dawling S: Gradual withdrawal of diazepam after long-term therapy. *Lancet* 1983;1:1402-1406.

Tyrer P, Rutherford D, Huggett T: Benzodiazepine withdrawal symptoms and propranolol. *Lancet* 1981;1:520-522.

Uhlenhuth EH, Balter MB, Lipman RS: Minor tranquilizers: clinical correlates of use in an urban population. *Arch Gen Psychiatry* 1978;35:650-655.

Van Oefele K, Wolf B, Ruther E: Poster presentation at 4th International Cong Sleep Res, Bologna, Italy, July 18-22, 1983.

WHO: Expert Committee on Drug Dependence. Sixteenth Report, World Health Org Tech Rep Ser No 407, Geneva, WHO, 1969.

WHO: Evaluation of dependence liability and dependence potential of drugs: Report of a WHO Scientific Group. Tech Rep Series No 577, Geneva, WHO, 1975.

WHO: Report of the Fifth World Health Organisation Review of Psychoactive Substances for International Control. Geneva, WHO, November 16-20, 1981.

WHO: Report of the Sixth World Health Organisation Review of Psychoactive Substances for International Control. Geneva, WHO, September 6-10, 1982.

Winokur A, Rickels K: Withdrawal and pseudo-withdrawal from diazepam therapy. *J Clin Psychiatry* 1981;42:442-444.

Woods JH: Experimental abuse liability of benzodiazepines. *J Psychoactive Drugs* 1983;15:61-66.

Woody GE, O'Brien CP, Greenstein R: Misuse and abuse of diazepam – an increasingly common medical problem. *Int J Addict* 1975;10:843-848.

14
Experimental Abuse Liability Assessment of Benzodiazepines

James H. Woods, PhD

The topic of this article is the experimental psychology and experimental pharmacology of benzodiazepines as applied to their abuse liability assessment.[1] The issues of physiological and psychological dependence on benzodiazepines are considered to be separate topics and will be examined as such.

Physiological dependence indicates a particular state of an organism during drug treatment such that discontinuation of treatment is followed by the development of a time-limited withdrawal reaction that can be prevented by continuing drug administration or reversed by resuming administration following interruption. Important in the definition is the time-limited nature of the withdrawal syndrome: in chronic drug treatment of certain disorders, discontinuation of medication may lead to the reappearance of those symptoms that originally indicated the need for medication. These symptoms, which may persist indefinitely following termination of drug treatment, should not be considered part of the withdrawal syndrome.

Physiological dependence is often contrasted with behavioral or psychological dependence. *Psychological dependence* is characterized by a tendency to repeatedly seek and self-administer a drug. Often, the term psychological dependence is used to denote a condition not necessarily involving physiological dependence, but characterized by a craving for a drug or drug effect that fulfills some psychological need of the individual. Much of what is connoted by the term is unnecessary in the evaluation of the behavioral effects of psychological dependence.

In terms of both historical descriptions and the current scientific view, the essential feature of psychological dependence is continued drug seeking or self-administration. Additionally, the most important aspect of drug self-administration is reinforcement, a process in which the probability that a person will engage in a particular behavior is increased or maintained by an environmental event that follows the behavior. For example, if changing physicians leads to drug procurement and this behavior becomes more frequent, then changing physicians may be said to be an instance of reinforced drug-seeking behavior. In addition, the act of taking the drug itself may be said to be reinforced by the drug effect, if, for example, the drug capsules are taken more frequently than placebo capsules. Obviously, in most clinical or experimental settings, drug-taking behavior is not attended to in great detail. Some of the experiments described below, however, were designed specifically to examine that behavior.

Finally, distinct from the definitions of physiological and psychological dependence is abuse liability. The *abuse liability* of a compound is defined as its capacity to produce physiological or psychological dependence in conjunction with the capacity to alter behavior in a manner that is detrimental to the individual or his/her social environment.

Two different kinds of procedures can be used to evaluate physiological dependence in animals. One procedure assesses cross-dependence between compounds: it assesses the capacity of one compound to suppress withdrawal from dependence on another compound. For instance, a barbiturate can be used to induce dependence in an animal, and once reliable measures of the withdrawal syndrome from the barbiturate have been established, another drug can be studied in terms of its capacity to suppress the syndrome in this animal. The second kind of procedure used to study physiological dependence in animals consists of the assessment of direct dependence to a compound following its chronic administration. This may be a more appropriate procedure than the assessment of cross-dependence. That is to say, the majority of cross-dependence studies in animals has found that indeed there is some cross-dependence among various kinds of propanediols, alcohol, barbiturates and benzodiazepines. However, some recent studies of direct- and cross-dependence suggest that these findings of cross-dependence may have overgeneralized the similarities among some of these compounds.

These recent studies have been reported by Martin, McNicholas and Cherian (1982) at the University of Kentucky. These investigators noted some differences in withdrawal signs seen after repeated administration of diazepam or pentobarbital. The signs that were specific to withdrawal from these drugs in rats were seizures and grand mal convulsions for pentobarbital, and what the authors called "explosive awakenings" (a rigid jump or turn that propelled the rat against the sides of the cage) for diazepam. Martin and colleagues concluded that the withdrawal syndromes produced by the two drugs were qualitatively different, though not as a result of differences in the pharmacokinetics of the drugs. They found that the most compelling argument for the qualitative nature of the difference was that while each drug partially suppressed the withdrawal syndrome of the other, the effects reached a plateau in their dose-effect evaluation. Thus, pentobarbital completely suppressed, in a dose-related manner, its own withdrawal syndrome. In contrast, the maximal extent to which diazepam suppressed pentobarbital withdrawal occurred at a dose of 10 mg/kg, and a four-fold increase in dose failed to produce any further suppression of withdrawal. Thus, despite the apparent cross-dependence of benzodiazepines and barbiturates, these investigators demonstrated an incomplete cross-dependence between pentobarbital and diazepam. What distinguishes these observations from those of previous investigators is that Martin and colleagues described the entire withdrawal syndrome in precise and detailed terms, whereas previous investigators tended to draw inferences about a state of dependence or cross-dependence based on observations of a single sign of withdrawal.

The largest series of studies to date on benzodiazepine dependence in animals has been conducted by Tomoji Yanagita (1981) at the Central Institute for Experimental Animals in Kawasaki, Japan. In these experiments, which have been carried out in Rhesus monkeys, withdrawal severity has been assigned three different grades. The first is a mild withdrawal syndrome, indicated by apprehension, hyperirritability, mild tremor, anorexia and piloerection. These signs continue in intermediate withdrawal, which is more specifically recognized by aggravated tremor, rigidity, impaired motor performance, retching, vomiting and a considerable amount of weight loss. The most severe withdrawal that can be observed is indicated by grand mal convulsions and some indication of delirium (as inferred from behavior directed toward what appears to be imaginary objects in the environment), nystagmus, some dissociation from the environment and a substantial hyperthermia. Thus, as the severity of the syndrome increases, signs of withdrawal include more extensive pathophysiology.

Based on his studies of the vast majority of benzodiazepines that are on the market in this country, in Europe and other parts of the world, as well as a number of experimental compounds, Yanagita concludes that all of the benzodiazepines are capable of producing at least mild and intermediate withdrawal syndromes. These experiments demonstrated qualitative and quantitative differences in the dependence produced respectively by benzodiazepines and barbiturates. Furthermore, they demonstrated that all the benzodiazepines studied to date apparently share the ability to produce some degree of physiological dependence. If there were qualitative differences among the benzodiazepines in this regard, it seems reasonable to assume that they would have emerged in Yanagita's studies.

Henry Swain (personal communication, 1982) at the University of Michigan has made some interesting observations relevant to low-dose physiological dependence. These contrast with Yanagita's studies, which tend to use very large doses of compounds, attempting to obtain very high levels of intoxication. Swain's experiments, on the other hand, used small doses: an eighth or a quarter of a milligram per kilogram of diazepam, delivered subcutaneously every 6 hours over a 5-month period, after which an examination of behavioral change was conducted over a 10-day period. Withdrawal signs were found under these conditions. The signs observed were twitching, tremor, irritability, some peculiar posture of the monkeys and considerable abdominal tenderness. These signs appeared on the first day, became slightly more severe on the second and third days, and persisted for a period of up to 10 days. These data suggest that there is a mild withdrawal syndrome from these lower doses of diazepam.

These data further present the opportunity, with the use of the recently described benzodiazepine antagonists, of designing experiments that approximate therapeutic dose conditions and might allow some of the issues described by Leo Hollister (1983) regarding the actual variables associated with dependence development at therapeutic dose levels to be unraveled.

There appears to be little doubt that chronic administration of high doses of some benzodiazepines can result in physiological dependence in humans, as demonstrated by withdrawal signs that can appear in approximately 4 to 10 days and continue up to 2 weeks (Hollister *et al.*, 1963; Hollister, Motzenbecker & Degan, 1961). Clearly documented instances of dependence development to therapeutic doses of benzodiazepines have also been provided by Winokur and colleagues (1980), although apparently only a small percentage of patients may actually develop such dependence. It is quite unclear as to what causes some people to develop dependence to therapeutic doses, although the possibility that concurrent or prior alcohol abuse may predispose to such dependence should be considered and evaluated.

Although such studies usually emphasize the capacity of benzodiazepines to produce physiological dependence, they do not indicate what the significance of this dependence might be. People who develop dependence often discover that fact for themselves only when they attempt to terminate drug administration. Thus, the state of physiological dependence is not a consequence of compulsive drug seeking with concomitant escalation of drug intake. Although the discomfort of withdrawal may prompt the individual to consider resuming drug administration, this distress could possibly be minimized with proper instruction on gradual reduction of drug dosage. Reports on benzodiazepine withdrawal rarely indicate that patients request more drugs.

The basic procedures for evaluating psychological dependence, as defined previously, consist of self-administration studies in animals and humans. This entails training an animal to make a specific response that will deliver the drug in some way: making the drug available either as a fluid for oral consumption or through an intragastric or intravenous cannula. With respect to these routes of administration, it is very interesting to note that the accumulated evidence makes it very difficult to contend that any of the benzodiazepines act as reinforcers when delivered by either the oral or the intragastric route of administration, which obviously represent the routes of most relevance to therapeutics as well as to virtually all cases of abuse. From the point of view of the scientists who study drug self-administration, the intravenous route is the best, in that animals will on occasion self-administer benzodiazepines when delivered intravenously. But even here, the results are not particularly striking. In these experimental procedures, it is difficult to induce amounts of drug by self-administration sufficient to produce significant degrees of intoxication.

The best evidence for strong reinforcing effects in animal self-administration procedures comes from studies (e.g., Lukas & Griffiths, 1982) of 2 short-acting benzodiazepines. One is midazolam, a compound that is being evaluated for potential use in anesthesia, and the other is triazolam.

Comparisons in animal studies suggest that barbiturates of intermediate or ultrashort durations of action are more often effective reinforcers in some experimental situations than any of the benzodiazepines. In direct preference studies, or in studies in which the rate of response is used as a measure of the strength of the reinforcing effect, barbiturates of equivalent duration of action tend to show a much stronger reinforcing effect (Griffiths et al., 1981).

Steven Paul (personal communication, 1982) has suggested that differences in receptor mechanisms might, in part, underlie differences in the pharmacological effects of benzodiazepines and barbiturates. Such receptor differences may be related to the differences in reinforcing properties of benzodiazepines and barbiturates. For the present, however, this is simply speculation.

There have been very few formal studies of human benzodiazepine self-administration. These have virtually been completely restricted to studies of diazepam and they have been of different types: either drug preference studies in normal volunteer subjects with significant sedative drug self-administration histories, or studies in special populations of patients, such as those in psychiatric wards or methadone patients.

First, in normal human subjects, a study done by Johanson and Uhlenhuth (1980) at the University of Chicago compared preference for diazepam in three different doses to a placebo. The same study also included amphetamine as a positive control. The subjects were given color-coded capsules on four occasions and asked to fill out questionnaires regarding mood states at various times after the drug administration. After experiencing each drug or placebo condition twice, subjects participated in five sessions at which they could choose between the capsules while other conditions remained the same. Diazepam was not selected in more than 50 percent of the trials in any of these sessions. In some preference tests, a placebo was chosen more often than diazepam. Nevertheless, amphetamine was preferred significantly to the placebo. Diazepam produced significant subjective effects that appeared to reflect decreases in vigor and arousal, and increases in fatigue or confusion.

The same investigative team (DeWit *et al.*, 1982) did some followup experiments with diazepam in anxious subjects and the results were no more positive than they were with normal subjects. That is to say, small doses of diazepam cannot really be said to be reinforcing in the sense that they would produce a preference. At large doses, placebo is preferred to diazepam. The point here is that in anxious subjects (at least those without histories of sedative abuse) it is difficult to show a reinforcing effect, despite the fact that diazepam reduces reported anxiety.

In sedative abusers, there have been two types of experiments involving either measurement of the direct maintenance of a response by a benzodiazepine or those involving measurement of a drug preference (a measurement of the capacity of the benzodiazepine to maintain self-administration behavior relative to another substance). In one study (Griffiths, Bigelow & Liebson, 1979), subjects had to ride a bicycle to produce the opportunity to self-administer 1 of the 2 doses (10 or 20 mg) of oral diazepam. Diazepam very weakly and transiently maintained self-administration behavior, but the behavior was much better maintained by 90 mg of pentobarbital. Preference studies (Griffiths *et al.*, 1980) in sedative abusers show that when diazepam is offered at the very high doses required to produce subjective effects comparable to those of pentobarbital at intermediate doses, there is a very clear preference for pentobarbital over diazepam in virtually all comparisons. These findings support the animal data rather convincingly.

Other studies, though not formal studies of drug self-administration, suggest that when patients in psychiatric wards or chronically anxious outpatients are allowed to self-regulate their doses of benzodiazepines, they tend to be reduced over long periods of time (e.g., in the range of 6 months). Finally, while there are a variety of case reports that indicate that high doses of benzodiazepines are indeed self-administered, these are almost invariably in the context of multiple drug use. It is difficult to draw the conclusion that the benzodiazepine involved is indeed the major culprit.

In conclusion, these experiments, taken as a whole, lead to a rather conservative view of the abuse liability of the various benzodiazepines. The amount of information on dependence liabilities of the increasing number of benzodiazepines varies quite dramatically among members of the class. Far more is known about the older members than about those that are very new, which makes it particularly difficult to draw rational, reasonable comparisons across members of the class when reviewing the literature.

As mentioned previously, all of the benzodiazepines show some capacity to produce physiological dependence. Even for the oldest compounds, about which there is considerable literature, there seems to be no compelling evidence that the dependence liability of these drugs is associated with significant individual or social detriment: abuse liability. In the absence of such evidence, it seems most appropriate to balance assessment of the risk of benzodiazepine abuse with evaluation of the public health and social benefits that accompany appropriate benzodiazepine use.

NOTE

1. This article is excerpted from a larger review that this author conducted together with two colleagues in pharmacology at the University of Michigan, Jonathan Katz and Gail Winger. One purpose of the review was for presentation to a World Health Organization committee on international drug control during their deliberations with respect to scheduling benzodiazepines under the United Nations Convention on Psychotropic Substances.

References

DeWit H, Johanson CE, Uhlenhuth EH, *et al*: The effects of two non-pharmacological variables on drug preference in humans. Paper presented at CPDD Meetings, Toronto, June 1982.

Griffiths RR, Bigelow GE, Liebson I: Human drug self-administration: double-blind comparison of pentobarbital, diazepam, chlorpromazine and placebo. *J Pharmacol Exp Ther* 1979;210:301-310.

Griffiths RR, Bigelow GE, Liebson I, *et al*: Drug preferences in humans: double-blind choice comparison of pentobarbital, diazepam and placebo. *J Pharmacol Exp Ther* 1980;215:649-661.

Griffiths RR, Lukas SE, Bradford LD, *et al*: Self-injection of barbiturates and benzodiazepines in baboons. *Psychopharmacology* 1981;75:101-109.

Hollister LE: Principles of therapeutic applications of benzodiazepines. *J Psychoactive Drugs* 1983;15:1-2.

Hollister LE, Bennett JL, Kimbell I, *et al*: Diazepam in newly admitted schizophrenics. *Dis Nerv Syst* 1963;24:746-750.

Johanson CE, Uhlenhuth EH: Drug preference and mood in humans: diazepam. *Psychopharmacology* 1980;71:269-273.

Lukas SE, Griffiths RR: Comparison of triazolam and diazepam in self-administration by the baboon. *Pharmacologist* 1982;24:133.

Martin WR, McNicholas LF, Cherian S: Diazepam and pentobarbital dependence in the rat. *Life Sci* 1982;31:721-737.

Winokur A, Rickels K, Greenblatt DJ, *et al*: Withdrawal reaction from long-term, low dosage administration of diazepam. *Arch Gen Psychiatry* 1980;37:101-105.

Yanagita T: Dependence-producing effects of anxiolytics, in Hoffmeister F, Stille G (eds): *Psychotropic Agents. Part II: Anxiolytics, Gerontopsychopharmacological Agents, and Psychomotor Stimulants*. New York, Springer-Verlag, 1981.

15
Abuse Liability of Benzodiazepines: A Review of Human Studies Evaluating Subjective and/or Reinforcing Effects

Roland R. Griffiths, PhD
John D. Roache, PhD

This chapter reviews human experiments pertinent to the abuse liability of benzodiazepines. These studies assess subjective and/or reinforcing effects in subjects with histories of drug abuse (Table 1). This review is limited to the assessment of reinforcing and/or subjective effects; no attempt is made to analyze the possible contribution of physiological dependence or the role of adverse effects. In the first section, methodological issues that bear on the assessment of the abuse liability of benzodiazepines are discussed. Section II reviews experiments in which benzodiazepines have been systematically compared to placebo; Section III reviews studies which compare benzodiazepines and phenothiazines; Section IV reviews studies comparing benzodiazepines and barbiturates; and Section V reviews comparisons between different benzodiazepines.

I. METHODOLOGICAL AND SUBJECT POPULATION CONSIDERATIONS

That there is some abuse liability associated with the benzodiazepines is suggested by numerous documented case reports of abuse and "psychological dependence" (cf. Marks, 1978). However, the limitations of an analysis based on case reporting are substantial. The best validated human experimental approach for providing information about the abuse liability of drugs is to utilize placebo controlled, double-blind methodologies to

Table 1 Human experiments assessing subjective and/or reinforcing effects of benzodiazepines in subjects with histories of drug abuse.

Agents examined	Dosage range	Study population	Study type	Primary dependent measures	Reference
Triazolam (TZ) Zopiclone (Z)	TZ: 0.25 mg Z: 3.75mg	Male alcoholic inpatients recently detoxified	Within-subject drug comparisons. Self-administration; multiple daily doses. Also, subject choice of TZ vs. Z.	Drug preference	Bechelli et al.,1983
Triazolam (TZ) Zopiclone (Z)	TZ: 0.25 mg Z: 3.75 mg	Male alcoholic inpatients recently detoxified	Within-subject drug comparisons. Self-administration: multiple daily doses. Also, subject choice of TZ vs. Z.	Subjective reports Drug preference	Boissl et al., 1983
Diazepam (DZ) Prazepam (PZ) Methaqualone (M) Placebo (PL)	DZ: 10 mg PZ: 20 mg M: 200–400 mg	Male and female casual sedative users	Two separate within-subject drug comparisons: DZ vs. PZ vs. PL, and M vs. PL.	Subjective reports	Cole et al., 1982a
Diazepam (DZ) Buspirone (B) Methaqualone (M) Placebo (PL)	DZ: 10–20 mg B: 10–40 mg M: 300 mg	Male and female casual sedative users	Within-subject drug comparisons: DZ vs. B vs. M vs. PL.	Subjective reports	Cole et al., 1982b
Diazepam (DZ) Lorazepam (LZ) Placebo (PL)	DZ: 10–40 LZ: 1.5–6.0 mg	Male recreational sedative users	Between-group drug comparisons with two groups: DZ vs. PL, and LZ vs. PL.	Subjective reports	Funderburk et al., 1983a

Drugs	Doses	Subjects	Design	Measures	Reference
Clorazepate (CZ) Diazepam (DZ) Lorazepam (LZ) Placebo (PL)	CZ: 7.5 mg DZ: 5.0 mg LZ: 1.0 mg	Male recreational sedative users	Between-group drug comparisons with four treatment groups: CZ, DZ, LZ, and PL.	Subjective reports	Funderburk et al., 1983b
Diazepam (DZ) Chlorpromazine (C) Pentobarbital (PB) Placebo (PL)	DZ: 10–20 mg C: 25–50 mg PB: 30–90 mg	Male drug users – documented histories	Single-subject design with data grouped into four treatment groups: DZ, C, PB, and PL. Drug self-administration multiple daily doses.	Self-administration rates	Griffiths, Bigelow, and Liebson, 1979
Diazepam (DZ) Pentobarbital (PB) Placebo (PL)	DZ: 50–100 mg PB: 200–400 mg	Male drug users – documented histories	Between-group drug comparisons with two groups: DZ vs. PL, and PB vs. PL.	Subjective reports	Griffiths et al., and Liebson, 1983
Diazepam (DZ) Pentobarbital (PB) Placebo (PL)	DZ: 50–400 mg PB: 200–900 mg	Male drug users – documented histories	Single-subject design: within-subject comparisons of DZ vs. PL, or PB vs. PL. Also within-subject drug comparisons and subject choice of DZ vs. PB vs. PL.	Subjective reports Drug preference	Griffiths et al., 1980
Diazepam (DZ) Oxazepam (OX) Placebo (PL)	DZ: 10–160 mg OX: 30–480 mg	Male drug users – documented histories	Within-subject drug comparisons: DZ vs. OX vs. PL.	Subjective reports	Griffiths et al., 1984a

211

Diazepam (DZ) Oxazepam (OX) Placebo (PL)	DZ: 40–160 mg OX: 480 mg	Male drug users – documented histories	Within-subject drug comparisons and subject choice of DZ vs. OX vs. PL. Three DZ doses (40, 80, 160 mg) were compared to a single dose of OX (480 mg) using between-group comparisons.	Subjective reports Drug preference Epidemiological data on DZ and OX abuse	Griffiths et al., 1984b
Diazepam (DZ) Pentobarbital (PB)	DZ: 2–40 mg PB: 30–50 mg	Male and female drug-dependent inpatients hospitalized for treatment	Single-subject design: within-subject choice of DZ vs. DZ or DZ vs. PB. Self-administration; multiple choices daily.	Drug preference	Healey and Pickens, 1983
Diazepam (DZ) Halazepam (HZ) Placebo (PL)	DZ: 20–40 mg HZ: 160–320 mg	Male alcoholic inpatients recently detoxified	Balanced incomplete block design for comparisons between drug doses: DZ, HZ, and PL.	Subjective reports	Jaffe et al., 1983
Chlordiazepoxide (CD) Diazepam (DZ) Pentobarbital (PB) Placebo (PL)	CD: 50–200 mg DZ: 10–40 mg PB: 120–240 mg	Male alcoholic and sedative users	Two separate within-subject drug comparisons: CD vs. PB vs. PL, and DZ vs. PB vs. PL.	Subjective reports	Jasinski et al., 1982

Chlordiazepoxide (CD) Pentobarbital (PB) Placebo (PL)	CD: 100–400 mg PB: 120–240 mg	Male alcoholic and sedative users	Within-subject drug comparisons: CD vs. PB vs. PL.	Subjective reports	Jasinski et al., 1983
Diazepam (DZ) Prazepam (PZ) Placebo (PL)	DZ: 10 mg PZ: 20 mg	Male and female casual sedative users	Within-subject drug comparisons: DZ vs. PZ vs. PL.	Subjective reports	Orzack et al., 1982
Diazepam (DZ) Oxazepam (OX) Triazolam (TZ) Pentobarbital (PB) Placebo (PL)	DZ: 10–160 mg OX: 30–480 mg TZ: 0.5–3.0 mg PB: 100–600 mg	Male drug users – documented histories	Two separate within-subject drug comparisons: DZ vs. OX vs. PL, and TZ vs. PB vs. PL.	Subjective reports	Roache and Griffiths 1983

characterize subjective effects and/or behavioral reinforcing properties in subjects with histories of drug abuse. This approach, pioneered by the U.S. Addiction Research Center of the National Institute on Drug Abuse starting more than 40 years ago, has been used to assess opioids (Jasinski, 1977), psychomotor stimulants (Griffith, 1976), and sedative–hypnotics (Fraser & Jasinski, 1977). With this experimental approach, the abuse liability of a drug is inferred from the ability of a drug: 1) to serve as a reinforcer (i.e. increase the probability of behavior which results in its administration), and/or 2) to produce pleasant subjective effects, sometimes called "euphoria" or "liking". Reinforcing effects can be assessed by using various drug self-administration procedures, while pleasant ("euphoric") subjective effects can be assessed by using various scale or item-based questionnaires. Because the term "euphoria" is defined differently in different studies, the term will be used in the present review only to indicate a "pleasant" subjective state. Although it is sometimes explicitly or implicitly assumed that the reinforcing effect of a drug is causally dependent on the subjective effects, such assumptions can be reasonably questioned (Schuster, Fischman & Johanson, 1981), and no position on this issue is taken in this review.

The appropriateness of using subjects with histories of drug abuse to assess the abuse liability of drugs is supported by its face validity as well as by the results of several experiments. One set of studies (Beecher, 1959) showed that there was a closer correspondence between experimental result and clinical observation when studies were conducted with "post-addict" populations rather than with "normals" or "patient populations". In these studies, normals and patients hospitalized for chronic disease consistently rated amphetamine as producing a fairly strong euphoric effect whereas heroin, morphine, pentobarbital, and placebo were all similarly rated as less euphoric or unpleasant. The "post-addict" subjects also rated amphetamine as producing euphoric effects but, in contrast to the other populations, these subjects rated the opioids as producing euphoric subjective effects. Studies with college students and full-time employees have also shown that normal volunteers may have a preference for amphetamine-induced effects rather than effects produced from sedatives or tranquilizers. In a series of experiments in which normal volunteers were allowed to choose between color-coded drug options, 5 mg *d*-amphetamine was consistently preferred to placebo or diazepam whereas placebo was preferred to 5 or 10 mg diazepam (Johanson & Uhlenhuth, 1980). The authors speculated that the lack of diazepam choice in these subjects may have been due to sedative effects of diazepam being an undesirable feature in students and individuals with daytime behavioral and cognitive requirements.

II. COMPARISONS OF BENZODIAZEPINES WITH PLACEBO

Using adequately controlled, double-blind experimental designs, fourteen studies compared a benzodiazepine to placebo in subjects with histories of drug abuse (Griffiths, Bigelow & Liebson, 1979, 1983; Griffiths *et al.*, 1980, 1984a, 1984b; Jasinksi *et al.*, 1982, 1983; Cole *et al.*, 1982a, 1982b; Orzack *et al.*, 1982; Jaffe *et al.*, 1983; Funderburk *et al.*, 1983a, 1983b; Roache & Griffiths, 1983). The results indicate that benzodiazepines produce reinforcing effects (i.e., maintain self-administration) and/or produce subjective effects indicating some abuse liability. These results have been obtained with a variety of different benzodiazepines (diazepam, triazolam, oxazepam, prazepam, halazepam, lorazepam, and chlordiazepoxide), representing compounds with different pharmacokinetic profiles (fast vs. slow onset; fast vs. slow elimination) and compounds used for different clinical indications (anxiolytic and hypnotic). No study that examined a reasonable range of doses failed to demonstrate such reinforcing/subjective effects of benzodiazepines.

III. COMPARISON OF BENZODIAZEPINES WITH PHENOTHIAZINES

The sensitivity of the human experimental methods in the evaluation of reinforcing/subjective effects of benzodiazepines is established using a pharmacologically inactive, negative control such as a placebo. However, it is also important to examine the effects induced by a pharmacologically *active*, negative control because it is plausible that subjects with histories of drug abuse may self-administer or indicate a liking for virtually any psychoactive substance, independently of actual abuse liability. One study tested this possibility by comparing diazepam to chlorpromazine, a drug considered to have little or no abuse liability.

Diazepam vs. chlorpromazine. In the one study which has used a pharmacologically active negative control (Griffiths, Bigelow & Liebson, 1979), subjects with histories of sedative drug abuse were allowed to orally self-administer placebo, diazepam (up to 100 or 200 mg per day in different groups of subjects), or chlorpromazine (up to 250 or 500 mg per day in different groups of subjects) for up to 15 consecutive days. Although both drugs produced subjective effects and observable signs of sedative intoxication, chlorpromazine was similar to placebo in that it did not maintain self-administration; diazepam showed dose-related increases in self-administration.

These results comparing diazepam and chlorpromazine are consistent with animal drug self-administration data and clinical information about the abuse of these drugs. Studies with non-human primates have shown that benzodiazepines, including diazepam, maintain modest self-administration in contrast to chlorpromazine which does not maintain self-administration

(Yanagita & Takahashi, 1973; Griffiths *et al.*, 1981). Clinically, there have been numerous documented cases of diazepam abuse (cf., Marks, 1978) while chlorpromazine abuse, in contrast, is almost nonexistent. The good correspondence between the human experimental results and the preclinical and clinical information help validate the human methods.

IV. COMPARISON OF BENZODIAZEPINES WITH PENTOBARBITAL OR METHAQUALONE

Eight studies have compared reinforcing/subjective effects of several benzodiazepines with those of the short-acting barbiturate, pentobarbital, and two studies have made limited comparisons of diazepam to methaqualone.

Diazepam vs. pentobarbital. Five studies compared the subjective/reinforcing effects of diazepam to pentobarbital administered orally to subjects with histories of sedative drug abuse. Using a double-blind crossover design, Jasinski *et al.* (1982) showed that diazepam produced typical pentobarbital-like subjective effects (including increases in a "euphoria" scale), with the onset, peak, and duration of effects similar for both diazepam (10, 20, and 40 mg) and pentobarbital (120 and 240 mg). Relative potency determinations indicated that diazepam was 10 times more potent than pentobarbital.

Another study (Healey & Pickens, 1983) utilized single subject designs and analysis to examine self-administration of diazepam and pentobarbital. Male and female drug-dependent subjects were told to self-administer unrestricted numbers of doses on an *ad libitum* basis in order to "remain comfortable and prevent withdrawal symptoms"; however, subjects were only allowed free access to drugs as long as they did not become intoxicated. In this study, subjects were allowed to select between a standard compound (diazepam and pentobarbital) and one of several doses of diazepam. Unfortunately, there were no orderly dose-related effects on preference across subjects. When given a choice between pentobarbital and several doses of diazepam, subjects most often alternated between the two available options. The inconsistency across subjects, the absence of placebo controls, and the instructional limitations on drug self-administration, make conclusions about relative reinforcing effects of diazepam and pentobarbital difficult to draw from this study.

In a third study (Griffiths, Bigelow & Liebson, 1983), different groups of subjects were given single daily doses of diazepam (50 or 100 mg) or pentobarbital (200 or 400 mg) for 5 consecutive days. Using a subject-rated liking scale, both drugs produced similar degrees of liking. However, diazepam, but not pentobarbital, produced dose-related decreases in staff ratings of subjects' mood and social interactions and increases in hostility and complaining, thus suggesting a possible "dysphoric" component to the diazepam effect.

The final two studies clearly suggest that diazepam has a lower abuse liability than pentobarbital. Using single subject designs and analysis, two groups of subjects received a substantially wider range of doses (than former studies) of diazepam (50–400 mg) and pentobarbital (200–900 mg), and a third group received both diazepam (200 mg) and pentobarbital (400 mg) for within–subject comparisons (Griffiths et al., 1980). In the across-group dose–effect comparison, pentobarbital consistently produced greater subject ratings of drug liking than diazepam. When subjects were allowed repeated opportunities to choose between different dose levels of drug, subjects in the pentobarbital group preferred higher doses over lower doses in contrast to the subjects from the diazepam group who did not consistently prefer higher doses of diazepam over lower doses. When the group of subjects receiving both drugs was allowed repeated opportunities to choose between 200 mg of diazepam and 400 mg of pentobarbital, all 6 subjects preferred the pentobarbital. In another study (Griffiths, Bigelow & Liebson, 1979), part of which has been described previously, subjects were allowed to orally self-administer placebo, diazepam (up to 100 or 200 mg per day in different groups of subjects) or pentobarbital (up to 300 or 900 mg per day in different groups of subjects) for up to 15 consecutive days. Both diazepam and pentobarbital maintained self-administration above placebo levels with the higher dose of each associated with higher average rates of self-administration than the lower dose. The high dose of pentobarbital was associated with higher rates of self-administration than the high dose of diazepam, again indicating the relatively greater reinforcing effectiveness of pentobarbital.

In conclusion, two studies found diazepam to be less reinforcing and/or to display reduced euphoric subjective effects in comparison to pentobarbital (Griffiths, Bigelow & Liebson, 1979; Griffiths et al., 1980). The apparent discrepancy between these studies and the three reports which did not show a relatively reduced euphoric/reinforcing effect of diazepam (Jasinski et al., 1982; Healey & Pickens, 1983; Griffiths, Bigelow & Liebson, 1983) may partly be a consequence of the doses selected for comparison. Additionally, differences in doses and dosing frequency may have resulted in different degrees of drug tolerance and/or accumulation of nordiazepam, the active metabolite of diazepam. The roles of tolerance development and nor-diazepam accumulation in the effects of repeated diazepam dose schedules are discussed in Griffiths et al., 1984a. The overall conclusion from these studies, that diazepam produces less euphoric/reinforcing effects than pentobarbital, is supported by: 1) the finding that no comparative study has shown a greater abuse liability of diazepam; 2) two studies have found a distinctly reduced abuse liability of diazepam; and 3) one study found diazepam produced deleterious changes in mood and behavior which plausibly could reduce the chronic self-administration of the drug.

Chlordiazepoxide vs. pentobarbital. Using the same double-blind, crossover design used in the diazepam/pentobarbital comparison, Jasinski *et al.* (1982, 1983) conducted two separate studies comparing pentobarbital (120 and 240 mg) and chlordiazepoxide (either 50, 100 and 200 mg or 100, 200, and 400 mg). The results showed that onset, peak and duration of chlordiazepoxide and pentobarbital were similar and both drugs produced elevations on a measure of euphoria. Except for the euphoria scale, valid relative potencies were obtained on all measures; pentobarbital was 2 times more potent than chlordiazepoxide. With the euphoria scale, chlordiazepoxide produced a flat dose–response curve suggesting that the abuse liability of chlordiazepoxide is less than that of pentobarbital.

Triazolam vs. pentobarbital. Using a double-blind Latin square design in subjects with histories of sedative drug abuse, Roache & Griffiths (1983) compared the effects of placebo, triazolam (0.5, 1.0, 2.0 and 3.0 mg) and pentobarbital (100, 200, 400 and 600 mg). The two drugs produced similar dose-related effects on area under the time–action curve (AUC) data from a variety of performance measures (psychomotor performance, digit-symbol substitution performance, staff ratings of drug effect); statistically valid relative potency estimates were obtained indicating triazolam was approximately 200 times more potent than pentobarbital. With subjective measures of drug effect and drug liking (AUC), however, valid relative potency estimates could not be obtained because, even though triazolam produced elevations in subjective effects and liking, pentobarbital produced substantially greater increases than did triazolam. This study, therefore, suggests that the abuse liability of triazolam is less than pentobarbital.

Diazepam vs. methaqualone. Using double-blind, crossover designs, two studies have compared diazepam with methaqualone. In one study, a single dose of diazepam (10 mg) was compared to placebo in one group of subjects and methaqualone (200 and 400 mg) was compared to placebo in another group of subjects (Cole *et al.*, 1982a). While statistical comparisons between the two drugs were not reported, the authors concluded that methaqualone produced greater increases in a euphoria measure and an abuse potential scale. In a second study, 2 doses of diazepam (10 and 20 mg) were compared with methaqualone (300 mg) (Cole *et al.*, 1982b). Although methaqualone and 20 mg diazepam were not statistically different on a euphoria measure, methaqualone did produce greater estimates of monetary street value and greater subject ratings on a visual analog scale on which subjects rated whether they "would definitely enjoy taking the drug again". Both of these studies should be considered preliminary because of the limited number of low doses examined. The results, however, suggest that diazepam may have a lower abuse liability than methaqualone.

The overall conclusion from this set of studies, that pentobarbital has greater abuse liability than several benzodiazepines, is consistent with preclinical, clinical and epidemiological information about relative abuse liability. First, intravenous and intragastric drug self-administration experiments with non-human primates have shown that short-acting barbiturates (including pentobarbital) are more effective than benzodiazepines (including diazepam and chlordiazepoxide) in maintaining self-administration (Yanagita & Takahashi, 1973; Griffiths *et al.*, 1981). Although the quickly eliminated benzodiazepines (midazolam and triazolam) maintain higher levels of self-injection than do benzodiazepines that are slowly eliminated or have active metabolites that are slowly eliminated (e.g., diazepam), these quickly eliminated compounds do not maintain the high consistent levels of self-injection maintained by short-acting barbiturates such as pentobarbital (Griffiths *et al.*, 1981, 1984c; Lukas & Griffiths, 1982). Second, clinicians familiar with drug abuse patients estimate that the "euphoria" produced by the short-acting barbiturates (including pentobarbital) is greater than that produced by diazepam and chlordiazepoxide (Wesson & Smith, 1977). Finally, epidemiological measures which are presumed to reflect actual drug abuse, uniformly rank the short-acting barbiturates (including pentobarbital) higher than the benzodiazepines (Jones, 1977; Cooper, 1977; Marks, 1978). As in the previous section, the good correspondence between the human experimental results and these various assessments of abuse liability support the validity of the human methods.

V. COMPARISON OF DIFFERENT BENZODIAZEPINES

Studies comparing diazepam with 6 other benzodiazepines (oxazepam, halazepam, lorazepam, chlordiazepoxide, prazepam, and clorazepate) suggest there are meaningful differences among benzodiazepines with respect to reinforcing/subjective effects.

Oxazepam vs. diazepam. Two studies have directly compared the subjective/reinforcing effects of diazepam and oxazepam using within-subject designs. One study systematically examined the effects of a wide range of diazepam (10–160 mg) and oxazepam (30–480 mg) doses using a double-blind, crossover design in which the order of exposure to the 2 drugs was counterbalanced across subjects (Roache & Griffiths, 1983; Griffiths *et al.*, 1984a). Dose effects with area under the time–action curve (AUC) data showed the 2 drugs produced similar effects on a variety of psychomotor, cognitive, staff-rated, and subjective measures. Determinations of relative potencies across measures showed diazepam to be relatively more potent than oxazepam in producing drug liking (5.68 times more potent) than in producing psychomotor and cognitive impairment (2.72 and 2.57 times more potent, respectively). Diazepam produced greater peak effects than oxazepam on a number of staff and subject rated measures, including drug liking. An analysis of time course showed that onset of effect was more rapid and time to maximal effect was shorter with diazepam (1–2 hr) than with oxazepam (4–12 hr). Diazepam was categorized as producing barbiturate-like subjective effects (38.3%) more frequently than was oxazepam (13.8%), while oxazepam was identified as placebo more often than diazepam (50% vs. 21.6%, respectively). Repeated administration of 160 mg diazepam and 480 mg oxazepam showed that AUC liking was greater for diazepam than oxazepam.

In a second study (Griffiths *et al.*, 1984b), the effects of and preference for placebo, oxazepam (480 mg) and diazepam (40, 80 and 160 mg) were examined. Under double-blind conditions and in counterbalanced order, subjects were given initial exposure to letter-coded drugs and then were exposed to a series of choice days on which subjects chose between 2 available drug alternatives. With this method, 3 sets of multiple 2-drug choices enabled the examination of subject preference for placebo, 480 mg oxazepam, and one of three doses of diazepam (40, 80 and 160 mg). Compared with oxazepam, diazepam produced greater drug liking (AUC), peak liking and euphoria, and was judged to be of greater monetary street value. Diazepam was categorized as producing barbiturate-like subjective effects more frequently than was oxazepam (54% vs. 21%), while oxazepam was identified as placebo more often than diazepam (32% vs. 4%). Diazepam was associated with a more rapid onset of effect than was oxazepam, and this rapid onset was repeatedly cited by subjects in post-study written comments as being a desirable feature of the drug effect. In the choice tests, 80 and 160 mg diazepam were preferred to 480 mg oxazepam on 62.5% and 91.7% of the choice tests, respectively. In the choice tests between drug and placebo, placebo was never preferred to diazepam (0%) while placebo was preferred to oxazepam on 21.4% of choice tests.

Overall, the results of these studies suggest that diazepam has a higher abuse liability than oxazepam. This conclusion is indicated by several measures including: relative potency comparisons, peak effect and time course analysis, estimated street value, drug identification, and finally by a demonstrated preference for diazepam when subjects were given a choice. In a double-blind crossover study with normal volunteers, Bliding (1974) showed that, relative to diazepam, oxazepam is slowly absorbed and associated with less intense or delayed onset of behavioral effects. The author speculated that the slow onset of action of oxazepam might be expected to reduce its appeal as a drug of abuse. The comments of subjects in the preference study (Griffiths *et al.*, 1984b), confirmed that the rapid onset of diazepam's action was, in fact, a desirable feature. The overall conclusions from these two studies are also compatible with an analysis of epidemiological data (Griffiths *et al.*, 1984b) showing that diazepam abuse uniformly exceeds oxazepam abuse on seven epidemiological measures of drug abuse (e.g. emergency room and medical examiner mentions, Drug Enforcement Administration (DEA) illicit drug cases, DEA theft and loss reports).

Chlordiazepoxide vs. diazepam. No study has compared the reinforcing/subjective effects of diazepam and chlordiazepoxide directly. However, Jasinski *et al*. (1982, 1983) conducted a set of 3 experiments, which has been described previously, in which diazepam and chlordiazepoxide were compared separately to pentobarbital using a double-blind crossover design. Relative to diazepam and pentobarbital, chlordiazepoxide produced a flat dose–response curve on the euphoria scale. The authors concluded that there may be qualitative differences between diazepam and chlordiazepoxide. The suggestion that diazepam may have a greater abuse liability than chlordiazepoxide is consistent with both preclinical and clinical observations. First, the authors of a drug self-administration study in monkeys concluded that diazepam was a more effective reinforcer than was chlordiazepoxide (Yanagita & Takahashi, 1973). Second, clinicians familiar with drug abuse patients estimate that the "euphoria" produced by diazepam is greater than that produced by chlordiazepoxide (Wesson & Smith, 1977).

Halazepam vs. diazepam. Using a double-blind, balanced, incomplete (3-way crossover) block design, Jaffe *et al*. (1983) compared the subjective effects of orally administered placebo, halazepam (160 and 320 mg), and diazepam (20 and 40 mg) in alcoholic subjects who had recently completed treatment of alcohol withdrawal. Examination of time-course showed that time to peak subjective effect was shorter with diazepam than with halazepam. Diazepam produced dose-related increases in a euphoria scale; the low dose of halazepam produced only modest increases in euphoria while the high dose was not different from placebo. Generally similar results were obtained with a visual analogue scale of drug liking; diazepam produced dose-related increases while only the high dose of halazepam produced significant increases in liking. Although the generality of the results of this study are limited because of the narrow (2-fold) dose range of the two drugs tested, the study suggests that halazepam may have a lower abuse liability than diazepam.

Lorazepam vs. diazepam. A parallel-group, double-blind design was used to compare diazepam (0, 10, 20 and 40 mg) and lorazepam (0, 1.5, 3 and 6 mg) on a series of psychomotor, cognitive and subjective tasks in subjects with histories of "recreational" sedative use (Funderburk *et al*., 1983a). Similar dose-related effects of the two drugs were reported on a drug-liking scale as well as a set of cognitive and psychomotor tasks. Lorazepam, however, tended to produce effects of longer duration than diazepam. The fact that the two drugs produce similar elevations in drug liking suggests that the abuse liability of lorazepam is similar to that of diazepam.

221

In a second study by these investigators (Funderburk *et al.*, 1983b), a parallel group design was used to compare the effects of placebo and therapeutic doses of diazepam (5 mg), lorazepam (1.0 mg) and clorazepate (7.5 mg) alone and in combination with alcohol in subjects with histories of "recreational" use of sedative drugs. The portion of the study relevant to relative abuse liability involved the morning administration of the drug without alcohol and the assessment of behavioral and subjective effects over a subsequent 4-hour period. The results showed that lorazepam and diazepam produced significantly higher subjective ratings of liking than did clorazepate and placebo. Although the use of only single dose levels is a serious limitation of this study, the results with diazepam and lorazepam are consistent with the previous study which examined a 4-fold range of doses suggesting that diazepam and lorazepam have similar abuse liability.

Clorazepate vs. diazepam. As previously described, Funderburk *et al.*, (1983b) conducted a study using a parallel group design to compare the effects of placebo and therapeutic doses of diazepam (5 mg), lorazepam (1.0 mg), and clorazepate (7.5 mg) in subjects with histories of "recreational" use of sedative drugs. Clorazepate did not produce increases in subjective ratings of drug-liking and drug effect in contrast to diazepam and lorazepam which did. Unfortunately, examination of only single dose levels of drugs provides insufficient grounds for drawing meaningful general conclusions about the relative abuse liability of clorazepate.

Prazepam vs. diazepam. Using a double-blind crossover design, a single dose of prazepam (20 mg) was compared to placebo and 10 mg diazepam (Cole *et al.*, 1982a; Orzack *et al.*, 1982). On a variety of subjective measures of sedation, both diazepam and prazepam produced effects different from placebo but the two drugs were not differentiable from each other. Both drugs tended to produce increases on a euphoria measure but the effects were not significantly different from placebo. While these data suggest that prazepam may produce effects similar to diazepam, no meaningful conclusions can be drawn because only a single low dose of both drugs was examined.

Triazolam vs. zopiclone. Two studies used similar experimental designs to compare the reinforcing effects of the benzodiazepine triazolam with zopiclone, a nonbenzodiazepine hypnotic with a putative site of activity at the benzodiazepine receptor (Bechelli *et al.*, 1983; Boissl *et al.*, 1983). Using a double-blind crossover design, chronic alcoholics who had just completed withdrawal treatment were permitted to self-administer capsules of either 0.25 mg triazolam or 3.75 mg zopiclone. After exposure to both color-coded treatments over the first 4 days of the experiment, subjects were permitted to choose which treatment (drug) they would receive on the next 2 days. Although significantly more subjects chose triazolam than zopiclone (25 vs. 15) in the Bechelli *et al.* study, this effect was not replicated in the Boissl *et al.* study (22 vs. 18). The implications of these results are quite limited. The lack of dose manipulations substantially limits the possible conclusion from the Bechelli study that triazolam is a more efficacious reinforcer than zopiclone. Furthermore, in absence of a placebo control, one cannot conclude with certainty that triazolam served as a positive reinforcer in this study. Finally, the failure to replicate the choice results in a similarly designed experiment further reduces confidence in the results.

VI. CONCLUSIONS

Over the last 4 years, human experimental studies have been conducted in subjects with histories of sedative drug abuse which provide information about the relative abuse liability of benzodiazepines. When compared to placebo, it is clear that benzodiazepines produce reinforcing effects and/or subjective effects indicating some liability for abuse. Studies comparing benzodiazepines (diazepam, chlordiazepoxide and triazolam) to pentobarbital (a drug widely accepted as having significant abuse liability) have suggested that pentobarbital has greater abuse liability than the benzodiazepines. One study also suggested that methaqualone may have a greater abuse liability than diazepam. A study comparing diazepam to chlorpromazine (a drug widely accepted as having little or no abuse liability) suggested that chlorpromazine has less abuse liability than diazepam. These results with pentobarbital and chlorpromazine correspond well to both animal drug self-administration data and clinical information about the relative abuse of benzodiazepines, barbiturates and phenothiazines, thus validating the human experimental methods.

Using these same methods, a series of studies has compared different benzodiazepines. Although conclusions from some studies have been limited because only a narrow range of doses was investigated, the results to date suggest that there are meaningful differences among benzodiazepines; lorazepam has been suggested to have an abuse liability similar to diazepam, while oxazepam, halazepam, and chlordiazepoxide may have abuse liability less than diazepam. The data on clorazepate, prazepam, triazolam, and zopiclone are too limited to draw any conclusions.

Acknowledgements

Preparation of this paper was supported in part by National Institute on Drug Abuse grants DA-01022 and DA-01147.

References

Bechelli LP, Navas F, Pierangelo SA: Comparison of the reinforcing properties of zopiclone and triazolam in former alcoholics. *Pharmacology* 1983;27:Supp2:235-241.

Beecher HK: *Measurement of Subjective Responses: Quantitative Effects of Drugs*. New York: Oxford University Press, 1959.

Bliding A: Effects of different rates of absorption of two benzodiazepines on subjective and objective parameters. *Eur J Clin Pharmacol* 1974;7:201-211.

Boissl K, Dreyfus JF, Delmotte M: Studies on the dependence-inducing potential of zopiclone and triazolam. *Pharmacology* 1983;27:Supp2:242-247.

Cole JO, Orzack MH, Benes FM, et al: Subjective effects of benzodiazepines and methaqualone in recreational sedative users. *Psychopharmacol Bull* 1982a;18:87-96.

Cole JO, Orzack MH, Beake B, et al: Assessment of the abuse liability of buspirone in recreational sedative users. *J Clin Psychiatry*, 1982b;43:69-74.

Cooper JE (ed): *Sedative-Hypnotic Drugs: Risks and Benefits*. DHEW Publication No. (ADM) 78-592. Washington, DC, U.S. Government Printing Office, 1977.

Fraser HF, Jasinski DR: The assessment of the abuse potentiality of sedative/hypnotics (depressants): methods used in animals and man, in Martin WR (ed): *Handbook of Experimental Pharmacology*. New York, Springer-Verlag, 1977, vol 45, pp 589-612.

Funderburk F, Griffiths RR, Bigelow G, et al: Behavioral differentiation of anxiolytic medication. Paper presented at the annual meeting of International Study Group Investigating Drugs as Reinforcers, Lexington, Kentucky, June 1983b.

Funderburk F, McLeod D, Griffiths RR, et al: Diazepam (DZ) and lorazepam (LZ): Comparison of behavioral and subjective effects. *The Pharmacologist* 1983a;25:199.

Griffith JD: Structure-activity relationships of several amphetamine-like drugs in man, in Ellinwood EH, Jr, Kilbey MM (eds): *Cocaine and Other Stimulants*. New York, Plenum Press, 1976, pp 705-715.

Griffiths RR, Lamb RJ, Roache JD, et al: Relative abuse liability of triazolam: experimental assessment in animals and humans. In press, 1984c.

Griffiths RR, Bigelow GE, Liebson I: Human drug self-administration: double-blind comparison of pentobarbital, diazepam, chlorpromazine and placebo. *J Pharmacol Exp Ther* 1979;210:301-310.

Griffiths RR, Bigelow GE, Liebson I: Differential effects of diazepam and pentobarbital on mood and behavior. *Arch Gen Psychiatry* 1983;40:865-873.

Griffiths RR, Bigelow GE, Liebson I, et al: Drug preference in humans: double-blind choice comparison of pentobarbital, diazepam and placebo. *J Pharmacol Exp Ther* 1980;215:649-661.

Griffiths RR, Lukas SE, Bradford LD, et al: Self-injection of barbiturates in baboons. *Psychopharmacology* 1981;75:101-109.

Griffiths RR, McLeod DR, Bigelow GE, et al: Relative abuse liability of diazepam and oxazepam: behavioral and subjective dose effects. *Psychopharmacology* (in press) 1984a.

Griffiths RR, McLeod DR, Bigelow GE, et al: Comparison of diazepam and oxazepam: preference, liking and extent of abuse. *J Pharmacol Exp Ther* 1984b;229:501-508.

Healey ML, Pickens RW: Diazepam dose preference in humans. *Pharmacol Biochem Behav* 1983;18:449-456.

Jaffe JH, Ciraolo DA, Nies A, et al: Abuse potential of halazepam and of diazepam in patients recently treated for acute alcohol withdrawal. *Clin Pharmacol Ther* 1983;34:623-630.

Jasinski DR: Assessment of the abuse potentiality of morphine-like drugs (methods used in man), in Martin WR (ed): *Handbook of Experimental Pharmacology*. New York, Springer-Verlag, 1977, vol 45, pp 197-258.

Jasinski DR, Haertzen CA, Henningfield JE, et al: Progress report of the NIDA Addiction Research Center, in Harris LS (ed): *Problems of Drug Dependence 1981: Proceedings of the 43rd Annual Scientific Meeting, The Committee on Problems of Drug Dependence, Inc.* National Institute on Drug Abuse Research Monograph No 41, National Technical Information Service No (TD) 82-190760. Washington, DC, U.S. Government Printing Office, 1982, pp 45-52.

Jasinski DR, Henningfield JE, Johnson RE: Progress report of the NIDA Addiction Research Center, Baltimore, Maryland, 1982, in Harris LS (ed): *Problems of Drug Dependence 1982: Proceedings of the 44th Annual Scientific Meeting, The Committee on Problems of Drug Dependence, Inc.* National Institute on Drug Abuse Research Monograph No 43, DHHS Publication No (ADM) 83-1264. Washington, DC, U.S. Government Printing Office, 1983, pp 92-98.

Johanson CE, Uhlenhuth EH: Drug preference and mood in humans: diazepam. *Psychopharmacology* 1980;71:269-273.

Jones BE: Predicting abuse liability of depressant drugs, in Thompson T, Unna K (eds): *Predicting Dependence Liability of Stimulant and Depressant Drugs*. Baltimore, University Park Press, 1977, pp 35-46.

Lukas SE, Griffiths RR: Comparison of triazolam and diazepam self-administration by the baboon. *The Pharmacologist* 1982;24:133.

Marks J: *The Benzodiazepines – Use, Overuse, Misuse, Abuse*. Baltimore, University Park Press, 1978.

Orzack MH, Cole JO, Ionescu-Pioggia M, et al: A comparison of some subjective effects of prazepam, diazepam and placebo, in Harris LS (ed): *Problems of Drug Dependence 1981: Proceedings of the 43rd Annual Scientific Meeting, The Committee on Problems of Drug Dependence, Inc.* National Institute on Drug Abuse Research Monograph No 41, National Technical Information Service No (TD) 82-190760. Washington, DC, U. S. Government Printing Office, 1982, pp 309-317.

Roache JD, Griffiths RR: Effects of diazepam (DZ), oxazepam (OX), triazolam (TZ), and pentobarbital (PB) on objective and subjective measures: assessment of abuse liability. *The Pharmacologist* 1983;25:214.

Schuster CR, Fischman MW, Johanson CE: Internal stimulus control and subjective effects of drugs, in Thompson T, Johanson CE (eds): *Behavioral Pharmacology of Human Drug Dependence*. National Institute on Drug Abuse Research Monograph No 37, DHHS Publication No (ADM) 81-1137. Washington, DC, U. S. Government Printing Office, 1981, pp 116-129.

Wesson DR, Smith DE: *Barbiturates: Their Use, Misuse and Abuse*. New York, Human Sciences Press, 1977.

Yanagita T, Takahashi S: Dependence liability of several sedative-hypnotic agents evaluated in monkeys. *J Pharmacol Exp Ther* 1973;185:307-316.

16
Acute and Chronic Toxicity of Benzodiazepines

Donald R. Wesson, MD
Susan Camber, MA

Benzodiazepines have a remarkably low frequency of allergic reactions, organ toxicity and overdose lethality. Acute toxicity is produced by drug interactions, idiosyncratic reactions, and overdose. Chronic toxcitity results from accumulation of the benzodiazepine or metabolites, from tolerance to therapeutic effects with subsequent escalation of dosage, and from the development of benzodiazepine dependence. As the benzodiazepine dependency syndromes and their treatment are described in detail in Chapter 17, they will not be addressed here.

DRUG INTERACTIONS

Additive Effects

The central nervous system depressant effects of ethyl alcohol and benzodiazepines are additive (Hansten, 1979). The combination can impair driving skills beyond that of a given level of blood alcohol – a fact of significant forensic consequences. Physicians should warn their patients to whom they prescribe benzodiazepines about the hazards of drinking alcohol while they are taking benzodiazepines. The sedative effects of benzodiazepines are also at least additive with barbiturates and other sedative–hypnotics. As with alcohol, the combination of a benzodiazepine and another sedative–hypnotic can be lethal in doses of drugs which would not be lethal if each were taken alone.

Metabolic Considerations

In the elderly and the very young, metabolism of desmethyldiazepam (the intermediate metabolite of diazepam, prazepam, chlordiazepoxide and clorazepate) is decreased, and desmethyldiazepam may accumulate.

As noted in detail in Chapter 17, benzodiazepines cross the placenta and are excreted in breast milk. An infant, who was nursed by a mother regularly taking 4–6 mg/day of diazepam, was dosed by the breast milk with both diazepam and desmethyldiazepam. The infant's serum was found to have 46 ng/ml of desmethyldiazepam which shows that even if the mother is using diazepam at low therapeutic levels the infant can be exposed to significant amounts of benzodiazepines (Wesson, Camber, *et al.*, 1985).

Some medications interact with benzodiazepines to decrease their rate of metabolism. For example, cimetidine (Tagamet R) inhibits demethylation of long-acting benzodiazepines (Desmond *et al.*, 1980), however cimetidine does not affect the duration of action of short-acting benzodiazepines (Klotz & Reimann, 1980).

Medications can also increase the rate of benzodiazepine metabolism. Oral contraceptive steroids containing estrogen significantly decrease diazepam half-life (Abernathy *et al.*, 1982).

ACUTE OVERDOSE

Because of their widespread availability, benzodiazepines are often ingested in accidental overdoses, suicidal gestures, and overdoses with suicidal intent. The low lethality of benzodiazepines is an important advantage over their sedative–hypnotic predecessors. Even when taken in 10–100 times the usually prescribed amounts, benzodiazepines, if taken alone, are rarely lethal. Most lethal overdoses involving benzodiazepines are due to combinations of benzodiazepines with alcohol or other drugs (Finkle, McCloskey and Goodman, 1979).

BEHAVIORAL TOXICITY

Motor Impairment

The motor-impairing effects of toxic amounts of benzodiazepines are common to other sedative–hypnotics, i.e. slurred speech, ataxia, nystagmus, and decreased facility with skilled motor movements. The effect of benzodiazepines on psychomotor performance in highly anxious patients is complex. The patient's psychomotor performance may already be impaired by high levels of anxiety. Reducing anxiety with low or moderate doses of benzodiazepines may improve psychomotor performance, however with increasing doses, a point will be reached where the toxicity of the benzodiazepine will add impairment. In a study comparing 5 and 10 mg doses of diazepam taken 3 times a day, psychomotor impairment was observed in both healthy volunteers and anxious patients with the 10 mg dosage level (Markku, *et al.*, 1983).

Cognitive Impairment

Many experimental studies that have used single dosing of healthy subjects with diazepam and other benzodiazepines have reported impairment of memory. Inferring impairment in anxious patients who take benzodiazepines over an extended time is tenuous because the effect of anxiety reduction in patients might enhance their memory and tolerance to memory-impairing effects of the benzodiazepine could occur. On the other hand, the accumulation of benzodiazepine metabolites that would be expected in patients who are taking long-acting benzodiazepines might produce increasing memory impairment over time.

Ghoneim *et al.* (1981) conducted a study which addressed the issues of tolerance and metabolite accumulation. Healthy subjects were administered 0.2 mg/kg of oral diazepam for 21 days. The investigators found that subjects had difficulty with retention of new information. With continued dosing, some tolerance to the memory impairment occurred in spite of accumulation of metabolites. When retested one week after stopping diazepam, complete recovery of memory function had occurred.

Idiosyncratic Rage or Depressive Reactions

Animals dosed with benzodiazepines show a striking reduction of aggressive behaviour. Humans dosed with benzodiazepines show variable effects on hostility, anger and agressiveness. Generally the effect on humans is in the direction of reducing hostility and anger, and the effect is used therapeutically. For example Abramson (1983) reported successful treatment of "narcissistic rage" with benzodiazepines. Some people, however, respond to usual therapeutic doses of benzodiazepines with a paradoxical increase in anxiety, and a few people respond with overt rage. DiMascio *et al* (1973) hypothesized that only in patients with poor impulse control could chlordiazepoxide release sufficient hostility to result in rage reactions. In experimental studies of hostility , he reported that one-week administration of chlordiazepoxide increased scores "on a test measuring assaultiveness, direct hostility, irritability and verbal hostility" in high and medium anxious males. Oxazepam did not show the same increase in hostility scores.

Rosenbaum *et al* (1984) reported eight cases (out of 80 treated) in whom alprazolam appeared to induce hostility. These authors noted the DiMascio study previously cited and commented that only one of their eight patients had been notably impulsive before treatment with alprazolam and that five patients seemed well able to "inhibit the expression of their significant chronic frustration and resentment." These authors also noted that the initial hostility reactions occurred within the first week of treatment. In two patients, the hostility emerged after a single dose of alprazolam.

We have observed patients who reported an emergence or intensification of suicidal impulses after taking a single dose of diazepam. With chronic, high-dose use, worsening of the mood component of depression is common.

Relapse in Individuals Recovering From Drug Dependency

The role of benzodiazepines in the aftercare treatment of individuals who have abused alcohol or other drugs is controversial. Recovery-oriented drug abstinence treatment of chemical dependency actively prohibits the use of all mind-altering drugs (generally excepting nicotine and caffeine) during recovery. There are three concerns about the use of sedatives. First, the use of any mood altering drug is a breach of the drug-free philosophy. Second, the reduction of both anxiety and guilt produced by the benzodiazepine may reduce the person's resolve to avoid drugs. Third, some benzodiazepines produce in some people a desirable subjective state which will substitute for the effect of the previous drug of abuse, and some of these people will become benzodiazepine abusers.

Benzodiazepines differ among themselves in their propensity to induce subjective alterations. Jaffe *et al.* (1983) compared halazepam and diazepam in a double-blind, three-way crossover, placebo-controlled study in 30 men recently treated for alcohol withdrawal. Using measures of euphoria, sedation, "drug-liking", and "feeling the drug", they found diazepam (in 20 and 40 mg doses) to have more euphoria, sedation and "drug-liking" than equipotent antianxiety doses of halazepam (160 and 320 mg), and concluded that halazepam should have a lower potential for abuse than diazepam.

Psychiatrically-oriented drug treatment programs recognize that some drug abusing patients need lithium, antidepressants or neuroleptics to control underlying psychopathology. The use of sedatives, including benzodiazepines, is generally discouraged. Not all physicians consider the prescription of a benzodiazepine contraindicated. Kolin and Linet (1981), for example, describe the use of benzodiazepines during the first month following detoxification to treat subacute symptoms of alcohol withdrawal. They found no difference between diazepam and alprazolam in terms of anxiety relief and side-effects.

Some physicians in alcohol or other drug treatment programs consider dependence on certain drugs acceptable if the access is medically controlled and use is not producing measurable organic pathology. In treating alcoholics, for example, such physicians consider chronic use of a benzodiazepine acceptable because it is less harmful than chronic alcohol abuse. Methadone maintenance treatment of heroin dependency is based on a similar rational.

Combining Stimulants and Benzodiazepines

Use of stimulants and depressants together is common in recreational drug abuse. Thus, the behavioral consequences of simultaneous use of cocaine (or amphetamine) with alcohol, methaqualone or a benzodiazepine frequently occurs. A person who ingests high doses of both a stimulant and a depressant shows psychomotor and judgmental impairment resulting from the sedative, coupled with a high energy level due to the stimulant. The combination sometimes leads to disastrous behavioral consequences.

References

Abernathy DR, Greenblatt DJ, Divall M, et al: Impairment of diazepam metabolism by low dose estrogen containing oral contraceptive steroids. N Eng J Med 1982;306:791-792.

Abramson R: Lorazepam for narcissistic rage. J Operat Psychiatry 1983;14:52-55.

Desmond PV, Patwardham RV, Schenker S, et al: Cimetidine impairs elimination of chloridiazepoxide (Librium) in man. Ann Int Med 1980;93:266-268.

DiMascio A: The effects of benzodiazepines on aggression: reduced or increased?, in Garattini S, Mussini E, Randall LO (eds.): The Benzodiazepines. New York, Raven Press, 1973.

Finkle BS, McCloskey KL, Goodman LS: Diazepam and drug associated deaths; J Am Med Assoc 1979;242:428-434.

Ghoneim MM, Mewaldt SP, Berie JL, et al.: Memory and performance effects of single and 3-week administration of diazepam. Psychopharmacology 1981;73:147-151.

Hansten PD: Drug Interactions. Philadelphia, Lea & Febiger, 1979.

Jaffe JH, Domenic AC, Nies A, Dixon RB, Monroe LL: Abuse potential of halazepam and of diazepam in patients recently treated for acute alcohol withdrawal. Pharmacol Ther 1983; 34:623-630.

Klotz U, Reimann I: Influence of cimetidine on pharmacokinetics of desmethyldiazepam and oxazepam. Eur J Clin Pharmacol 1980;18:517-520

Kolin IS, Linet OT: Double-blind comparison of alprazolam and diazepam for subchronic withdrawal from alcohol. J Clin Psychiatry 1981;42:169-173.

Markku L, Erwin AB, Brendle A, Simpson D: Psychomotor effects of diazepam in anxious patients and healthy volunteers. J Clin Psychopharmacology 1983;3:88-96.

Rosenbaum JF, Woods SW, Groves JE, Klerman GL: Emergence of hostility during alprazolam treatment. Am J Psychiatry 1984;141:792-793.

Wesson DR, Camber S, Harkey M, Smith DE: Diazepam and desmethyldiazepam in breast milk. J Psychoactive Drugs 1985; in press.

IV. Dependence

17
Benzodiazepine Dependency Syndromes

David E. Smith, MD
Donald R. Wesson, MD

Benzodiazepines, like other sedative–hypnotics, can induce tolerance and physical dependence. This chapter reviews three types of physical dependence that can occur with benzodiazepines: a high-dose dependency of the barbiturate type, a low-dose dependency that may occur with therapeutic doses, and dependency that may occur in the neonate from placental or breast-milk transfer of a benzodiazepine.

HIGH-DOSE DEPENDENCY OF THE BARBITURATE TYPE

Hollister and colleagues showed that after diazepam (Hollister *et al.*, 1963) and chlordiazepoxide (Hollister, Motzenbecker & Degan, 1961), had been taken for a month in dosages 2–3 times the maximum recommended daily therapeutic dose a withdrawal syndrome of the barbiturate type occurred when the benzodiazepine was abruptly stopped. (Since meprobamate, glutethimide, methyprylon, alcohol and methaqualone and other sedative–hypnotics have a similar withdrawal syndrome to barbiturates, the more general term, "sedative–hypnotic withdrawal syndrome" is often used.) Thus, for over 2 decades it has been established that diazepam and chlordiazepoxide could produce physical dependence if taken in high-doses for a month or more.

The severity of sedative–hypnotic withdrawal syndrome is a function of both time and dose. The time required to develop physical dependency is inversely related to dose. If barbiturates are given to patients in sufficient quantity to produce continuous sleep, one week is a sufficient period to induce profound physical dependence. For people who are ambulatory, at least some time of the time, several weeks of daily dosing with a barbiturate is required. The same is probably true with benzodiazepines.

The sedative–hypnotic withdrawal syndrome is traditionally divided into major and minor. Minor withdrawal consists of anxiety, insomnia, tremor, and nightmares. A major withdrawal syndrome includes all the symptoms of minor withdrawal and, in addition, may include grand mal seizures, psychosis, hyperpyrexia, and death.

Benzodiazepines suppress alcohol and other sedative–hypnotic withdrawal syndromes, therefore benzodiazepines, alcohol, barbiturates and other sedative–hypnotics are cross-tolerant. The mechanisms for the development of central nervous system tolerance and physical dependency for sedative–hypnotics are not known. Unlike benzodiazepines, which occupy specific receptor sites in many central nervous system nerve cells, the effects of barbiturates cannot be be produced by direct receptor-site binding because specific binding sites for barbiturates and other non-benzodiazepine sedative–hypnotics do not occur.

Untreated, the high-dose sedative–hypnotic withdrawal syndrome peaks in intensity as blood-levels of the sedative drop, and signs and symptoms subside over a period of a few days.

LOW-DOSE DEPENDENCY WITH THERAPEUTIC DOSES

Physicians have reported case studies claiming that signs and symptoms developing after a patients abruptly stopped long-term use of thera-peutically prescribed doses of benzodiazepines were due to benzodiazepine withdrawal (e.g. Bant, 1975; Pevnick *et al.*, 1978; Berlin & Conell, 1983; Lader, 1983; LeBellec, 1980; Levy, 1984). Several review articles describing low-dose benzodiazepine withdrawal have been published (Schöph, 1983; Mackinnon & Parker, 1982; Owen & Tyrer, 1983).

Symptoms which have been attributed to benzodiazepine withdrawal include anxiety, tension, agitation, restlessness, irritability, tremor, nausea, insomnia, panic attacks, impairment of memory and concentration, perceptual alterations (hyperacusis, hypersensitivity to touch, pain), parathesias, feelings of unreality, visual hallucinations, psychosis, tachycar-dia, and increased blood pressure. Unfortunately, there are no pathog-nomonic signs or symptoms, and such a broad range of non-specific symptoms could be produced by a number of illnesses including agitated depression, generalized anxiety disorder, panic disorder, partial complex seizures, and schizophreniform disorders.

The validity of the low-dose withdrawal syndrome is controversial. Many people, who take benzodiazepines in therapeutic doses for months-to-years, can abruptly discontinue taking their benzodiazepine without developing symptoms. Other people, who take similar amounts of a benzodiazepine believe themselves to have developed physical dependency on the benzodiazepine, and they cannot tolerate the symptoms that develop following cessation or dosage reduction of the benzodiazepine. Some physicians believe that the symptoms that emerge during the immediate withdrawal period can be explained solely on the basis of symptom return, whereas other physicians propose that at least some of the symptoms are the product of a withdrawal reaction.

There are four possible etiologies for the symptoms that emerge when benzodiazepines are stopped: "symptom re-emergence", "symptom emergence", "symptom generation", and "symptom overinterpretation".

(1) Symptom Re-emergence (or Recrudescence): The patient's symptoms of anxiety, insomnia or muscle tension abate during benzodiazepine treatment, and the patient forgets how severe the symptoms were before beginning benzodiazepine treatment. As discomfort in the present seems more real than that experienced in the past, present discomfort may be believed to be more severe when, in fact, symptoms are of equal severity to those experienced before treatment.

(2) Symptom Emergence: If the patient's initial symptoms were secondary to a progressive disease, symptom progression may have been masked during benzodiazepine therapy. When the benzodiazepine is stopped, the symptoms that emerge are, in fact, more severe in intensity than the symptoms experienced before taking the benzodiazepine, but the etiology of the symptom intensification is due to progression of disease.

(3) Symptom Generation or True Withdrawal Syndrome: Signs or symptoms may develop as a result of receptor site alterations due to the benzodiazepine exposure.

(4) Symptom Overinterpretation: Everyone on occasion experiences anxiety, variations in sleep pattern, and musculo-skeletal discomfort. Most people accept such symptoms as reasonable consequences of everyday stresses, overexertion, or minor viral infections. They may self-medicate their symptoms with over-the-counter medications or alcohol, but they do not generally go to a physician for treatment of the symptoms. In contrast, people who are stopping benzodiazepines may expect the development of withdrawal symptoms because of the widespread publicity about Valium[R] withdrawal. These patients may assume that any symptoms occurring during the withdrawal period are due to benzodiazepine withdrawal and that they require medical attention. Merz and Ballmer (1983) studied the frequency with which symptoms and symptom combinations attributed to minor barbiturate or low-dose benzodiazepine withdrawal occur in an untreated, healthy population. They report that many of the non-specific

symptoms attributed to withdrawal are common among non-patients who do not use drugs.

Clearly, assigning *causality* to a patient's symptoms that emerge after discontinuance of a benzodiazepine is subject to uncertainty. This is especially the case when a patient is evaluated after "dependence" is already established. Unfortunately, this is the usual clinical situation and is the circumstance of most reported case studies of benzodiazepine dependence.

The time course of symptom resolution is the primary differentiating feature between symptoms generated by withdrawal and symptom re-emergence, emergence, or overinterpretation. Withdrawal symptoms subside with continued abstinence, whereas symptoms of other etiologies persist. Figure 1 compares the intensity of symptoms in the barbiturate type withdrawal and the low-dose benzodiazepine withdrawal. The "intensity" label on the ordinate axis of Figure 1 indicates a global measure of symptoms. The time course shown is for a long-acting benzodiazepine.

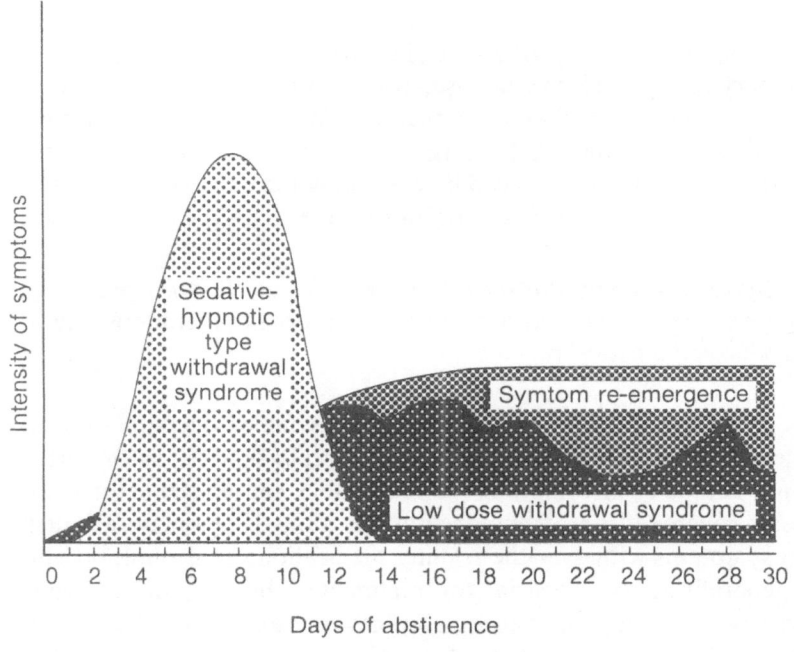

Figure 1 Comparison of intensity and time course of sedative–hypnotic and low-dose benzodiazepine withdrawal syndromes. The "Intensity of Symptoms" is a global scale of all symptoms. Symptom re-emergence is the return of symptoms that were present before a benzodiazepine was taken. Times shown are for a long-acting benzodiazepine. Short-acting benzodiazepines would have an accelerated time course.

Short-acting benzodiazepines have an accelerated time course for the sedative–hypnotic type withdrawal syndrome, and the peak intensity of sedative–hypnotic type withdrawal for the short-acting benzodiazepines (e.g. oxazepam, alprazolam, and triazolam) occurs in 2–4 days. The fluctuation of symptom intensity of the low-dose withdrawal syndrome illustrates the waxing and waning of symptoms which often occurs without apparent psychological cause. The time of emergence is variable, and it may not coincide with the time-course illustrated in Figure 1.

We believe that the waxing and waning of symptoms is an important marker to distinguish low-dose withdrawal from symptom reemergence. Table 1 shows salient features of benzodiazepine withdrawal, anxiety disorders, and symptoms re-emergence.

Table 1 Comparison of syndromes related to benzodiazepine withdrawal

	Sedative–Hypnotic Type Withdrawal	Low-Dose Benzodiazepine	Symptom Re-emergence
Symptoms	Anxiety insomnia, nightmares, seizures, psychosis, hyperpyrexia, death	Anxiety, including somatic manifestations, insomnia, muscle spasm, psychosis	Variable, but should be same as symptoms present prior to taking benzodiazepines
Time course	Begin 1–2 days after stopping short-acting benzodiazepines, and 2–4 days after stopping long-acting benzodiazepines.	Begin 1 day after stopping. Symptoms may continue weeks-to-months, but improve with time.	Emerge when benzodiazepine is stopped. Continue unabated with time.
Response to reinstitution of benzodiazepine	Reversal of symptoms 2–6 hours after reinstituting hypnotic level doses.	Reversal within 45–90 minutes of small doses of benzodiazepine.	Responsive in 45–90 minutes to usual therapeutic doses of benzodiazepine..

Chronicity of use, dosage, concurrent drug use and individual susceptibility all interact in the development of low-dose physical dependency. Continuous exposure to the benzodiazepine fosters development of physical dependence of the sedative–hypnotic type and probably also fosters the development of low-dose dependency. Thus, short-acting benzodiazepines are no less prone to development of physical dependence if taken *on a daily basis* than are long-acting benzodiazepines. Once physical dependence develops, the sedative–hypnotic type withdrawal syndrome produced by short-acting benzodiazepines would be expected to be more intense because of the more rapid drop in tissue levels of these drugs (Hollister, 1980).

Since the reports of specific benzodiazepine binding sites in rat brain by Mohler and Okada (1977) and Squires and Braestrup (1977), attempts to characterize the benzodiazepine receptor site have been the subject of intense research. Localized in synaptic contact regions in the cerebral cortex, cerebellum and hippocampus in association with GABA receptor sites, the benzodiazepine receptor sites affect GABA's affinity for binding to its specific site and modify the permeability of the cell membrane to the chloride ion. We have hypothesized that low-dose benzodiazepine withdrawal is receptor site mediated (Wesson & Smith, 1982). A receptor site mediated withdrawal syndrome would offer a plausible explanation why symptom resolution takes more time than for non-benzodiazepine sedative-hypnotic withdrawal.

The specific benzodiazepine antagonist (Ro 15-1788) will precipitate withdrawal reactions in animals dependent upon benzodiazepines (Cumin, Bonetti *et al.*, 1982; also see Haefely's discussion in Chapter 1). The availability of a specific benzodiazepine antagonist opens the possiblity of testing the benzodiazepine low-dose withdrawal syndrome by inducing withdrawal in the same way that naloxone can be used to test for opiate dependence.

The development of physical dependence may also be influenced by exposure to drugs or medications other than the benzodiazepine. For example, pentobarbital has been shown to increase affinity of diazepam to benzodiazepine receptors (Skolnick *et al.*, 1981; Olsen and Loeb-Lundberg, 1980). Pretreatment with barbiturates may affect the development of withdrawal symptoms as demonstrated in a study by Covi *et al.* (1973). They randomly assigned 92 patients to a 10 week pre-chlordiazepoxide treatment with either phenobarbital or diphenylhydantoin. During the subsequent 2 weeks, subjects were given 15 mg chlordiazepoxide 3 times per day, then switched to an identical-appearing placebo for 2 weeks, and then returned to a final 2-week treatment period of 15 mg chlordiazepoxide 3 times a day. Although the mean distress levels during chlordiazepoxide treatment were no different in the two groups, the mean distress levels while on placebo were significantly greater for the phenobarbital pretreated group than the diphenylhydantoin pretreated group.

Case Studies of Benzodiazepine Dependency

In a placebo crossover study, Tyrer *et al.*, (1981) found that patient's symptoms were related to the rate of fall of desmethyldiazepam. Patients whose desmethyldiazepam levels decreased more rapidly had a greater number of symptoms.

We have reported a series of case studies of patients who believed themselves to be physically dependent on therapeutic doses of diazepam and other benzodiazepines (Smith & Wesson, 1983). We studied patient's perception of being benzodiazepine dependent and how their physicians responded to the patient's assertion of having developed benzodiazepine dependency.

Few of the patients we studied used only benzodiazepines. Regardless of which benzodiazepine or other medication they had been taking, they claimed Valium^R dependency. Most patients used multiple psychotropic medications, and even patients who used other sedative–hypnotics or benzodiazepines in addition to Valium^R concluded that they were Valium^R dependent. Other drug use commonly associated with the development of benzodiazepine dependency in our subjects was chronic opiate use (e.g., codeine and methadone), barbiturates or other sedatives, or daily alcohol use – not necessarily alcoholism. Daily use of alcohol or family history of alcoholism may be risk factors in the development of low-dose benzodiazepine dependency.

Most patients were focused on their symptoms and preoccupied with determining the cause. They sought reassurance that the symptoms were not indicative of irreversible tissue damage. Rarely were their episodes of withdrawal untreated. Their physicians provided symptom treatment with a variety of medications, and some patients treated themselves with over-the-counter medications, street drugs, or home remedies. Because of the widespread publicity about Valium^R dependence, the patients' physicians frequently switched their Valium^R dependent patients to a short-acting benzodiazepine, using the rational that short-acting benzodiazepines are less likely to produce physical dependency. (This is contrary to the prediction of some authors who believe that short-acting benzodiazepines will induce a more intense withdrawal syndrome.)

Prospective Studies

Prospective placebo-controlled studies of patients whose symptoms would normally be treated with benzodiazepines are needed to separate symptom recurrence from withdrawal symptoms. The researcher must measure symptoms before treatment, during treatment with the benzodiazepine, and after crossover to placebo. A study described by Chouinard et al. (1983) collected this type of data. The observations reported in this study are not comforting. Forty-eight patients were treated for 3 weeks with identical capsules which contained either bromazepam (16 patients dosed with 18 mg/day), diazepam (16 patients dosed with 15 mg/day) or placebo (16 patients). At the end of three weeks, half of each benzodiazepine treated group (8 subjects on bromazepam and 8 subjects on diazepam) were switched to placebo and half were gradually withdrawn. Subjects whose benzodiazepines were abruptly withdrawn faired worse than subjects treated with placebo. Seven of the 16 patients who were abruptly withdrawn had increases of 10% or more above baseline on both the Hamilton Anxiety and self-rating symptom scales during the immediate withdrawal period. The authors called this effect "rebound anxiety."

Current Understanding of the Low-Dose Dependency Syndrome

The low-dose benzodiazepine dependency syndrome is not well understood or well characterized. The dose–response relationship is not established, and the development of dependency appears idiosyncratic. Based on our studies, we believe that risk factors include a family or personal history of alcoholism, daily alcohol use or concomitant use of other sedatives. The low-dose withdrawal syndrome probably has a different mechanism than the sedative–hypnotic type withdrawal syndrome as the time course and spectrum of signs and symptoms are different than for typical sedative–hypnotic withdrawal. For this reason, we object to calling the low-dose benzodiazepine withdrawal syndrome a "minor" sedative–hypnotic withdrawal syndrome. We believe that a low-dose benzodiazepine withdrawal syndrome is different from non-benzodiazepine sedative–hypnotic withdrawal for the following reasons:

1. The benzodiazepine withdrawal syndrome is not completely suppressed by phenobarbital.
2. Symptoms are rapidly reversed by doses of benzodiazepines below those that would be expected to be effective in treating symptoms.
3. The time needed for symptom resolution appears much longer in the low-dose withdrawal syndrome than in classic sedative-hypnotic withdrawal. Symptoms typically takes 6 months to a year to completely subside.
4. Symptoms are most intense during withdrawal of the last few milligrams of benzodiazepine.

PHYSICAL DEPENDENCE IN THE NEONATE

Pregnant women who take benzodiazepines may cause intrauterine benzodiazepine dependency in the fetus and benzodiazepine withdrawal in the neonate. Diazepam and its first metabolite, desmethyldiazepam, cross the placenta (Errkola, Kangas & Pekkarinen, 1973; McCarthy, O'Connell & Robinson, 1973; Cavanaugh & Condo, 1964). Withdrawal signs in

242

neonates have been attributed to intrauterine exposure to diazepam (Mazzi, 1977: one case; Rementeria & Bhatt, 1977: three cases). The mothers' diazepam dosages ranged from 5 to 20 mg per day during the last 4 weeks of gestation. Neonates were hypertonic, irritable, hyperreflexic and tremulous. Although vigorous suckers, they were subject to vomiting. Serum levels of benzodiazepines in the neonates were not reported, and diazepam withdrawal as the causal etiology for the neonates' signs was inferential.

TREATMENT OF BENZODIAZEPINE DEPENDENCE

If the formulation of two withdrawal syndromes is correct, withdrawal strategies must be tailored to the three possible dependency situations:

1. With low-dose, daily usage of therapeutic doses of benzodiazepines for more than 6 months, only a low-dose benzodiazepine withdrawal syndrome would be expected.
2. With high-dose usage, greater than recommended therapeutic doses for more than 1 month and less than 6 months, a classical sedative–hypnotic withdrawal syndrome would be anticipated.
3. If daily high doses of benzodiazepine were continued more than 6 months, both a sedative–hypnotic withdrawal syndrome and a low-dose withdrawal syndrome would be anticipated.

Table 2 Benzodiazepines' "High Dose"/"Low Dose" Designations

| | Total Daily Dose | |
Generic Name	Low dose (mg)	High dose (mg)
Alprazolam	0.75–4	>4
Chlordiazepoxide	15–100	>100
Clonazepam	1.5–20	>20
Clorazepate	15–60	>60
Diazepam	4–40	>40
Flurazepam	15–30	>30
Halazepam	60–160	>160
Lorazepam	1–10	>10
Oxazepam	10–30	>30
Prazepam	20–60	>60
Temazepam	15–30	>30
Triazolam	0.25–0.5	>0.5

Table 2 shows our designation of high and low-doses of some benzodiazepines.

Treatment: Low-Dose Benzodiazepine Withdrawal Syndrome

Since seizures, hyperpyrexia and other life-threatening medical complications are not expected, gradual reduction of the benzodiazepine is pharmacologically rational. On an outpatient basis, we recommend a stepwise reduction of the benzodiazepine by the smallest unit dose each week for a patient who is physically dependent but still in control of medication use. The person who has lost the ability to control drug usage and escalates dosage as symptoms emerge requires inpatient treatment. During withdrawal, patients manifest multiple, shifting symptoms, and psychometric assessment is useful in establishing trends. We use a mini-computer to administer a symptom check-list. This interactive method of test administration where the patient sits at a terminal and enters responses has proven to be a time-efficient method of tracking symptom changes in patients. Interviews with these patients tend to be lengthy as they are preoccupied with their symptoms and seek endless assurance that the symptoms are not the result of irreversible physiological changes.

Propranolol (20 mg every 6 hours) is used starting on the 5th day of withdrawal. Propranolol has been found to reduce symptom intensity (Tyrer et al., 1981). This schedule of propranolol is continued for 2 weeks and then discontinued. Afterwards, propranolol is used as needed for control of tachycardia, increased blood pressure and anxiety. Continuous propranolol therapy for more than 2 weeks is not recommended as propranolol itself may result in symptom rebound when discontinued after prolonged therapy (Snyder, 1981; Glaubiger & Lefkowitz, 1977; Harrison & Alderman, 1976).

Treatment: Sedative–Hypnotic Type Benzodiazepine Withdrawal

A phenobarbital substitution technique (Smith & Wesson, 1970) is preferred for withdrawal from any of the benzodiazepines for two reasons: (1) None of our patients have had a withdrawal seizure when phenobarbital was used for withdrawal, whereas two patients being withdrawn using gradual reduction of the benzodiazepine have had withdrawal seizures; and (2) in the treatment of drug dependence, we prefer not to administer the drug of dependence to the patient during treatment.

An estimate of the patient's daily benzodiazepine usage during the month before treatment is used to compute the detoxification starting dose of phenobarbital. The benzodiazepine is converted to phenobarbital withdrawal equivalence by using Table 3. The computed phenobarbital equivalence is given daily, divided into 3 or 4 doses. If other sedative–hypnotics (including alcohol) are used, the phenobarbital conversion for the other sedative–hypnotic is added to the amount computed for the benzodiazepine. However, regardless of the total computed conversion, the maximum phenobarbital dose is 500 mg/day. After 2 days of stabilization on phenobarbital, the patient's daily phenobarbital dosage is then decreased 30 mg each day.

Table 3 Phenobarbital withdrawal conversion for benzodiazepines and other sedative–hypnotics

Generic name	Dose (mg)	Phenobarbital withdrawal Conversion (mg) *
Benzodiazepines		
alprazolam	1	30
chlordiazepoxide	25	30
clonazepam	2	15
clorazepate	15	30
diazepam	10	30
flurazepam	15	30
halazepam	40	30
lorazepam	1	15
oxazepam	10	30
prazepam	10	30
temazepam	15	30
Barbiturates		
amobarbital	100	30
butabarbital	100	30
butalbital	50	15
pentobarbital	100	50
secobarbital	100	30
Glycerols		
meprobamate	400	30
Piperidinediones		
glutethimide	250	30
Quinazolones		
methaqualone	300	30

*Withdrawal doses of phenobarbital are sufficient to supress most withdrawal symptoms, but are not the same as therapeutic dose equivalency.

Before each dose of phenobarbital, the patient is checked for the presence of sustained horizontal nystagmus, slurred speech and ataxia. If sustained nystagmus is present, the scheduled dose of phenobarbital is withheld. If all three signs are present, the next two doses of phenobarbital are withheld and the total daily dose of phenobarbital for the following day is cut in half.

Figure 2 shows how we sequence pharmacological treatment when both a sedative–hypnotic and low-dose syndrome are expected.

FUTURE RESEARCH

The physiological signs we attribute to low-dose benzodiazepine withdrawal (e.g. dilated pupils, increased pulse rate and increased blood pressure) are the same as those observed in human subjects when beta-carboline-03-carboxylic acid is injected. Since these symptoms of beta-carboline are *blocked* by the benzodiazepine antagonist Ro 15-1788, it may be that the antagonist

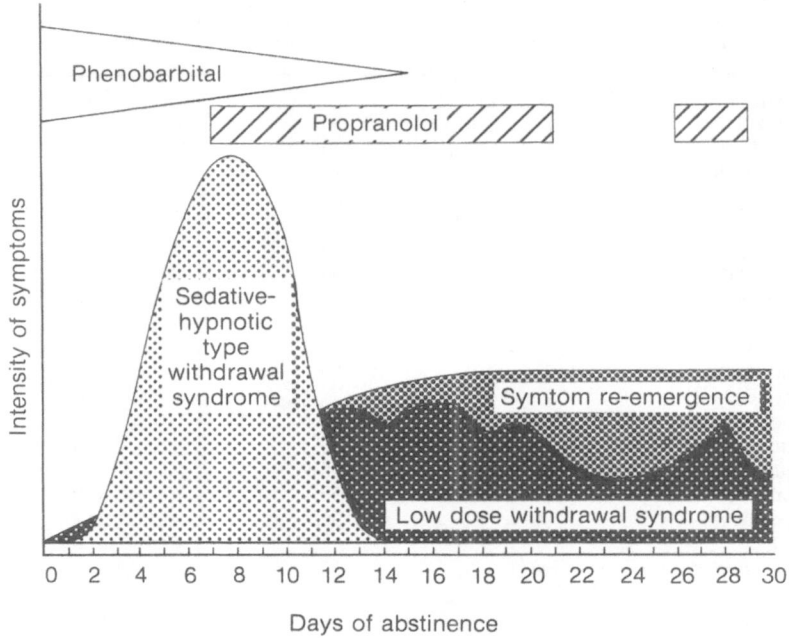

Figure 2 Treatment of Benzodiazepine withdrawal. The time course shown would be for a long-acting benzodiazepine. The sequencing would be compressed for a short-acting benzodiazepine.

would be the treatment of choice for low-dose withdrawal – perhaps more specific than propranolol. Antagonists have two different roles depending on the state of the receptor site when given: (1) If given while benzodiazepines (agonists) were still on the receptor sites, the result would be to precipitate withdrawal, but (2) if given after the receptor sites were clear (but perhaps hypersensitive to effects of endogenous agonists), the antagonist, by binding to the receptor site, may decrease sensitivity. Further research in the area of benzodiazepine receptor-antagonist interaction is urgently needed.

References

Berlin RM, Conell, LJ: Withdrawal symptoms after long-term treatment with therapeutic doses of flurazepam: A case report. *Am J Psychiatry* 1983;140:488-490.

Bant W: Diazepam withdrawal symptoms. (letter) *Br Med J* 1975;4:285.

Cavanaugh D, Condo DS: Diazepam - a pilot study of drug concentrations in maternal blood, amniotic fluid and cord blood. *Curr Ther Res* 1964;6:122.

Chouinard G, Labonte A, Fontaine R, Annable L: New concepts in benzodiazepine therapy: rebound anxiety and new indications for the more potent benzodiazepines. *Prog. Neuro-Psychopharmacol & Biol. Psychiat.* 1983;7:669-673.

Covi L, Lipman RS, Pattison JH, *et al*: Length of treatment with anxiolytic sedatives and response to their sudden withdrawal. *Acta Psychiatr Scand* 1973;49:51-64.

Cumin R, Bonetti EP, Scherschlicht R, Haefely WE: Use of the specific benzodiazepine antogonist, Ro 15-1788, in studies of physiological dependence on benzodiazepines. *Experientia* 1982;38:833-834.

Errkola R, Kangas L, Pekkarinen A: The transfer of diazepam across the placenta during labor. *Acta Obstet Gynecol Scand* 1973;52:167-170.

Glaubiger G, Lefkowitz RJ: Elevated beta-adrenergic receptor number after chronic propranolol treatment. *Biochem Biophys Res Commun* 1977;78:720-725.

Harrison DC, Alderman EL: Discontinuation of propranolol therapy: Cause of rebound angina pectoris and acute coronary events. *Chest* 1976;69:1-2.

Hollister LE: Benzodiazepines 1980: Current update. *Psychosomatics* 1980;21:1-5.

Hollister LE, Bennett JL, Kimbell I Jr, *et al*: Diazepam in newly admitted schizophrenics. *Dis Nerv System* 1963;24:746-750.

Hollister LE, Motzenbecker FP, Degan RO: Withdrawal reactions from chlordiazepoxide ('Librium'). *Psychopharmacologia* 1961; 2:63-68.

Iversen LL, Bloom FE: Studies of the uptake of 3H-GABA and (3H)glycine in slices and homogenates of rat brain and spinal cord by electron microscope autoradiography. *Brain Res* 1972;41:131-143.

Johnston GAR, Willow MB: Barbiturates and GABA receptors, in Costa E, DiChiari G, Gessa GL (eds): *GABA and Benzodiazepine Receptors*. New York, Raven Press, 1981.

Kales A, Scharf MB, Kales JD, *et al*: Rebound insomnia: A potential hazard following withdrawal of certain benzodiazepines. *J Am Med Assoc* 1979;241:1692-1695.

Lader M: Dependence on benzodiazepines. *J Clin Psychiatry* 1983;44:121-127.

LeBellec M, Bismuth CH, Lagier G, *et al*: Severe withdrawal symptoms after benzodiazepines are discontinued: Six clinical cases. *Therapie* 1980;35:113-118.

Levy A: Delirium and seizures due to abrupt alprazolam withdrawal: Case report. *J Clin Psychiatry* 1984;45:38-39.

MacKinnon, GL, Parker, WA: Benzodiazepine withdrawal syndrome: A literature review and evaluation. *Am J Drug Alcohol Abuse* 1982;9:19-33.

Mazzi E: Possible neonatal diazepam withdrawal: A case report. *Am J Obstet Gynecol* 1977;129:586-587.

Merz WA, Ballmer U: Symptoms of the barbiturate/benzodiazepine withdrawal syndrome in healthy volunteers: Standardized assessment by a newly developed self-rating scale. *J Psychoactive Drugs* 1983;15:1-2.

McCarthy GT, O'Connell B, Robinson AE: Blood levels of diazepam in infants of two mothers given large doses of diazepam during labor. *J Obstet Gynecol Br Comm* 1973;80:349-352.

Mohler H, Okada T: Benzodiazepine receptors. *Science* 1977;198:849-851.

Olsen RW, Leeb-Lundberg F: Convulsant and anticonvulsant drug binding sites related to GABA-regulated chloride ion channels, in Costa E, DiChiari G, Gessa GL (eds.): *GABA and Benzodiazepine Receptors*. New York, Raven Press, 1981.

Owen RT, Tyrer, P: Benzodiazepine dependence: A review of the evidence. *Drugs* 1983;25:385-398.

Pevnick JS, Jasinski DR, Haertzen CA: Abrupt withdrawal from therapeutically administered diazepam. *Arch Gen Psychiatry* 1978;35:995-998.

Rementeria JL, Bhatt K: Withdrawal symptoms in neonates from intrauterine exposure to diazepam. *J Pediatrics* 1977;90:123-126.

Rickels K, Case G, Downing RW, *et al*: Long-term diazepam therapy and clinical outcome. *J Am Med Assoc* 1983;250:767-771.

Schöph J: Withdrawal phenomena after long-term administration of benzodiazepines: A review of recent investigations. *Pharmacopsychiat* 1983;16:1-8.

Skolnick P, Moncada V, Barker JL, *et al*: Pentobarbital: Dual actions to increase brain benzodiazepine receptor affinity. *Science* 1981;211:1448-1450.

Smith DE, Wesson DR: A new method for treatment of barbiturate dependence. *J Am Med Assoc* 1970;213:294-295.

Snyder SH: Benzodiazepine receptors. *Psychiatric Annals* 1981; 11:19-23.

Snyder SH: Receptors, neurotransmitters and drug responses. *N Engl J Med* 1979;300:465-472.

Squires RF, Braestrup C: Benzodiazepine receptors in rat brain. *Nature* 1977;266:732-734.

Tyrer P, Rutherford D, Huggett T: Benzodiazepine withdrawal symptoms and propranolol. *Lancet* 1981;1:520-522.

Wesson DR, Smith DE: Low dose benzodiazepine withdrawal syndrome: Receptor site mediated. *NEWS: California Society for the Treatment of Alcoholism and Other Drug Dependencies* 1982;9:1-5.

Winokur A, Rickels K, Greenblatt DJ, *et al*: Withdrawal reaction from long-term, low-dose administration of diazepam: A double-blind placebo-controlled case study. *Arch Gen Psychiatry* 1980; 37:101-105.

V. Social-Cultural Issues

18

The Benzodiazepines: Public Health, Social and Regulatory Issues. An Industry Perspective

Bruce H. Medd, MD

Any review during the past decade of the public health, social and regulatory issues surrounding medications developed by the U.S. pharmaceutical industry has tended to focus on the benzodiazepines, particularly Valium[R]. Never before in the history of this industry has a medication drawn more attention from the political arena, the medical community and the public media than Valium[R]. No pharmaceutical agent has had more written about it either in the professional or lay press. No medicine has had so many public personalities heralding its potential risks, or conversely, has demonstrated such widespread safety and effectiveness as documented in thousands of articles in the worldwide scientific literature or evidenced by countless millions of satisfied patients over a 20-year period. If the present review is subjected to careful scrutiny and each issue is examined individually against a background of available scientific data and other documented evidence rather than against unsubstantiated or anecdotal information, rational public and regulatory policy should ultimately result.

When Dr. Mitchell Balter, of the National Institute of Mental Health (NIMH), first presented data from his large-scale international survey on the use of psychotherapeutic medication at the Fifth World Conference of Psychiatry in November 1982, critics were voicing the opinion that the United States, and perhaps the world, was overmedicated. And, although Dr. Balter's painstaking research clearly refuted this accusation, the critics refused to listen. When arguing the point, Dr. Balter would respond, "Look at the data". This tenet can be applied to all the issues which have surrounded the benzodiazepines over the past 15 years, for nothing is more conclusive than well-documented data. A brief review of the major issues and the available data appears here.

PUBLIC HEALTH ISSUES

The Overmedicated Society

The term "overmedicated society" began to appear in the mid-1960's and became the battle cry of critics to raise public concern over what they perceived as growing overuse of antianxiety medications. Benzodiazepine, and particularly Valium[R], usage received great public attention as the number of prescriptions increased through the late 1960's and early 1970's. It is important, however, when examining usage levels (see Table 1) to relate these figures to the prevalence of the disorders for which these medications are prescribed, at any given time (point prevalence) as well as annually (Dohrenwend *et al.*, 1980; Pardes, 1979; Regier, Goldberg & Taube, 1978; Kohn & White, 1976).

Table 1 Prevalence of Disorders vs. Use: General Adult Population

	Point prevalence	*Annual prevalence*
Incidence of emotional disorders	15%	20%
Use of prescribed anxiolytic drugs	2%	11%

There has never been any question regarding the effectiveness of Valium[R] in its indicated areas of use. Many thousands of references in the worldwide medical literature clearly reflect the remarkable benefits obtained with this agent. Still, critics have repeatedly suggested that benzodiazepines are imprudently used for the problems of everyday life and portray anxious patients as rushing to physicians in large numbers to demand prescriptions for tranquilizer medication. A 1971 survey, supported by grants from the Public Health Service and the National Institute of Mental Health (NIMH), found that Americans to a great degree had considerable doubts about the virtue of using tranquilizers (Manheimer, Davidson & Balter, 1973). These concerns were reported by persons of all ages, incomes, education, occupations and sex. The survey respondents felt that, although antianxiety medications *were efficacious*, they *were not* a cure and that using them was generally a sign of weakness.

Who Uses Benzodiazepines?

Two national NIMH surveys provide data on patients who received antianxiety medications. Results of a 1970–1 study population of 2,552 patients showed that only 15 percent took minor tranquilizers in a 12-month period (Mellinger *et al.*, 1978); and a 1979 survey of 3,161 adults showed the number of respondents using anxiolytics was 11 percent (Mellinger, Balter

& Uhlenhuth, 1984). The 1979 survey, a largely older and sicker population, found that contrary to popular belief regular long-term use of anxiolytics was *relatively rare* (15% of users) and that the *annual increase in the number of such users is small.*

The data suggest an increasingly cautious attitude on the part of many toward using medication despite a legitimate basis for use. In their conclusions, based on the 1979 survey, the authors (Mellinger *et al.*, 1978) state: "Our inquiry had addressed one prominent social concern about the prescribing and use of psychotherapeutic medications, namely that these medications are commonly prescribed for persons with minor and transient disturbances of small consequence. This widely held belief is not borne out by data from our national study of psychotherapeutic drug use as reported here."

Referring to the later study, the authors (Mellinger & Balter, 1981) observed: "With respect to... minor tranquilizers, long-term continuous use raises important questions about potential for physical dependence, as well as efficacy. These concerns sometimes overshadow the fact that under some conditions, *under-use* of psychotherapeutic drugs can pose health risks that are no less serious than over-use".

When tranquilizer usage in the United States was compared with similar data from nine Western European countries, the results showed that Americans were neither unique nor atypical in their usage patterns. One large-scale, cross-national study on the extent of tranquilizer use applied a household survey plus sampling techniques and compared the results with similar data available in the United States (Balter, Levine & Manheimer, 1974; Parry *et al.*, 1973). The average tranquilizer usage ranged from 10 percent in Spain to 17 percent in Belgium and France. A more recent study of ten Western European countries conducted in 1981 revealed average tranquilizer usage ranging from 7 percent in the Netherlands to 18 percent in Belgium with United States usage in the middle (Balter *et al.*, 1984).

Since 1973, the National Center for Health Statistics in the United States has conducted an annual National Ambulatory Medical Care Survey (NAMCS). It is an important source of detailed data concerning the medical care provided in physicians' offices. Each year NAMCS contacts a representative sample of physicians with office-based practices. These physicians submit, on a random-sample basis, records of their office visits. In 1980, for the first time since NAMCS began, physicians were asked to report the names of the specific medicines that they had prescribed. During visits where patients complained chiefly of anxiety, 79 percent received treatments other than medication and 61 percent received a prescription. More importantly, at visits where anxiety was the principal diagnosis, 75 percent received nonmedication therapy while only 58 percent received medication. Many patients who were treated for anxiety of course received both types of therapy (see Table 2).

Table 2 Therapy provided to anxious patients as compared to all patients

	Nonmedication*	Medication	Benzodiazepines
Visits with anxiety as most important complaint	79%	61%	25%
Visits with anxiety as principal diagnosis	75%	58%	37%
All visits	47%	63%	2%

*Primarily psychotherapy and counselling

Compared to data for all visits, the diagnosis of anxiety substantially increased the likelihood that patients would receive additional therapies: most frequently psychotherapy and/or counseling. Where physicians recorded a principal diagnosis of anxiety, 37 percent of patients were prescribed a benzodiazepine. Over half of this group also received nonmedication therapy. It appears, therefore, that benzodiazepine prescribing is frequently lower than one might expect, since anxiety represents the diagnostic category for which benzodiazepines accounted for only a small fraction of all types of prescriptions written during office visits.

It has been shown that new therapy with benzodiazepines is almost as likely to be directed to patients as adjunctive therapy for anxiety associated with an organic disorder, as it is to patients with a primary diagnosis of anxiety. Typically, they might be prescribed for persons suffering from cardiovascular disorders, ulcers, painful arthritic conditions and other ailments. Roughly 10 to 15 percent of the prescriptions for Valium[R] are for disorders related to peripheral muscle spasm or central nervous system (CNS) spasticity. Approximately 2 to 5 percent of Valium[R] prescriptions are for certain convulsive disorders (see Table 3).

Table 3 Principal diagnoses at visits where benzodiazepines are prescribed

Mental	36%
Anxiety	16%
Circulatory	17%
Musculoskeletal injuries	14%
Digestive	5%
Respiratory	4%
Nervous	4%
Genitourinary	3%

Therefore, the issue of the United States being an overmedicated society does *not* appear to be supported by scientific data. On the contrary, the evidence seems to indicate that the majority of prescribers and users of benzodiazepines tends to be extremely conservative.

Patient Usage Patterns

Many of the articles that have appeared in the lay media have suggested that patients generally tend to increase their dosage of Valium[R], but the reverse appears to be true in most cases. Scientific studies have shown that users of Valium[R], if they alter their prescribed dosage at all, are more likely to *decrease* the dosage. One study (Tessler, Stokes & Pietras, 1978) revealed that 91 percent of patients receiving Valium[R] either decreased the dose or followed their physician's dosage instruction accurately (see Table 4). Of the 6 percent increasing dosage, most had been prescribed medication on an "as needed" basis. The investigators also reported that none of these patients increased dosage above recommended levels.

Table 4 Summary of Valium[R] use patterns by patients; University of Massachusetts Survey, 1977; Central and Western Massachusetts

Total study population	Followed MD directions	Decreased dose	Increased dose	Unknown
236 (100%)	108 (45.8%)	106 (44.9%)	15 (6.4%)	7 (3.0%)

A study of the social effects of Valium[R] use (Caplan *et al.*, 1983) was conducted by the Institute for Social Research, University of Michigan. Data gathered from a heterogeneous group of adults showed that these users, too, actually tended to take less Valium[R] than prescribed.

Sex Bias and Prescribing

Since twice as many women as men receive prescriptions for antianxiety medications, the accusation has arisen that this is due to a sex bias by a predominantly male medical profession. This has generated great interest and creative speculation, particularly on the part of the public media. Many surveys and investigations comparing the prevalence of anxiety in men and women have demonstrated that, for whatever reasons, women do indeed have higher levels. Ilfeld (1978), in a study supported by the NIMH, evaluated 2,300 individuals in the Chicago area, and the findings reported that women suffered almost twice as many symptoms of anxiety as men.

Table 5 summarizes data from two national surveys regarding the respective annual use of anxiolytic medication by women and men (Mellinger & Balter, 1981; Parry *et al.*, 1973). Although these figures show that women do receive twice as many prescriptions compared to men, the most recent overall prevalence of use by women during a one-year period was only 14 percent.

Table 5 Summary of women usage studies

Study and years	Total study population	Study population Female	Male	Anxiolytic Rx users Female	Male
National Household Survey 1970-1	2,552 (100%)	1,503 (59%)	1,049 (41%)	300 (20%)	84 (8%)
National Patterns of Psychotherapeutic Drug Use 1979	3,161 (100%)	1,827 (58%)	1,334 (42%)	258 (14%)	100 (8%)

Dr. Gerald L. Klerman (1980), a past administrator of the Alcohol, Drug Abuse and Mental Health Administration, perhaps best explained this situation at the Second Annual Women in Crisis Conference:

Some have held that women who are in distress are too often prescribed medications for the symptoms they present to physicians. The fact is, that in proportion to the number of times women and men seek help, men and women receive the same percentage of prescriptions for medications. This holds true for tranquilizers, for cardiovascular medications and other drugs as well.

Women represent approximately 60 percent of the population which seek help from the health and mental health care system. The women also receive only slightly over 60 percent of all medications.

So while women are overrepresented in the health and mental health care system, they are not overrepresented in terms of receiving prescription drugs.

Dr. Klerman also suggested that women may be using the health care system more appropriately than men, in that women seek help "before they have a chronic and continuous disease". He noted that it would be interesting to conduct a study on "whether women live longer partly because they are good health consumers, seeking services before they have irreversible damage and before a disease is untreatable".

Acute Overdosage

The benzodiazepines, like all psychotherapeutic medications prescribed for patients with severe emotional disorders, have frequently been implicated in situations of acute overdosage. A review of the scientific data in this area clearly and substantively documents the remarkable safety of this class of medications.

One long-term retrospective study reviewed 773 admissions to Massachusetts General Hospital between 1962 and 1975 that were attributable to accidental or deliberate overdosage with a psychoactive medication (Greenblatt *et al.*, 1977). Of the 99 admissions for benzodiazepine overdosage, only 12 were attributed to a benzodiazepine taken alone. None of these patients developed serious CNS depression or required respiratory assistance. The most seriously intoxicated group included 31 cases who took benzodiazepines in combination with barbiturates, with or without alcohol. The authors concluded: "This report and a review of the literature suggest that serious intoxication following overdosage with a benzodiazepine derivative alone is unusual.... The severity of intoxication in cases of multiple drug ingestion probably depends largely on the type and quantity of nonbenzodiazepines or other agents involved".

Table 6 Summary of acute overdosage studies

Study & years	Number of Valium^R overdosage patients reviewed†	Death due to Valium^R alone
Massachusetts General Hospital Acute overdose cases with psychotropics 1962–1975*	99	0
Drug-associated deaths in 24 major U.S. cities and 3 Canadian provinces 1971–1976**	1,239	2
Yale-New Haven Hospital Emergency Room 1968–1975***	93	0
Los Angeles County and U.S.C. Medical Center 1977****	139	0
Totals	1,570	2

†Case reports in some of these studies could be duplicated.
*Greenblatt *et al.* (1977).
**Finkle, McCloskey & Goodman (1979).
***Jatlow, Dobular & Bailey (1979).
****Ungerleider *et al.* (1980).

Another large-scale survey (Finkle, McCloskey & Goodman, 1979) recorded the number of deaths over a five-year period in 24 sites in the United States, with a combined population of 62.9 million people, and in three provinces of Canada. Of the total 79.2 million people, 1,239 cases of overdosage involved diazepam, and of these, only two deaths (0.2%) *appeared* to have resulted from the use of diazepam alone. This survey, too, showed that the cause of death in the majority of situations was attributable to other substances rather than to diazepam.

SOCIAL ISSUES

Abuse Potential

During their first 10 years of use, the phenomenon of addiction to the benzodiazepines was basically unknown, except for one study that demonstrated that after high doses (well above those recommended) and sudden discontinuation, withdrawal symptoms could occur (Hollister, Motzenbecker & Degan, 1961). During the latter part of the 1960's and the 1970's, many drug abuse treatment centers that had initiated detoxification and maintenance programs (with or without methadone) utilized a variety of CNS-acting medications to relieve the discomforting anxiety that many patients experienced, usually when methadone dosages were reduced to 30 mg or less. The phenothiazines, barbiturates, meprobamate and other medications were tested, but proved unsuccessful. However, the benzodiazepines, and particularly Valium[R], were found to greatly relieve the anxiety that many of these patients experienced during methadone withdrawal. Since the medical and scientific evidence was still quite unclear regarding the abuse and addictive potential of the benzodiazepines, it was felt that they would not be a problem in these patients. Unfortunately, the exposure to Valium[R], along with the relief that this medication provided, caused some individuals who had been previously addicted to other substances to seek it for nontherapeutic uses. This gradually resulted in the media's onerous reference to Valium[R] as a street drug. However, it was also found that many of these individuals utilized Valium[R] as a therapeutic agent to overcome many of the drug-related problems that they experienced with agents such as amphetamines, hallucinogens, PCP and others. At a 1981 meeting of the Drug Abuse Advisory Committee for the Food and Drug Administration (FDA), authorities declared that although Valium[R] could be found on the street, it was "not a drug of primary abuse".

An additional 15 years of clinical and epidemiological research into the abuse of the benzodiazepines has shown that those who are at risk of psychological and physical dependence have had previous histories of dependence to other chemicals, primarily alcohol. Clearly, the last 20 years have proven most informative in understanding the addictive disease process.

In the early 1960's, minor tranquilizers were recommended not only for detoxification of the alcoholic patient, but also for their maintenance during recovery. Medicine has learned that any CNS-acting medication may be misused by the patient who has a previous history of alcohol dependence, and should be avoided. The principal belief of Alcoholics Anonymous of the chemically-free state reflects the current understanding of how these individuals should be managed and how problems arising from the ingestion of other chemicals can be avoided. It is incumbent on all who are involved with health care delivery to be aware of the problems of the alcoholic patient, and to help them during their life-long recovery from this disease.

A 22-week study partially funded by the U.S. Public Health Service sought to determine the benefits and/or abuse potential of prolonged use of diazepam in chronically anxious patients (Rickels *et al.*, 1983). During the study period, tolerance did not develop in any patients as evidenced by the fact that they did not increase daily diazepam dosage but rather "often decreased drug intake on their own". The average dosage was 25 mg/day. It appears that when problems do arise in individuals who have been taking recommended doses of benzodiazepines, there are various factors involved. High doses (within the recommended range) and long periods of therapy are important characteristics that must be considered when evaluating an individual who has been receiving benzodiazepine therapy. Although there are those who state that individuals may become dependent in short periods of time, the scientific literature is hard put to support any specific time frame in which a patient may be at risk. Most of the documented cases of benzodiazepine dependence are of individuals who have received *continuous* therapy for at least six months to a year and, in most cases, much longer. A key factor here is *continuous* therapy, since the majority of benzodiazepine use is intermittent.

Another consideration that must be kept in mind by the therapist is the schedule for discontinuing benzodiazepine therapy in individuals who have received it for prolonged periods of time. As in the case of most CNS-acting and thyroid medications, steroids, beta-blockers and others, a slow tapering dosage over a period of time will prevent the onset of withdrawal symptoms in most patients. Specific schedules have been recommended by a number of authorities, and a physician who is dealing with a patient that has been receiving continuous benzodiazepine therapy for long periods of time and/or at high doses, should seek expert help in developing a tapered and titrated schedule of dosage reduction that will be most beneficial to the patient.

There have been some reports in the recent medical literature regarding withdrawal phenomena in patients receiving doses of benzodiazepines in the low to middle therapeutic dosage range. In most of the reports, these are individuals who have been on long-term therapy and admittedly had difficulty discontinuing their medication. Thus the results are biased from the beginning. It is hoped that as further study of this phenomenon is carried out over the next decade, the medical profession and the pharmaceutical industry will gain greater insight into the types of patients that are at risk and so improve diagnosis. As knowledge of addictive disease increases, the physician will be able to make more informed medication decisions regarding dosage, duration and discontinuance of therapy. Attention must also be paid to the personal and family history of the patient with an addictive disease.

Illness Potential

The possibility that Valium[R] might enhance the growth of cancer was raised by one investigator in 1981, based on a laboratory study of tissue culture and three small-scale rat studies of transplanted mammary tumors. Over the years, epidemiological data have been used as the most frequent means of determining human risk of cancer associated with the use of medicines. Since Valium[R] has been in widespread use around the world for the past 20 years, this medication provides an excellent opportunity for such epidemiological research. One large-scale study (Kaufman et al., 1982) supported by the FDA, the National Institute of Child Health and Human Development and Hoffman-La Roche, examined the relationship of breast cancer to Valium[R] use. Almost 2,000 women admitted to major hospitals in several large metropolitan areas in the United States, Canada and Israel between 1976 and 1980 for breast, female and other cancers were interviewed regarding their use of Valium[R] and length of therapy (i.e., less than six months, more than six months, and others). A total of 1,236 women with breast cancer and 728 control subjects with other types of malignancies were evaluated (see Table 7). Results of the study showed that patients using diazepam regularly for either short or long periods of time had the same or lower incidence of all types of malignancies as the control patients. In summary, the authors concluded that the "results of this study suggest that diazepam does not increase the risk of breast cancer relative to other cancer, either as a promoter or as an initiator".

Table 7   Diazepam use among women with breast cancer and controls

Diazepam use	Breast cancer (N = 1,236)	Female cancer (N = 436)	Other cancer (N = 292)
Regular (more than 6 months)	3%	3%	3%
Regular (less than 6 months)	2%	3%	3%
Other	20%	19%	15%
None	75%	75%	79%

A second epidemiological study (Friedman & Ury, 1980), conducted at the Kaiser–Permanente Medical Center in California and supported by the National Cancer Institute (NCI), was reported in the October 1980 issue of the *Journal of the National Cancer Institute*. The study followed almost 13,000 patients receiving Valium[R] for up to six years. Among these patients, the incidence of all forms of cancer was slightly less compared to those not receiving this medication. Table 8 summarizes the results of these two studies.

Table 8 Summary of cancer risk studies

Study & years	Study population	Risk with Valium[R]
Hospital case study survey in metropolitan areas of U.S., Canada and Israel 1976–1980	1,964	No evidence
Kaiser-Permanente Medical Program San Francisco 1969–1976	12,961	No evidence

In another study, using a large prescription data base, Danielson and colleagues (1982) found that the rate of cancer of the breast among women who had used Valium[R] in the previous six months was identical to that of women who had not used Valium[R]. Additionally, the NCI has also published a large case-controlled study (Kleinerman *et al.*, 1981) in which the risk of cancer of the breast was slightly (but not significantly) greater among women who had never taken Valium[R]. More detailed analysis showed that risk of breast cancer did not increase with increasing duration of Valium[R] use or the length of time since first use. Investigators concluded: "Our results thus fail to demonstrate a relation between Valium[R] use and risk of breast cancer".

Other case-controlled studies have been reported by Wallace *et al.* (1982) for breast cancer, and by Adam and Vessey (1981) for melanoma. None have shown any increased risk associated with Valium[R] use. The studies capable of addressing the issue of whether or not Valium[R] might act as a "promoter" of preexisting cancer are unanimous in their negative findings.

The results of all these important large-scale studies in humans, as well as animal data, fulfill the most rigid criteria currently available to experts to ensure that a medicine is free from any association with cancer. Even the most conservative assessment of the combined findings of these studies failed to provide any evidence of a *possible* link between Valium[R] and cancer.

Oral Clefts

A possible association between the development of fetal oral clefts and the use of Valium[R] during the first trimester of pregnancy was suggested by investigators in the 1970's. The Finnish Register of Congenital Malformations provided data on the incidence of this anomaly, and information concerning intake of various classes of medication was procured, both from records on file and by retrospectively questioning the mothers (Saxen, 1975). A total of 599 infants with oral clefts were born during the study period (1967–71) and compared to 590 matched controls. Consumption of salicylates, antipyretic analgesics, antineurotics (mainly Valium[R]) sulfonamides and antibacterials was noted.

Generally, drug consumption was more frequent among mothers of children with oral malformations than that occurring in the control group. When examining antineurotic medications (mainly Valium[R]), although data showed usage was almost two times as much in the first trimester by mothers of affected infants as compared to controls, it was more difficult to evaluate the significance due to a lack of similar studies. Factors other than drug consumption that might have affected results were not measured such as possibility of memory bias, chance correlations and effects of other drugs administered. As a matter of fact, when data from the next two years (1972–73) were examined, association of antineurotic drugs with the occurrence of cleft malformation was *approximately half that found originally, even though association of oral defects with overall intake of drugs remained significant* (Saxen, 1975).

An association between Valium[R] usage in the first trimester and incidence of oral clefts was suggested in studies conducted in Norway and the United States as well as the Finnish Study. Investigators concluded, after reviewing all three studies, that the data did not demonstrate a causal relationship between maternal exposure to Valium[R] and the occurrence of oral clefts and recommended further research be done (Safra & Oakley, 1976).

A more recent large-scale epidemiological study, funded jointly by Roche Laboratories and the FDA, was conducted by investigators at Boston University, Harvard and Tufts University Medical Schools and the findings presented are based on data collected from mothers of 3,109 children born with birth defects (Rosenberg *et al.*, 1983).

The authors conclude that '...diazepam use during the first trimester of pregnancy does not increase the risk of giving birth to a child with an oral cleft', and '...there is little reason on the basis of the available evidence to believe that in utero exposure to diazepam, in the way it is commonly used in pregnancy, materially influences the occurrence of oral clefts'.

In addition to refuting any connection between use of Valium[R] during pregnancy and development of the two major types of oral-cleft anomalies,

262

the authors also found that previous studies in this area "had methodological problems that limited their interpretability". These findings do not change the fact that all medication should be avoided during pregnancy.

REGULATORY ISSUES

Over the past three years, the United States and other governments, international organizations and interested parties have debated the merits of placing all or some of the benzodiazepines in Schedule IV of the Convention of Psychotropic Substances. Behind this debate appears to be the desire on the part of some individuals and organizations to do something about a perceived problem of benzodiazepine abuse. A widely held belief is that the mere fact of regulating a substance will solve a particular problem, or that by scheduling a drug or drugs under an international treaty something has been done to reduce abuse. This is not necessarily the case.

There has been little discussion on the practical effects of controlling the benzodiazepines internationally. Indeed, while lip service has been paid to the need to balance the costs versus the benefits of international scheduling, there has been little attention paid to attempting to quantify those benefits and costs, or to determining whether, in fact, this action will help governments fulfill the aims of the Psychotropic Convention. International control is only justified if it can be shown that national efforts are insufficient to deal with the problem, and the health and social consequences of the abuse of a medication outweigh the therapeutic benefits of its ready availability. It also must be shown that international control will, in fact, help governments attain the aims of the Convention. These considerations notwithstanding, the Commission on Narcotic Drugs voted in February 1984 to include 33 benzodiazepines in Schedule IV of the Psychotropic Convention.

Information/Education Needs

Historically, the primary responsibility of the pharmaceutical industry has been the research and development of safe and effective prescription medications. However, it is now quite clear that the industry's responsibility extends beyond this to the communication of appropriate and accurate information on these medications to physicians and other health care professionals. Nowhere is this more important than with the issue of the abuse potential of the benzodiazepines. As has been presented to various government and international agencies, any attempt to differentiate the abuse potential for members of the benzodiazepine class is one fraught with dangerous consequences. New benzodiazepines, claiming to have a lower potential for abuse, have quickly been shown to have problems once used in the clinical setting. Therefore, if the medical profession would accept the premise that all benzodiazepines have some potential for abuse (although low, and primarily in individuals who are at high risk), future problems with newer benzodiazepines will be avoided. It is hoped that the Valium[R] experience has made a major contribution to the understanding of when these medicines should and should not be used.

Most authorities agree that because of the widespread therapeutic value of benzodiazepines, both within the United States and throughout the world, any problems associated with their use cannot be successfully addressed on a regulatory basis. Information and education is clearly the most effective method of conveying, to both professional and nonprofessional audiences, the appropriate use of this significant class of medications. Patients and the public at large have expressed an intense interest in learning more about all prescription medications, and it is strongly recommended that the pharmaceutical industry assume responsibility for providing the necessary information. By doing so, the industry can play a major role in improving the delivery of health care.

References

Adam S, Vessey M: Diazepam and malignant melanoma. *Lancet* 1981;2:1344.

Balter MB, Levine J, Manheimer DI: Cross-national study of the extent of anti-anxiety/sedative drug use. *N Engl J Med* 1974;290:769.

Balter MB, Manheimer DI, Mellingel GD, *et al*: A cross-national comparison of anti-anxiety sedative drug use. *Curr Med Res Opin* 1984;8:5.

Caplan RD, Abbey A, Abramis DJ, Tranquilizer use and well-being: a longitudinal study of social and psychological effects. Technical report, Institute for Social Research, The University of Michigan. Research Report Series, 1984.

Danielson DA, Jick H, Hunter JR, *et al*: Nonestrogenic drugs and breast cancer. *Am J Epidemiol* 1982;116:329.

Dohrenwend BP, Dohrenwend BS, Gould MS, *et al*: *Mental Illness in the United States.* New York, Praeger, 1980.

Finkle BS, McCloskey KL, Goodman LS: Diazepam and drug associated deaths. *J Am Med Assoc* 1979;242:428.

Friedman GD, Ury HK: Initial screening for carcinogenicity of commonly used drugs. *J Nat Can Inst* 1980;65:723.

Greenblatt DJ, Allen MD, Noel BJ, *et al*: Acute overdose with benzodiazepine derivatives. *Clin Pharmacol Ther* 1977;21:497.

Hollister LE, Motzenbecker FD, Degan RO: Withdrawal reactions from chlordiazepoxide (Librium[R]). *Psychopharmacol* 1961:2:63.

Ilfeld FW: *Clinical Anxiety/Tension In Primary Medicine*. Amsterdam, Excerpta Medica, 1978.

Jatlow P, Dobular K, Bailey D: Serum diazepam concentrations in overdose. *Am J Clin Pathol* 1979;72:571.

Kaufman DW, Slone D, Shapiro S, *et al*: Diazepam and the risk of breast cancer. *Lancet* 1982;1:537.

Kleinerman RA, Rinton RA, Hoover R, *et al*: Diazepam and breast cancer. *Lancet* 1981;1:1153.

Klerman GL: Government funding. Paper presented at Second Annual Women in Crisis Conference. New York, June, 1980.

Kohn R, White KL: *Health Care – An International Study*. Oxford, England, Oxford University Press, 1976.

Manheimer DI, Davidson DT, Balter MB: Popular attitudes and beliefs about tranquilizers. *Am J Psychiatry* 1973;130:1246.

Mellinger GD, Balter MB: Prevalence and patterns of use of psychotherapeutic drugs. Paper presented at International Seminar: Epidemiological Impact of Psychotropic Drugs. Milan, Italy, June 1981.

Mellinger GD, Balter MB, Manheimer DI, *et al*: Psychic distress, life crisis and the use of psychotherapeutic medications. *Arch Gen Psychiatry* 1978;35:1045.

Mellinger GD, Balter MB, EH, *et al*: Uhlenhuth Prevalence and correlates of the long–term regular use of anxiolytics. *J Am Med Assoc* 1984;251:375.

Pardes H: Future needs of psychiatrists and other mental health personnel. *Arch Gen Psychiatry* 1979;36:1401.

Parry JH, Balter MB, Mellinger GD, *et al*: National patterns of psychotherapeutic drug use. *Arch Gen Psychiatry* 1973;28:769.

Regier DA, Goldberg ID, Taube CA: The de facto U.S. mental health service system. *Arch Gen Psychiatry* 1978;35:685.

Rosenberg L, Mitchell AA, Parsels JL, *et al*: Lack of relation of oral clefts to diazepam use during pregnancy. *N Engl J Med* 1983;309:1281.

Safra MJ, Oakley GP, Jr: Valium: an oral cleft teratogen. *Cleft Palate J* 1976;13:198.

Saxen I: Associations between oral clefts and drugs taken during pregnancy. *Int J Epidemiol* 1975;4:37.

Tessler R, Stokes R, Pietras M: Consumer response to Valium^R. *Drug Ther* 1978;9:178.

Ungerleider JT, Lundberg GD, Sunshine I, *et al*: The Drug Abuse Warning Network (DAWN) program. *Arch Gen Psychiatry* 1980;37:106.

Wallace RB, Sherman BM, Bean JA: A case control study of cancer and psychotropic drug use. *Oncology* 1983;39:279.

19
Benzodiazepines: International Legislation and Relation to the Convention on Psychotropic Substances 1971

John Marks, MD

INTRODUCTION

Dependence and abuse of any substance can produce public health and social problems. Health authorities must be concerned with such problems and attempts to solve them often involve the use of legislation. Where the problem is local, legislation should equally be local. When there is a more general, international problem, then the question arises whether local legislation enacted by individual countries is adequate or whether a broader internationally based control system represents a more appropriate solution. The benzodiazepines are substances for which there is a dependence risk and some abuse. This is considered in Chapter 13. Hence it is important to examine their relationship to local and international legislation and the present chapter attempts this task.

LOCAL CONTROL OF PSYCHOTROPICS – CURRENT SITUATION

The majority of countries, both industrially developed and those of the Third World, now have local laws which cover control of benzodiazepine use in clinical medicine. In about two-thirds of the countries, the benzodiazepines are themselves specifically mentioned within the legislation (e.g., the United States); in the others, the regulations are such that although the group of benzodiazepines are not mentioned by name, the regulations nevertheless apply to these substances (e.g., the United Kingdom).

In the majority of the countries where benzodiazepines are controlled, the legislation applies to every member of the therapeutic group, and it is rare to find special controls restricted to individual substances. The regulations nearly always demand availability only on prescription. However, there are differences between countries on whether the prescriptions are not repeatable (about one-third); limited in the number of repeats; or limited as to the period over which repeats may be dispensed by pharmacists. In about half the countries, in addition to prescription requirements, some form of local reporting system exists. The details on the exact reporting systems vary considerably.

While there is considerable uniformity in the *requirement* of prescription in the majority of countries, a considerable gap exists in many countries between the legal requirement and the implementation. Thus, for example, in about one-third of countries that have been studied, national legislation does not appear to be implemented effectively. Usually this stems from a lack of economic resources and personnel rather than from any active desire to avoid the implementation of the existing laws.

INTERNATIONAL CONTROL OF PSYCHOTROPICS – GENERAL CONSIDERATIONS

In 1971, a new international convention for the control of drugs that are liable to abuse was adopted in Vienna following extensive discussion (United Nations, 1971a).

This Convention complements the existing legislative and control measures for narcotics, is concerned with the psychoactive substances and is known as the United Nations Convention of Psychotropic Substances, 1971. This Convention entered into force on August 16th, 1976, when it had been signed by 40 governments. More governments have added their signatures since then, although the number of signatories is still substantially less than for the equivalent convention that deals with narcotics.

As a result of this Convention, the signatory states, both industrially developed and in the Third World, are committed to formulating, implementing and enforcing national legislation which gives local force to the terms of the international convention.

The Convention itself (United Nations, 1971a), the commentary to the Convention (United Nations, 1971b) which analyses the wording and provisions of the articles in detail, and various World Health Organisation, United Nations and other reports (Lande, 1970; Kramer, 1978; Addiction Research Foundation, 1980; WHO, 1981a) provide valuable information on the way that the Convention is being interpreted in practice. All these documents should be consulted by those interested in the subject.

The conditions under which a substance may be included in one of the schedules of the Convention are clearly defined, viz:

"the substance has the capacity to produce of state of dependence" *and* "Central nervous system stimulation or depression, resulting in hallucinations or disturbances in motor function or thinking or behaviour or perception or mood",

or "Similar abuse and similar ill effects as a substance in Schedule I, II, III or IV".

That is to say, a psychoactive drug with a capacity to produce a state of dependence or similarity of abuse to a substance already controlled *may* be scheduled under this Convention.

However, the scope of control is limited with the objective of protecting public health. Hence an additional criterion is that

"there is sufficient evidence that the substance is being or is likely to be abused so as to constitute a public health or social problem warranting the placing of the substance under international control".

The meaning of this criterion and the extent of the public health and social problem requiring that control be exercised within the Convention was considered by the World Health Organisation Expert Committee at its sixteenth meeting (WHO, 1969) and confirmed at the twenty-first meeting (WHO, 1978). It was deemed necessary for the drug dependence to cause behavioral problems that adversely affect others *and* to be 'widespread in the population or have a significant potential for becoming widespread'. When this applies, a public health problem exists and society must then take the responsibility for deciding on the need for the control of the drug.

Another important criterion relating to controls is whether "international control" as opposed to national "are suitable to solve or at least alleviate the problem" (Commentary p 47 para 8 (United Nations, 1971b)).

THE ROLE OF INTERNATIONAL LEGISLATION IN THE PSYCHOTROPIC SUBSTANCE ABUSE FIELD

Any legislation within the drug field must take full account of the general framework of the nation's public health policy. This applies particularly to the 1971 Convention in which Schedules III and IV contain several substances with extensive and valid medical use. It is important, therefore, that the laws should attempt to treat the reasons behind the phenomenon of drug abuse rather than just impose strict controls on supply.

There is no single cause for the development of abuse of any particular drug – rather there are many factors that play a varying role. These lie within the realm of the drug itself, the personality of the individual and the external environment.

Drug specific factors – direct, e.g., dependence potential; as well as indirect drug related circumstances (e.g., availability and accessibility which influence demand), may be of great importance. The desire to relieve personal problems constitutes an important element underlying the onset or continuation of drug misuse. Thus the ability of drugs to produce euphoria, inner contentment, excitement, or at the other end of the scale, oblivion in sleep, represent drug specific causes of misuse.

According to current theory, certain people are more likely to develop dependence for *personality* reasons. The personal characteristics that appear to present the greatest risk are social inadequacy or psychopathology. Moreover, patients with a severe chronic and intractable psychoneurosis, e.g., phobia, are likely to receive long-term sedative or tranquillizer therapy and may become dependent on the agent that is prescribed.

The external environment is thought to play a vital role in the genesis of dependence. Social stress factors include poverty, boredom, urban conditions and trends in behaviour patterns. Cultural factors include the presence of deviant behaviour groups and teenager rebellion.

Legislation should try to take full account of the multifactorial aetiology. However, it is important to realise that there is a need for further study. Thus, the WHO Expert Committee on drug dependence stated (WHO, 1981b):

"Recognising the limits of available knowledge and understanding of the causes of the non-medical use of drugs and drug dependence, the Committee urged that further research be initiated to characterize those persons most vulnerable to various forms of drug dependence".

So far as the factors related to the *personality* of the individual are concerned, legislation can only have a rather limited role. Personality cannot.be changed by legislation and though the laws will have some deterrent effects, the unprincipled, the weak willed and the psychopath are unlikely to be influenced by norms imposed on them by others. Moreover, the mere existence of publicised legal constraints may encourage experimentation in the young.

How far it is possible to influence *environmental factors* by legislation must be a matter of dispute. In so far as drug abuse represents a reaction to social change and technology, legislation can do little. However, it is possible for the state to influence certain aspects of the environment, e.g., urbanisation, pollution, economics, the rights of minorities, etc. However these matters achieve scant attention in current international legislation.

Rather, the main force of drug laws has been directed against the *product related* causes of drug abuse. In the absence of a clearer understanding of how to deal with the other causes, this is likely to remain the pattern for a considerable time. Thus, the main emphasis is placed on controls of availability of products of abuse and of their movement. However, the importance of recognition, treatment and rehabilitation of those who are dependent is also recognised.

It is abundantly clear that drug abuse cannot be effectively prevented by legislative controls of the drugs and of their supply alone. A further aim must be to exert an influence on demand. Criminal legislation represents a costly, ineffective and ambivalent means of achieving this. Thus, in addition to the controls of movement and supply, preventive measures are desirable. These are recommended within Article 20 of the Convention (United Nations, 1971a). Both technical and financial assistance are available under the auspices of the United Nations to this end. As experience is gained, so the technical information that is available improves. Unfortunately, the international financial assistance that is available does not develop at a similar rate.

Among preventive measures that should be considered are education for medicals, paramedicals and the public in the correct use of drugs and in the dangers of misuse and abuse: the creation of constructive alternative uses of leisure, particularly for adolescents: adequate treatment, rehabilitation and reintegration facilities.

THE PROCESS BY WHICH A PSYCHOTROPIC IS PUT UNDER INTERNATIONAL CONTROL

The final decision on whether a substance is controlled under the Convention of Psychotropic Substances, 1971 rests with the United Nations, based upon a decision taken by the Commission on Narcotic Drugs of the Economic and Social Council. If any country, or the World Health Organisation, has information which suggests that a substance should be controlled, then it notifies the Secretary General of the United Nations and furnishes him with the appropriate supporting information. This notification is then forwarded formally to the World Health Organisation which, with the advice of an Expert Committee, established at the invitation of WHO considers the available medical and scientific evidence that a problem exists. WHO also seeks information on the therapeutic uses; the extent of the dependence and abuse and its international implications.

If the WHO considers that the situation covered by Article 2 para 4 (a) and (b) of the Convention applies, then WHO communicates to the Commission

"... an assessment of the substance, including the extent or likelihood of abuse, the degree of seriousness of the public health and social

271

problem and the degree of usefulness of the substance in medical therapy, together with recommendations on control measures, if any, that would be appropriate in the light of its assessment".

This implies that WHO must take account of the balance between medical usefulness of the substance and the level of public health and social problems involved in any abuse. The Commentary to the 1971 Convention stresses that WHO is required to cover "all the points".."under paragraph 4" in a written communication.

"But only those "assessements" of WHO "as to medical and scientific matters" contained in that Organisation's communications pursuant to paragraphs 4 and 6 are "determinative", and not the views of the Organisation's representative at meetings of the Commission, or those of other of its official spokesmen expressly on other occasions..." (Commentary para 15 p 69).

The Commission considers the WHO report which is submitted to it. The Report is "determinative as to medical and scientific matters". However, in reaching a decision, the Commission should bear in mind "economic, social, legal, administrative and other factors it may consider relevant" and "may seek further information from the World Health Organisation or from other Appropriate sources". The question of the determinative aspect of the WHO Report on medical and scientific matters is considered in some detail in the Commentary to the Convention and it is considered (paragraph 24 on page 71) that this includes "the view of WHO on the therapeutic usefulness of the substance".

WHO is required to express both the "public health and social problem" and the "usefulness" in terms of "degree", which implies some measure of quantification. The Commentary (page 69 para 18) indicates that the Commission has the right to examine the data for such an assessment and "the WHO views on the reliability or importance of statistical data, estimated figures etc., not being 'medical and scientific matters' would not be determinative" (United Nations, 1971b).

Moreover, those [WHO] reasons which are not "medical or scientific"-..."may be replaced by the Commission's own establishment of facts"..."while [WHO] reasons whether 'medical, scientific or other'"-..."may be outweighed by such economic, social, legal, administrative or other factors as the Commission may consider relevant" (Commentary, para 19 page 70).

Hence, it is clear that the Commission may review the evidence on whichWHO reaches its conclusions and also seek for and look at its own evidence on any of these matters that do not come strictly within the framework of "medical and scientific".

Having considered the evidence presented by WHO, together with any evidence that it may itself seek in the light of "economic, social, legal, administrative or other factors", the Commission then decides by a vote whether the substance shall be controlled and if so in which Schedule. Normally, the voting is on the individual substances.

The decisions of the Commission "shall be taken by a two-thirds majority of the members of the Commission". Up to and including the meetings of the Commission in 1983, the Commission consisted of 30 states, hence a decision to control required 20 assenting votes (abstentions being equivalent in this respect to a dissent). At the UN Economic and Social Council on 25 May, 1983, a decision was taken to enlarge the membership of the Commission from 30 to 40 members. Hence, now and in the future, 27 assenting votes will be required for control to be imposed by a decision of the Commission.

THE PROBLEMS INHERENT IN INTERNATIONAL CONTROL

The Reliability of the Data Upon Which Decisions Are Based

As is explained above, the decision to place a substance within the schedules of the Convention is taken by the Narcotics Commission of the United Nations but the scientific and medical evidence is furnished as a report by the WHO.

The overall principles for international control under the 1971 Convention was stated in the Sixteenth Report of the WHO Expert Committee on Drug Dependence (WHO, 1969) and are restated with great clarity in the Twenty-first Report (WHO, 1978).

> "In contrast to the established narcotic control treaties, the 1971 Convention required that the therapeutic value of psychotropic substances be balanced against the risk to public health and social well-being arising from their use..." and

> "the need, type and degree of international control must be based on two considerations: a) the degree of risk to public health and b) the usefulness of the drug in medical therapy. The drug's usefulness must be weighed against the potential or established risks that arise from any abuse. The resulting ratio determines both the need for control and the degree of control. Because of the established therapeutic usefulness and the necessary and legitimate use of many of the [psychotropic] drugs...WHO must make every effort to ensure that the inclusion of drugs in the schedules is justified by the appropriate assessment of the balance between risk and benefit."

The Division of Mental Health of the WHO is responsible for determining the facts and for preparing the report and is advised by an expert international committee on drug dependence, the members of which are chosen by WHO.

The findings on the existence of dependence and of the psychoactive nature of the effects in humans are relatively easy to determine when there is extensive experience of clinical use. However, it is the aim of the Convention to *prevent* problems of dependence rather than deal with those that are already established. Thus, some recommendations are made by WHO from predictions from animal pharmacological and toxicological data, substantiated by limited information from man. The test methods and their relevance are reviewed in the Twenty-first Report of the WHO Expert Committee (WHO, 1978).

The determination of the abuse potential on the other hand has to be made as a value judgement, of the balance between "the degree of risk to public health" and "the usefulness of the drug in medical therapy". It must also consider the relevance of international control in avoiding an abuse problem, an aspect that will be considered later. The WHO Expert Committee on Drug Dependence in their Twenty-first Report (1978) stressed the difficulties that must exist due to the lack of adequate means of measuring or expressing several of the criteria in quantitative terms. This would include the risk of abuse and the estimate of the social and public health problems both of which should be expressed in quantitative terms.

The question of the validity of the data on which the advice is given was a matter of concern to the members of the Expert Committee and was dealt with extensively in their Twenty-first Report (1978). There is considerable agreement among those involved in drug abuse control that further information is needed in order to reach correct decisions.

Since there are problems relating to the validity of data, it follows, in the author's opinion, that

> a. the evidence upon which the decisions are reached should be published fully with the report so that the Commission and any interested parties may examine and question its factual validity as allowed within the Convention (Commentary to Article 2 paras 5 and 6 of the Convention – p 69 (United Nations, 1971b)).

> b. all decisions for scheduling should be reviewed periodically as new methods produce fresh data. The Convention allows for such reviews, initiated either by WHO or a signatory state. It is to be hoped that adequate use will be made of this review procedure.

Since many aspects considered by the Expert Committee are based upon opinions rather than scientific facts, it is essential that the selection and working of the Expert Committee should be undertaken in as open a fashion as possible. This in no way implies criticism of the nature or integrity of the Committee but stresses that "not only must justice be done, but it must be seen to be done". At present, it would appear that this is not being achieved and, in consequence, unnecessary and unfortunate suspicions exist. For example, the selection of the Expert Committee appears to lie within a narrow central group within the WHO secretariat, with no apparent appeal procedure, while the Expert Committee meetings are held in private. In the opinion of the author, such an arrangement by its nature breeds suspicion, not least of political influence. The excellent scientific name of WHO would best be served by a more open style of decision making.

Controls Lead To Restriction For Therapeutic Use

An essential feature of the 1971 Convention is that the therapeutic use of the substances shall be adequately preserved. This implies that the legislation that arises locally as a result of the Convention should not reduce authorised therapeutic use.

Although it is the clear intention of the Convention that local legislation should allow for appropriate medical access to drugs within the less stringent schedules, this does not always follow in practice. Within the industrially developed nations, where there are adequate facilities and personnel, few difficulties exist, but in some developing countries the penal and medical resources are inadequate. Here, in practice, the placing of a substance in even the least stringent schedule often leads to its total removal from the licit therapeutic armamentarium while there is relative ease of access within a "black market" (Zarco & Almonte, 1977; Soueif, 1981).

This problem of therapeutic availability of some of the important psychoactive substances is one that has so far been given inadequate attention in considerations of the practical implications of the 1971 Convention.

Variability of Application of the Controls

Legislation by its very nature is only as good as the will and ability that exists to apply it. For international conventions, this implies the legislative powers and enforcement facilities that exist within the individual countries. Hence, while the concept will be uniform, the details will vary.

In addition, there are major national differences in the way that laws are enforced and the economic ability to enforce them. Thus, it is apparent that terms of the Convention cannot be applied in an entirely uniform fashion at present.

Unfortunately, some countries do not exercise at present all the controls under the Single Convention and several countries that are already Parties to the Psychotropic Substances Convention are not operating the prescribed controls under this new treaty. In a few cases, the fundamental problem is cultural, but usually the problem is an economic one. This may be the result of the effect that it is believed that the export controls would have on trade; or a low gross national product which allows too low a funding for health matters. Unfortunately, this is a problem which has not been totally solved yet. More funds and a greater level of technical assistance must be made available. Since drug control measures tend to produce the greatest social cost when they are inadequately enforced, the inability to enforce the appropriate legislation may be a good reason for hesitation about becoming a signatory to the Psychotropic Convention. Yet the Convention will only be effective with majority support. Hence nations must be convinced that the control decisions that are taken have clear benefit.

The Relation of Controls to the Rights of Society

Although there is general agreement that the best answer would be a society in which none of the members resorted to the use of psychoactive agents, this must be regarded as a dream of Utopia, not least because some level of mental sickness is as inevitable as physical sickness.

At the present, despite a wide range of social conditions and political ideologies, there is no community in the world which has no substance dependence problem. Some of this abuse has even been accorded the privilege of social acceptability in some communities (e.g., alcohol, nicotine, coffee).

Criminal legislation is a form of social control which aims to contain within tolerable limits deviant behaviour. Normally, criminal laws imply that the deviant behaviour damages others. Contravention of some aspects of the drug laws, on the other hand, often affects no person other than the one who is directly involved. This applies particularly to those parts that relate to possession and consumption. It is in this area that legislators have to exercise the greatest caution.

Thus, there is a conflict of interest between the desire of the State to protect the health of the individual and the freedom for the individual that is specifically recognised in Article 29:2 of the United Nations Universal Declaration of Human Rights (UN Document A/811):

"In the exercise of his rights and freedoms, everyone shall be subject to such limitations as are determined by law solely for the purpose of securing due recognition and respect for the rights and freedoms of others and of meeting the just requirements of morality, public order and the general welfare in a democratic society".

This aspect is fully covered in the 1971 Convention, for drugs can only be scheduled if there is a "public health and social problem" which warrants international control. This implies that the abuse by the individual has had repercussions that have extended beyond his own confines and affected society in general. In these circumstances, the rights of the individual, though considered, are subservient to the good of the community. Nevertheless, when international controls as defined within the 1971 Convention are translated into national laws, it is important to ensure that the rights of the individual are preserved as fully as possible.

The Relevance of the Controls

The emphasis on product related aspects of control places great importance on correct scheduling by the Commission, advised by WHO. It also implies that the level of control, be it national or international, is appropriate to deal with the level of risk. Over control can be just as undesirable as under control. Legal measures which are out of step with accepted norms of the society can undermine respect for the law. Moreover, since many of the products controlled by the Convention on Psychotropic Substances are valuable therapeutic agents, it is important to ensure that the medical advantages are still available at reasonable cost.

The imposition of tight controls may cause misusers to transfer to alternative substances. It is important to ensure that too rigorous controls on low risk drugs do not encourage movement to drugs of higher risk that may be more readily available in the illegal sector or to substances that are present as everyday household substances (e.g., industrial solvents).

However, even relevant controls can produce problems. If the specific drug habit deviates from the socially acceptable behaviour, the consumers concerned may be rejected by the general public. The self-perception of the user varies with the social response. He may well withdraw further from society, founding or joining a subculture of like-minded individuals, thus increasing the distance between user and established society. In consequence, the activity of legislators may perpetuate the abuse that they wish to prevent. The greater the alienation, the less is the tolerance displayed by society towards the dissidents. The efforts of the legislator must be directed to achieving relevant controls without alienation.

When the level of risk of a drug is perceived to be high by the general public, then the chance of a large subculture developing is small. When the general public does not *perceive* a great risk – even if one exists – then the subculture may be large and enforcement of legislation difficult (e.g., alcohol in prohibition days, cannabis currently in the USA). On the other hand, the greater the risk and the greater the level of law enforcement, the greater the tendency for a tighter though smaller subculture.

Moreover, if the law is violated widely and by consensus no victims complain, the law enforcement officers may be forced to adopt practices which cause considerable resentment among the public. Enforcement of the law is difficult and costly unless the public broadly accepts its wisdom and necessity. Legislators should bear this in mind.

Another significant problem of drug control is that it can lead to a drug producing and dealing network which can also take part in other organised crime. Large profits within the illicit trade can in their turn lead to police corruption. Within this illicit trade, the drug price rises and, in its turn, this leads to the user being forced into crime to cope with his dependence. This is a difficult problem because, by their very nature, it is the drugs with the highest dependence risk that need the most control but are the most likely to lead to criminal activity. The police authorities will be given the greatest chance to concentrate on the most difficult problems if legislators are careful not to include too wide a range of drugs in the controls and particularly to exclude those that can be dealt with by lesser regulations. This principle is inherent in the Convention on Psychotropic Substances.

Benefit–Cost Aspects of the Controls

Drug misuse, in addition to the effects on the individual, will often impose social and economic costs on the community. However, the imposition of controls also leads to social and economic costs.

It is essential that the social cost and benefits be equated with care. However, it is at present very difficult to produce such an equation in the Psychotropic Substances legislation area because the science of cost–benefit analysis in the field of health care is still only in its infancy. Some of the readily defined costs are easy to compute. Less readily quantified are some of the social costs and most of the health benefits. The whole matter has been considered in the Report of the WHO Expert Committee (1978); in chapter 14 of the UN Social Defense and Research Institute (1973); in an article by Kramer (1978) and in paragraph 4.2.3 (p 40) of the 1981 Report of the WHO Expert Committee (WHO, 1981b).

The fact that narcotic abuse is regarded as a serious problem and that the costs involved are fully justified by the benefits is attested to by the very large number of signatories to the Single Convention. The number of governments who are also signatories to the Convention on Psychotropic Substances is also encouraging. It would appear that one reason for some other countries not becoming parties is concern about the benefit–cost ratio of this later Convention. It is therefore essential that the Commission constantly keeps this matter of cost–benefit under consideration if the Convention is to be effective. That this is accepted as a principle is shown by the importance accorded it in the Convention (United Nations, 1971a), the

Commentary (1971b) and the recent WHO Expert Committee Report (1981b). It is hoped that the principle is followed in practice in the deliberations of the Commission.

An outline of the current views of some of the costs and benefits, both social and economic, that should be considered is given in Table 1. It is important to appreciate that while the economic costs occur to a greater or lesser extent once a decision is taken to impose controls, the benefits only occur from reduction of drug damage – to the individual, to the family and to society. However, drug use does not invariably lead to damage. This is particularly true to therapeutic substances and this is therefore highly relevant for a consideration of therapeutically useful substances in the least stringent Schedules (III & IV) of the Psychotropic Substances Convention.

Table 1. Outline of some of the social and economic costs and benefits of drug legislation.

	Cost of Controls	Benefits from Controls*
SOCIAL	For the individual	For the Individual
	1. Personal freedoms restricted 2. Difficult licit drug supply or costs of alternative treatment	1. Improved physical and mental health 2. Improved family relationships
	For society	For society
	1. Rebel subcultures 2. Corruption	1. Reduced accidents 2. Reduced drug contagion risk 3. Reduced criminality 4. Altered social attitudes
ECONOMIC	For the individual	For the individual
	1. Burden of illicit drug costs 2. Higher costs of licit drugs	1. Improved work performance
	For society	For society
	1. Smuggling, black market 2. Drug security and distribution costs 3. Record keeping 4. Law enforcement 5. Initial treatment costs	1. Ultimately reduced medical and welfare costs 2. Reduced criminality and private security costs

* Mainly the results of costs of drug abuse.

279

THE HISTORY OF CONSIDERATION OF INTERNATIONAL CONTROL OF THE BENZODIAZEPINES

The benzodiazepines that were then available were first considered for inclusion in Schedule IV during the plenipotentiary conference at which the Psychotropics Convention was established (UNO, 1971a). After considerable discussion, they were excluded from the list that would be controlled.

It was not until 1981 that the matter was raised again. In that year, the World Health Organisation was requested to study 12 benzodiazepines. The WHO Expert Committee in its 5th Review recommended that *all* currently marketed benzodiazepines and detailed 23 of the group (i.e. the 12 originally defined in the request and a further 11 for which review had not been requested) be placed in Schedule IV of the Convention on Psychotropic Substances. This decision was based on the conclusion that:

> "the evidence reviewed so far is insufficient to allow differentiation among the various benzodiazepines as to dependence potential, abuse liability, and risk to public health and"..."that at this time all benzodiazepines should be scheduled similarly".

The Director General of WHO proposed to the UN Commission on Narcotic Drugs (Session 2nd to 8th February 1982 in Vienna) that the 23 mentioned benzodiazepines be put in Schedule IV of the Convention of Psychotropic Substances. The proposal (i.e., that all 23 then available be controlled) departed from the United Nations request as the notification from the Secretary General concerned only the review of 12 benzodiazepines he had detailed. The UN Commission on Narcotic Drugs, partly for procedural reasons, took the decision: "to postpone consideration of the matter until the 30th Session of the Commission in February, 1983". The Commission further invited the Expert Committee to present further information relating to all the benzodiazepines for this 30th Session.

The WHO 6th Review of Psychoactive Substances for International Control in September 1982 (WHO, 1982) considered that it "had the liberty to further review the twelve substances in the light of new data made available to them" but that their main task was to consider the 15 additional benzodiazepines defined in the Secretary General's request. The Expert Committee's recommendation was to place 26 of the 27 benzodiazepines considered in Schedule IV of the Convention on Psychotropic Substances but to "defer the decision to place halazepam under control".

At their meeting in February 1983, the Commission rejected the recommendation for each of the 26 benzodiazepines and requested further consideration by the WHO Expert Committee.

The Eighth Review by the WHO Expert Committee (WHO, 1983) recommended that 33 of the 39 benzodiazepine type substances which they had been asked to examine should be subjected to international control in Schedule IV of the Convention on Psychotropic Substances. Five of the remaining six substances that were not recommended for control showed significant pharmacological and clinical differences which suggested that they are not benzodiazepine-like therapeutically; the sixth, zopiclone, is not a benzodiazepine. The Expert Committee suggested that the dependence and abuse potential of all the benzodiazepines must, on present evidence, be regarded as equivalent, for:

> "The abuse liabilities...were found to be in the range of low to moderate...extremely difficult to differentiate among these substances..."

The WHO Report *neither suggested nor produced evidence that the situation had worsened in the last year.* Since, in the vote in the United Nations Commission on Narcotic Drugs in 1983, no benzodiazepine was voted as needing to be controlled it would be thought, on logical grounds, that the recommendation should be rejected again.

Nevertheless, the United Nations Commission on Narcotic Drugs, at its Eighth Special Session in February 1984, decided to place all 33 benzodiazepines in Schedule IV of the 1971 Convention on Psychotropic Substances, the decision being taken on a substance by substance basis. Schedule IV requires that the distribution of the benzodiazepines shall be made under license only. They can be dispensed only on the basis of medical prescription. Schedule IV also implies some reporting requirements on the quantities exported and imported.

This decision does not even now cover all the benzodiazepines that are currently available, though not on the basis that they have been excluded as safe. As Smith and Marks have pointed out elsewhere in this book (Chapter 13), this will encourage the substitution of these other substances in the mistaken belief that they carry a lower dependence liability.

INTERNATIONAL CONTROL OF THE BENZODIAZEPINES IN PERSPECTIVE

From what has been said in this chapter, it should be apparent that the author regards Schedule III and IV of the Convention on Psychotropic Substances 1971 as one of the least useful portions of international drug legislation. Equally, the author still considers that international control of the benzodiazepines is neither necessary nor desirable for the following reasons:

1.   The dependence is low.

2. The benzodiazepines are not drugs of primary abuse.

3. A high benefit to cost ratio for control has not been demonstrated.

4. There is no evidence that international control will improve the situation above that achieved by local legislation.

5. There will be a reduction in availability for therapeutic purposes in some countries but illicit supplies will not be affected.

6. Dependence is most likely to occur with inappropriate long-term therapeutic administration. This can be dealt with best by medical, paramedical and lay education.

7. Resources will be diverted from the control of more dangerous substances, particularly narcotics.

Table 2. "Costs" of use of benzodiazepines compared with tobacco and alcohol.

	Tobacco	Alcohol	Benzodiazepines
Therapeutic value	Nil	Nil	Great
Population point level of use	50%	75%	2%
Dependence risk	High	High	Low
Mental deterioration	Nil	Often high	No clinical evidence
Physical damage	Very great	Great	Nil
Family breakdown	Nil	Great	Nil
Work situation	Nil	Great reduction	Can improve
Criminality	Nil	Great	Nil
Overdose risk	Nil	Large	Negligible
Accidents	Nil	Very great	Small
Drug contagion	High	High	Negligible
Total social cost	Great from physical illness	Great from physical and mental illness	Small or negligible

Attention is specifically drawn to the fact that two widely abused substances (alcohol and tobacco) are not subjected to control. A comparison of the benzodiazepine situation with that for these two socially acceptable substances of abuse is given in Table 2. This demonstrates that control of either of these substances would produce an infinitely greater medical and social benefit than the control of benzodiazepines.

SUMMARY AND CONCLUSIONS

An account is given of the principles and practice of legislation for the control of psychotropic substances. The role of international legislation is considered and the process by which a psychotropic substance is considered for international control is described. The problems inherent in international control are described.

A history is given of the extensive consideration of the control of the benzodiazepines by both the World Health Organisation and the United Nations Commission on Narcotic Drugs. The 33 benzodiazepines that have been considered have recently been placed on Schedule IV of the Convention on Psychotropic Substances 1971. On the basis of the whole appraisal, the following conclusions are drawn:

1. The views expressed by both the UNO and WHO that the methodology on various aspects of the consideration of substances for control needs considerable study can be fully endorsed. Specific attention is directed to the need expressed by the WHO for further research on both the economic and social effects of the therapeutic use and abuse of different classes of psychotropic drugs.

2. The Convention gives clear guidelines on the principles governing scheduling, assuming that the substance comes within the definition of "Psychotropic" (Article 2 para 4 (a) & (b) viz:

a. The extent of therapeutic use must be considered and ease of access for therapy maintained.

b. The balance between dependence/abuse risk with public health and social damage compared with the costs of control must be assessed.

c. There should be a need for *international* as opposed to local control.

The Commission also has the task *inter alia* of determining the *economic* and *political* wisdom of any scheduling decision.

3. There are substantial worries about the control of therapeutically valuable substances particularly in relation to the restriction of use of various countries; the cost–benefit ratio is poor; controls will reduce resources that are needed for the control of more dangerous substances.

4. If the benzodiazepines are viewed against these criteria, it is suggested that:

a. They have wide, and in some developing countries life-saving (e.g., tetanus), therapeutic value; that there are currently no appropriate therapeutic alternatives.

b. In certain countries, any scheduling will lead to a lack of availability for therapeutic use but instead to a thriving black market for abuse.

c. The dependence/abuse risk, though it exists, is small.

d. There are negligible medical, family, social or public health costs and hence the benefits from scheduling will be minimal.

e. Some commonly defined general benefits (e.g., reduced criminality) are illusory.

f. The costs of control will be substantial and use the resources which are already currently inadequate to ensure effective control of substances with greater risks (e.g., narcotics).

g. There would be far more medical logic in utilising resources for the control of tobacco and alcohol.

5. The recent decision by the Commission to place the benzodiazepines in Schedule IV is, in consequence, regarded as inappropriate. Education for medical and paramedical personnel and the general public on the appropriate use of this group of drugs would, in the author's opinion, be more effective.

References

Addiction Research Foundation: Report of the "International Working Group on the Convention on Psychotropic Substances, 1971". Alcohol and Drug Addiction Research Foundation, Toronto, September 8-12, 1980.

Kramer JC: Social benefits and social costs of drug control laws. *J Drug Issues* 1978;8:1-7.

Lande A: Principles of effective drug abuse control. Papers presented at the International Institute on the Prevention and Treatment of Drug Dependence, 1970, pp 51-79.

Lind RC: Benefit-cost approach to evaluation of programs, in *Controlling Drugs: International Handbook for Psychoactive Drug Classification*. United Nations Social Defence Research Institute, Rome. London, Jossey-Bass, 1974.

Soueif MI: The Psychotropic Convention in Egypt, in Smart R, Murray GF, Archibald HD (eds): *Psychotropic Substances and Their International Control*. Toronto, Alcohol and Drug Addiction Research Foundation, 1981.

United Nations: *United Nations Convention on Psychotropic Substances 1971*. New York, United Nations, 1971a.

United Nations: *Commentary on the Convention on Psychotropic Substances 1971*. New York, United Nations, 1971b.

United Nations: *Psychoactive Drug Control: Issues and Recommendations*. Rome, United Nations Social Defence Research Institute, 1973.

United Nations: *Report of the Seventh Special Session of the Commission on Narcotic Drugs*. Vienna, United Nations Organisation, 1982.

United Nations: *Report of the Thirtieth Session of the Commission on Narcotic Drugs*. Vienna, United Nations Organisation, 1983.

WHO: *Expert Committee on Drug Dependence: Sixteenth Report*, World Health Org Tech Rep Ser No 407. Geneva, WHO, 1969.

WHO: *World Health Organisation Expert Committee on Drug Dependence: Twenty-first Report*, Tech Rep Ser No 618. Geneva, WHO, 1978.

WHO: *Assessment of Public Health and Social Problems Associated with the Use of Psychotropic Drugs: Report of the WHO Expert Committee on the Implementation of the Convention on Psychotropic Substances, 1971*, World Health Org Tech Rep Ser No 656. Geneva, WHO, 1981a.

WHO: *Report of the Fifth World Health Organisation Review of Psychoactive Substances for International Control*. Geneva, WHO, November 16-20, 1981b.

WHO: *Report of the Sixth World Health Organisation Review of Psychoactive Substances for International Control*. Geneva, WHO, September 6-10, 1982.

Appendix 1
Cross-Reference of Research, Generic and Trade Names of Benzodiazepines

Table 1. Benzodiazepine research designations with corresponding generic names

Research Designation	Generic Name
lactam	demoxepam
methyloxazepam	temazepam
A 101	nordazepam
AB 35616	clorazepate
AB 39083	clorazepate
AH 3232	clorazepate
CB 4261	tetrazepam
CB 4306	clorazepate
CB 4311	clorazepate
CGS 8216	(antagonist)
CI 683	ripazepam
CS 370	cloxazolam
CS 430	haloxazolam
D 40TA	estazolam
EGYT 341	tofisopam
ER 115	temazepam
HR 158	loprazolam
HR 376	clobazam
HR 4723	clobazam
HR 930	fosazepam
K3917	temazepam

Research Designation	Generic Name
LA 111	diazepam
LM 2717	clobazam
ORF 8063	triflubazam
Ro 4-5360	nitrazepam
Ro 5-0690	chlordiazepoxide
Ro 5-0883	desmethylchlordiazepoxide
Ro 5-2092	demoxepam
Ro 5-2180	desmethyldiazepam
Ro 5-2807	diazepam
Ro 5-2925	desmethylmedazepam
Ro 5-3059	nitrazepam
Ro 5-3350	bromazepam
Ro 5-3438	fludiazepam
Ro 5-4023	clonazepam
Ro 5-4200	flunitrazepam
Ro 5-4556	medazepam
Ro 5-5345	temazepam
Ro 5-6789	oxazepam
Ro 5-6901	flurazepam
Ro 15-1788	(antagonist)
Ro 21-3981	midazolam
RU 31158	loprazolam
S 1530	nimetazepam
SAH 1123	isoquinazepam
SAH 47603	temazepam
SB 5833	camazepam
SCH 12041	halazepam
SCH 16134	quazepam
U 28774	ketazolam
U 31889	alprazolam
U 33030	triazolam
W 4020	prazepam
We 352	triflubazam

Research Designation	Generic Name
We 941	brotizolam
Wy 2917	temazepam
Wy 3467	diazepam
Wy 3498	oxazepam
Wy 3917	temazepam
Wy 4036	lorazepam
Wy 4082	lormetazepam
Wy 4426	oxazepam
Y 6047	clotiazepam

Table 2. Benzodiazepine generic names with corresponding trade names

Generic Name	Trade Name(s)
alprazolam	Xanax
bromazepam	Compendium, Lectopam, Lexatin, Lexomil, Lexotan, Lexotanil
brotizolam	Lendorm, Lendormin
camazepam	Albego, Limpidon, Paxor
chlordiazepoxide	Ansiacal, A-Poxide, Benzodiapin, Binomil, Cebrum, Chlortran, Corax, C-Tran, Decacil, Diazepina, Disarim, Eden-psich, Endequil, Elenium, Equibral, Helogaphen, Huberplex, Klopoxid, Labican, Liberans, Librium, Libritabs, Lixin, Medilium, Menrium, Mesural, Multum, Nack, Normide, Novopoxide, O.C.M., Omnalio, Philicorium, Psicofar, Psicoterina, Raysedan, Reposal, Relaxil, Reliberan, Risachief, Risolid, Seren, Silibrin, Sintesedan, Smail, Solium, SonimenTrilium, Tropium, Viansin, Zeisin, Zetran
clobazam	Castilium, Frisin, Frisium, Karidium, Noiafren, Sentil, Urbadan, Urbanol, Urbanyl

Generic Name	Trade Name(s)
clonazepam	Clonopin, Iktorivil, Landsen, Rivotril
clorazepate	Azene, Belseren, Covengar, Enadine, Justum, Mendon, Moderane, Nansius, Tencilan, Transene, Tranxen, Tranxene, Tranxilen, Tranxilene, Tranxilium, Uni-Tranxene
clorazolam	see triazolam
clotiazepam	Rize, Trecalmo
cloxazolam	Enadel, Lubalix, Olcadil, Sepazon, Tolestan
diazepam	Aliseum, Alupram, Amiprol, Ansiolin, Apaurin, Apozepam, Armonil, Atenex, Atensine, Atilen, Avex, Best, Bialzepam, Calmpose, Ceregulart, Cuadel, Cyclopam, Diaceplex, Diapam, Diatran, Diazemuls, Dipam, Dipezona, Dizam, Doval, Drenian, D-Tran, Ducene, E-Pam, Eridan, Euphorin, Evacalm, Faustan, Gradual, Gubex, Lembrol, Levium, Lorinon, Meval, Morostan, Neo-Calme, Neurolytril, Noan, Notense, Novodipam, Pacitran, Pax, Paxate, Paxel, Plidan, Pro-pam, Quetinil, Quievita, Relanium, Relivan X, Saromet, Scriptopam, Sedapam, Sedaril, Seduxen, Serenack, Setonil, Solis, Somasedan, Sonacon, Stesolid, Stesolin, Stess-Pam, Tensium, Tranimul, Tranquase, Tranquirit, Tranquo-Tablinen, Valitran, Valium, Valrelease, Vatran, Vival, Vivol
estazolam	Domnamid, Esilgan, Eurodin, Nuctalon
fludiazepam	Erispan
flunitrazepam	Darkene, Narcozep, Primun, Rohipnol, Rohypnol, Roipnal, Valsera

Generic Name	Trade Name(s)
flurazepam	Benozil, Dalmane, Dalmadorm, Dalmate, Domodor, Dormodor, Felison, Felmane, Flunox, Fordrim, Insumin, Lunipax, Midorm AR, Natam, Niotal, Remdue, Somlan, Valdorm
flutazolam	Coreminal
halazepam	Paxipam
haloxazolam	Somelin
ketazolam	Anxon, Contamex, Loftran, Solatran, Unakalm
loprazolam	Avlane, Dormonoct
lorazepam	Almazine, Aplacasse, Ativan, Control, Emotical, Emotival, Kalmalin, Loraus, Lorax, Lorsilan, Lorenin, NIC, Orfidal, Placidia, Psicopax, Quait, Securit, Sedarkey, Sedatival, Sidenar, Tavor, Temesta, Trapax, Wypax
lormetazepam	Loramet, Noctamid
medazepam	Ansilan, Anxitol, Azepamid, Benson, Diepin, Elbrus, Esmail, Lerisum, Medazepol, Megasedan, Metonas, Mezepan, Narsis, Navizil, Nivelton, Nobrium, Pazital, Psiquium, Raporan, Resmit, Rudotel, Serenium, Siman, Templane, Tranquilax
mexazolam	Melex
midazolam	Dormicum
nimetazepam	Elimin, Erimin, Hypnon

Generic Name	Trade Name(s)
nitrazepam	Apodorm, Arem, Benzalin, Calsmin, Dormicum, Dumolid, Eatan, Eunoctin, Hipsal, Hypnotin, Mitidin, Mogadan, Mogadon, Nelbon, Neuchlonic, Nipam, Nitrados, Nitrenpax, Noctene, Pacisyn, Paxisyn, Pelson, Persopir, Prosonno, Quill, Radedorm, Relact, Remnos, Sindepres, Somnased, Somnibel, Somnite, Sonebon, Sonnolin, Surem, Unisomnia
nordazepam	Calmday, Demadar, Madar, Stilny
oxazepam	Adumbran, Aplakil, Benzotran, Enidrel, Isodin, Limbial, Murelax, Nesontil, Nulans, Oxadin, Oxepam, Praxiten, Psiquiwas, Purata, Quen, Quilibrex, Sedokin, Serax, Serenal, Serenid-D, Serenid Forte, Serepax, Seresta, Serpax, Sobile, Sobril, Wakazepam
oxazolam	Convertal, Hializan, Serenal Tranquit
oxazolazepam	see oxazolam
pinazepam	Domar, Duna
prazepam	Centrax, Demetrin, Equipaz, Lysanxia, Mono Demetrin, Prazene, Reapam, Sedapran, Trepidan, Verstran
temazepam	Cerepax, Euhypnos, Lenal, Levanxene, Levanxol, Mabertin, Maeva, Normison, Planum, Remestan, Restoril, Signopam
tetrazepam	Clinoxan, Musaril, Myolastan
tofisopam	Grandaxin, Grandaxine, Seriel
tofizopam	see tofisopam
triazolam	Halcion

Table 3. Benzodiazepine trade names with corresponding generic names

Trade Name	Generic Name
Adumbran	oxazepam
Albego	camazepam
Aliseum	diazepam
Almazine	lorazepam
Alupram	diazepam
Amiprol	diazepam
Ansiacal	chlordiazepoxide
Ansilan	medazepam
Ansiolin	diazepam
Anxitol	medazepam
Anxon	ketazolam
Apaurin	diazepam
Aplacasse	lorazepam
Aplakil	oxazepam
Apodorm	nitrazepam
A-Poxide	chlordiazepoxide
Apozepam	diazepam
Arem	nitrazepam
Armonil	diazepam
Atenex	diazepam
Atensine	diazepam
Atilen	diazepam
Ativan	lorazepam
Avex	diazepam
Avlane	loprazolam
Azene	clorazepate
Azepamid	medazepam
Belseren	clorazepate
Benozil	flurazepam
Benson	medazepam
Benzalin	nitrazepam

Trade Name	Generic Name
Benzodiapin	chlordiazepoxide
Benzotran	oxazepam
Best	diazepam
Bialzepam	diazepam
Binomil	chlordiazepoxide
Calmday	nordazepam
Calmpose	diazepam
Calsmin	nitrazepam
Castilium	clobazam
Cebrum	chlordiazepoxide
Centrax	prazepam
Ceregulart	diazepam
Cerepax	temazepam
Chlortran	chlordiazepoxide
Clinoxan	tetrazepam
Clonopin	clonazepam
Compendium	bromazepam
Contamex	ketazolam
Control	lorazepam
Convertal	oxazolam
Corax	chlordiazepoxide
Coreminal	flutazolam
Covengar	clorazepate
C-Tran	chlordiazepoxide
Cuadel	diazepam
Cyclopam	diazepam
Dalmane	flurazepam
Dalmadorm	flurazepam
Dalmate	flurazepam
Darkene	flunitrazepam
Decacil	chlordiazepoxide
Demadar	nordazepam
Demetrin	prazepam

Trade Name	Generic Name
Diaceplex	diazepam
Diapam	diazepam
Diatran	diazepam
Diazemuls	diazepam
Diazepina	chlordiazepoxide
Diepin	medazepam
Dipam	diazepam
Dipezona	diazepam
Disarim	chlordiazepoxide
Domar	pinazepam
Domnamid	estazolam
Domordor	flurazepam
Dormicum	midazolam, nitrazepam
Dormodor	flurazepam
Dormonoct	loprazolam
Doval	diazepam
Drenian	diazepam
D-Tran	diazepam
Ducene	diazepam
Dumolid	nitrazepam
Duna	pinazepam
Eatan	nitrazepam
Eden-psich	chlordiazepoxide
Edenquil	chlordiazepoxide
Elbrus	medazepam
Elenium	chlordiazepoxide
Elimin	nimetazepam
Emotical	lorazepam
Emotival	lorazepam
Enadel	cloxazolam
Enadine	clorazepate
Enidrel	oxazepam
E-Pam	diazepam

Trade Name	Generic Name
Equibral	chlordiazepoxide
Equipaz	prazepam
Eridan	diazepam
Erimin	nimetazepam
Erispan	fludiazepam
Esilgan	estazolam
Esmail	medazepam
Euhypnos	temazepam
Eunoctin	nitrazepam
Euphorin	diazepam
Eurodin	estazolam
Evacalm	diazepam
Faustan	diazepam
Feliston	flurazepam
Felmane	flurazepam
Flunox	flurazepam
Fordrim	flurazepam
Frisin	clobazam
Frisium	clobazam
Gradual	diazepam
Grandaxin	tofisopam
Grandaxine	tofisopam
Gubex	diazepam
Halcion	triazolam
Helogaphen	chlordiazepoxide
Hializan	oxazolam
Hipsal	nitrazepam
Huberplex	chlordiazepoxide
Hypnon	nimetazepam
Hypnotin	nitrazepam
Iktorivil	clonazepam
Insumin	flurazepam
Isodin	oxazepam

Trade Name	GenericName
Justum	clorazepate
Kalmalin	lorazepam
Karidium	clobazam
Klopoxid	chlordiazepoxide
Labican	chlordiazepoxide
Landsen	clonazepam
Lectopam	bromazepam
Lembrol	diazepam
Lenal	temazepam
Lendorm	brotizolam
Lendormin	brotizolam
Lerisum	medazepam
Levanxene	temazepam
Levanxol	temazepam
Levium	diazepam
Lexatin	bromazepam
Lexomil	bromazepam
Lexotan	bromazepam
Lexotanil	bromazepam
Liberans	chlordiazepoxide
Limbial	oxazepam
Librium	chlordiazepoxide
Libritabs	chlordiazepoxide
Limpidon	camazepam
Lixin	chlordiazepoxide
Loftran	ketazolam
Loramet	lormetazepam
Loraus	lorazepam
Lorax	lorazepam
Lorinon	diazepam
Lorsilan	lorazepam
Lorenin	lorazepam
Lubalix	cloxazolam

Trade Name	Generic Name
Lunipax	flurazepam
Lysanxia	prazepam
Mabertin	temazepam
Madar	nordazepam
Maeva	temazepam
Medazepol	medazepam
Medilium	chlordiazepoxide
Megasedan	medazepam
Melex	mexazolam
Mendon	clorazepate
Menrium	chlordiazepoxide
Mesural	chlordiazepoxide
Metonas	medazepam
Meval	diazepam
Mezepan	medazepam
Midorm AR	flurazepam
Mitidin	nitrazepam
Moderane	clorazepate
Mogadan	nitrazepam
Mogadon	nitrazepam
Mono Demetrin	prazepam
Morostan	diazepam
Multum	chlordiazepoxide
Murelax	oxazepam
Musaril	tetrazepam
Myolastan	tetrazepam
Nack	chlordiazepoxide
Nansius	clorazepate
Narcozep	flunitrazepam
Narsis	medazepam
Natam	flurazepam
Navizil	medazepam
Nelbon	nitrazepam

Trade Name	Generic Name
Neo-Calme	diazepam
Nesontil	oxazepam
Neuchlonic	nitrazepam
Neurolytril	diazepam
NIC	lorazepam
Niotal	flurazepam
Nipam	nitrazepam
Nitrados	nitrazepam
Nitrenpax	nitrazepam
Nivelton	medazepam
Noan	diazepam
Nobrium	medazepam
Noctamid	lormetazepam
Noctene	nitrazepam
Noiafren	clobazam
Normide	chlordiazepoxide
Normison	temazepam
Notense	diazepam
Novodipam	diazepam
Novopoxide	chlordiazepoxide
Nuctalon	estazolam
Nulans	oxazepam
O.C.M.	chlordiazepoxide
Olcadil	cloxazolam
Omnalio	chlordiazepoxide
Orfidal	lorazepam
Oxadin	oxazepam
Oxepam	oxazepam
Pacisyn	nitrazepam
Pacitran	diazepam
Pax	diazepam
Paxate	diazepam
Paxel	diazepam

Trade Name	Generic Name
Paxipam	halazepam
Paxisyn	nitrazepam
Paxor	camazepam
Pazital	medazepam
Pelson	nitrazepam
Persopir	nitrazepam
Philicorium	chlordiazepoxide
Placidia	lorazepam
Planum	temazepam
Plidan	diazepam
Praxiten	oxazepam
Prazene	prazepam
Primun	flunitrazepam
Pro-Pam	diazepam
Prosonno	nitrazepam
Psicofar	chlordiazepoxide
Psicopax	lorazepam
Psicoterina	chlordiazepoxide
Psiquium	medazepam
Psiquiwas	oxazepam
Purata	oxazepam
Quait	lorazepam
Quen	oxazepam
Quetinil	diazepam
Quievita	diazepam
Quilibrex	oxazepam
Quill	nitrazepam
Radedorm	nitrazepam
Raporan	medazepam
Raysedan	chlordiazepoxide
Reapam	prazepam
Reposal	chlordiazepoxide
Relact	nitrazepam

Trade Name	Generic Name
Relanium	diazepam
Relaxil	chlordiazepoxide
Reliberan	chlordiazepoxide
Relivan X	diazepam
Remdue	flurazepam
Remestan	temazepam
Remnos	nitrazepam
Resmit	medazepam
Restoril	temazepam
Risachief	chlordiazepoxide
Risolid	chlordiazepoxide
Rivotril	clonazepam
Rize	clotiazepam
Rohipnol	flunitrazepam
Rohypnol	flunitrazepam
Roipnal	flunitrazepam
Rudotel	medazepam
Saromet	diazepam
Scriptopam	diazepam
Securit	lorazepam
Sedapam	diazepam
Sedapran	prazepam
Sedaril	diazepam
Sedarkey	lorazepam
Sedativil	lorazepam
Sedokin	oxazepam
Seduxen	diazepam
Sentil	clobazam
Sepazon	cloxazolam
Serax	oxazepam
Seren	chlordiazepoxide
Serenack	diazepam
Serenal	oxazepam, oxazolam

Trade Name	Generic Name
Serenid-D	oxazepam
Serenid Forte	oxazepam
Serenium	medazepam
Serepax	oxazepam
Seresta	oxazepam
Seriel	tofisopam
Serpax	oxazepam
Setonil	diazepam
Sidenar	lorazepam
Signopam	temazepam
Silibrin	chlordiazepoxide
Siman	medazepam
Sindepres	nitrazepam
Sintesedan	chlordiazepoxide
Smail	chlordiazepoxide
Sobile	oxazepam
Sobril	oxazepam
Solatran	ketazolam
Solis	diazepam
Solium	chlordiazepoxide
Somasedan	diazepam
Somelin	haloxazolam
Somlan	flurazepam
Somnased	nitrazepam
Somnibel	nitrazepam
Somnite	nitrazepam
Sonacon	diazepam
Sonebon	nitrazepam
Sonimen	chlordiazepoxide
Sonnolin	nitrazepam
Stesolid	diazepam
Stesolin	diazepam
Stess-Pam	diazepam

Trade Name	Generic Name
Stilny	nordazepam
Surem	nitrazepam
Tavor	lorazepam
Temesta	lorazepam
Templane	medazepam
Tencilan	clorazepate
Tensium	diazepam
Tolestan	cloxazolam
Tranimul	diazepam
Tranquase	diazepam
Tranquilax	medazepam
Tranquirit	diazepam
Tranquit	oxazolam
Tranquo-Tablinen	diazepam
Transene	clorazepate
Tranxen	clorazepate
Tranxene	clorazepate
Tranxilen	clorazepate
Tranxilene	clorazepate
Tranxilium	clorazepate
Trapax	lorazepam
Trecalmo	clotiazepam
Trepidan	prazepam
Trilium	chlordiazepoxide
Tropium	chlordiazepoxide
Unakalm	ketazolam
Unisomnia	nitrazepam
Uni-Tranxene	clorazepate
Urbadan	clobazam
Urbanol	clobazam
Urbanyl	clobazam
Valdorm	flurazepam
Valitran	diazepam

Trade Name	Generic Name
Valium	diazepam
Valrelease	diazepam
Valsera	flunitrazepam
Vatran	diazepam
Verstran	prazepam
Viansin	chlordiazepoxide
Vival	diazepam
Vivol	diazepam
Wakazepam	oxazepam
Wypax	lorazepam
Xanax	alprazolam
Zeisin	chlordiazepoxide
Zetran	chlordiazepoxide

Appendix 2:
Books on Benzodiazepines

Costa E (ed): *The Benzodiazepines: From Molecular Biology to Clinical Practice.* New York, Raven Press, 1983.

Costa E, Di Chiari G, Gessa GL (eds): *GABA and Benzodiazepine Receptors.* New York, Raven Press, 1981.

Costa E, Greengard P (eds): *Mechanisms of Action of Benzodiazepines.* New York, Raven Press, 1975.

Garattini S, Mussini E, Randall LO (eds): *The Benzodiazepines.* New York, Raven Press, 1973.

Greenblatt DJ, Shader RI: *Benzodiazepines in Clinical Practice.* New York, Raven Press, 1974.

Marks, J: *The Benzodiazepines: Use, Overuse, Misuse, Abuse.* 2nd Edn. Lancaster, England, MTP Press Limited, 1985.

Priest RG, Vianna Filho U, Amrein R, *et al.* (eds): *Benzodiazepines Today and Tomorrow.* Lancaster, England, MTP Press Limited, 1980.

Skolnick P, Tallman JF, Jr., *et al.* (eds): *Pharmacology of Benzodiazepines.* London, The Macmillan Press, Ltd., Scientific and Medical Division, 1982.

Szara SI, Ludford JP: *Benzodiazepines: A Review of Research Results, 1980.* NIDA Research Monograph 33. Rockville, Maryland, National Institute on Drug Abuse, 1981.

Index